Health Effects of
the New Labour Market

Health Effects of the New Labour Market

Edited by

Kerstin Isaksson
Christer Hogstedt
National Institute for Working Life
Solna, Sweden

Charli Eriksson
National Institute for Public Health
Stockholm, Sweden

and

Töres Theorell
National Institute for Psychosocial Factors and Health
Stockholm, Sweden

Kluwer Academic / Plenum Publishers
New York, Boston, Dordrecht, London, Moscow

Library of Congress Cataloging-in-Publication Data

Health effects of the new labour market / edited by Kerstin Isaksson ... [et al.].
    p. cm.
    Includes bibliographical references and index.
    ISBN 0-306-46300-8
    1. Unemployed--Health and hygiene--Congresses. 2. Unemployment--Health
aspects--Congresses. 3. Downsizing of organizations--Health aspects--Congresses. 4. Job
stress--Congresses. 5. Unemployed--Health and hygiene--Sweden--Congresses. 6.
Unemployment--Health aspects--Sweden--Congresses. 7. Downsizing of
organizations--Health aspects--Sweden--Congresses. 8. Job stress--Sweden--Congresses.
I. Isaksson, Kerstin, 1952- II. International Conference on Health Hazards and
Challenges in the New Working Life (1st : 1999 : Stockholm, Sweden)

HD5708 .H388 1999
158.7'2--dc21
                                                                99-047995

Proceedings of the First International Conference on Health Hazards and Challenges in the New Working
Life, held January 11–13, 1999, in Stockholm, Sweden

ISBN 0-306-46300-8

©2000 Kluwer Academic/Plenum Publishers, New York
233 Spring Street, New York, New York 10013

http://www.wkap.nl

10 9 8 7 6 5 4 3 2 1

A C.I.P. record for this book is available from the Library of Congress

CONTRIBUTORS

Arnell-Gustafsson Ulla, National Institute for Working Life, S-112 79 Stockholm, Sweden, e-mail: ulla.arnell-gustafsson@niwl.se

Axelsson John, The National Institute for Psychosocial Factors and Health (IPM), Box 230, 171 77 Stockholm, Sweden, e-mail: john.axelsson @ipm.ki.se

Bejerot Eva, National Institute for Working Life, S-112 79 Stockholm, Sweden, e-mail: eva.bejerot@niwl.se

de Witte Marco, University of Groningen, PO Box 800, Groningen, The Netherlands, e-mail: m.e.de.vitte@bdk.rug.nl

Eriksson, Charli, National Institute for Public Health, S-103 52 Stockholm, Sweden, e-mail: charli.eriksson@fhinst.se

Ertel Michael, Bundesanstalt fur Arbeitsschutz und Arbeidsmedizin, PO Box 5, 102 66 Berlin, Germany, e-mail: ertel@baua.de

Freese Charissa, WORC, Katholike University, PO Box 90153, 5000 LE Tilburg, The Netherlands

Fryer, David, University of Stirling, Psychology Department, Stirling, Scotland FK94LA, e-mail: d.m.fryer@stir.ac.uk

Gallagher Daniel G., James Madison University, Harrisonburg, VA, USA

Gallie Duncan, Nuffield College, Oxford OXI 1NF, Great Britain, e-mail: duncan.gallie@nuffield.ox.ac.uk

Hagström Tom, National Institute for Working Life, S-112 79 Stockholm, Sweden, e-mail: tom.hagstrom@niwl.se

Hellgren Johnny, Department of Psychology, Stockholm University, S-106 91 Stockholm, Sweden, e-mail: jhn@psychology.su.se

Härenstam, Annika, Department of Occupational Health, Norrbacka, 171 76 Stockholm, Sweden, e-mail: annika.harenstam@mailbox.swipnet.se

Hogstedt, Christer, National Institute for Working Life, S-112 79 Stockholm, Sweden, e-mail: christer.hogstedt@niwl.se

Isaksson, Kerstin, National Institute for Working Life, S-112 79 Stockholm, Sweden, e-mail: kerstin.isaksson@niwl.se

Jahoda Marie, 17 The Crescent, Keymer, Hassocks, Sussex, BN6 8RB, Great Britain, e-mail: m.jahoda@virgin.net

Johansson Kerstin, Department of Occupational Health, Norrbacka, 171 76 Stockholm, Sweden

Karlkvist Monica, Department of Occupational Health, Norrbacka, 171 76 Stockholm, Sweden

Kecklund, Göran, The National Institute for Psychosocial Factors and Health (IPM), Box 230, 171 77 Stockholm, Sweden, e-mail: goran.kecklund @ipm.ki.se

Kjellberg, Anders, National Institute for Working Life, S-112 79 Stockholm, Sweden, e-mail: anders.kjellberg@niwl.se

Kraut, Allen, Department of Internal Medicine, University of Manitoba, 5112 Bannatyne, Winnipeg MB, Canada, e-mail: akraut@ms.umanitoba.ca

Levi, Lennart, Sweden, The National Institute for Psychosocial Factors and Health (IPM), Box 230, 171 77 Stockholm, Sweden, e-mail: lennart.levi@ipm.ki.se

Loewenson Rene, Training and Research Support Center, 47 Van Praagh Ave, Milton Park, Harare, Zimbabve, e-mail: rloewenson@healthnet.zw

Lowden, Arne, The National Institute for Psychosocial Factors and Health (IPM), Box 230, S-171 77 Stockholm, Sweden, e-mail: arne.lowden@ipm.ki.se

Mayhew, Claire, Worksafe Australia, National Occupational Health & Safety Commission,92 Parramatta Road, Camperdown NSW 2050 GPO, Box 58, Sydney, Australia, e-mail: cmayhew@worksafe.gov.au

Murray Åsa, Stockholm Institute of Education, Box 47308, S-100 74 Stockholm, Sweden, e-mail: asa.murray@lhs.se

Mustard, Cam, Department of Community Health Sciences, University of Manitoba, 5112 Bannatyne, Winnipeg MB, Canada,

Olsson, Birgitta, The National Institute for Psychosocial Factors and Health (IPM), Box 230, 171 77 Stockholm, Sweden, e-mail: birgitta.olsson @ipm.ki.se

Pech, Eberhard, Bundesanstalt fur Arbeitsschutz und Arbeidsmedizin, PO Box 5, 102 66 Berlin, Germany,

Pettersson Pär, Department of Psychology, Stockholm University, S-106 91 Stockholm, Sweden, e-mail: pep@psychology.su.se

Quinlan Michael, University of New South Wales, School of Industrial Relations, Sydney, NSW, Australia, e-mail: m.quinlan@unsw.edu.su

Rydbeck Anna, Regionsjukhuset i Örebro, Department of Occupational Health and Medicine, S-701 85 Örebro, Sweden, e-mail: anna.rydbeck@orebroll.se

Schalk, René, WORC, Katholike University, PO Box 90153, 5000 LE Tilburg, The Netherlands, e-mail: m.j.d.schalk@kub.nl

Schouteten Roel, University of Groningen, PO Box 800, Groningen, The Netherlands, e-mail: r.s.schouteten@bdk.rug.nl

Sverke, Magnus, Department of Psychology, Stockholm University, S-106 91 Stockholm, Sweden, e-mail: mse@psychology.su.se

Söderfeldt Björn, Center for Oral Health Sciences, Carl Gustafs väg 34, S-214 21 Malmö, Sweden, e-mail: bjorn.soderfeldt@odsmhod.lu.se

Söderfeldt Marie, National institute for Working Life, S-112 79 Stockholm, Sweden, e-mail: marie.soderfeldt@niwl.se

Tate, Robert, Department of Community Health Sciences, University of Manitoba, 5112 Bannatyne, Winnipeg MB, Canada,

Theorell, Töres, The National Institute for Psychosocial Factors and Health (IPM), Box 230, 171 77 Stockholm, Sweden, e-mail: tores.theorell@ipm.ki.se

Ullsperger Peter, Bundesanstalt fur Arbeitsschutz und Arbeidsmedizin, PO Box 5, 102 66 Berlin, Germany,

Walld, Randy, Department of Community Health Sciences, University of Manitoba, 5112 Bannatyne, Winnipeg MB, Canada,

Westerlund Hugo, The National Institute for Psychosocial Factors and Health (IPM), Box 230, 171 77 Stockholm, Sweden, e-mail: hugo.westerlund@ipm.ki.se

Wiklund Per, Department of Occupational Health, Norrbacka, 171 76 Stockholm, Sweden, e-mail:perwik@ymed.ki.se

Åkerstedt, Torbjörn, The National Institute for Psychosocial Factors and Health (IPM), Box 230, 171 77 Stockholm, Sweden, e-mail: torbjorn.akerstedt@ipm.ki.se

PREFACE

The background for the international research conference "Health Hazards and Challenges in the New Working Life" was the emerging questions concerning the health and social effects of the rapid changes in the labour market leading to increasing long-term unemployment, temporary employment and irregular employment contracts.

We knew that other countries have had this development at the labour market for a much longer time than Sweden has and it seemed a good idea to invite interested researchers and practitioners to an international seminar to share the relevant research findings and discuss future research needs.

Thus, the first international, interdisciplinary research conference on "Health Hazards and Challenges in the New Working Life" was arranged in Stockholm during the last year of the 2nd millennium but was directed towards the foreseen development during the next millennium. We were very pleased that more than 200 participants came to a cold and dark country just after New Year's Eve, and that it was a truly multidisciplinary setting.

It became very obvious that it is necessary for the occupational health and safety research community to reach out to the public health research community as well as to the social and political sciences in order to understand the determinants and to perform comprehensive analyses at several levels in this new labour market situation.

The conference was organised by the Swedish National Institute for Working Life in collaboration with and financially supported by the National Institute of Public Health, the Council for Work Life Research and the Swedish National Institute for Psychosocial Factors and Health (IPM).

We are grateful to Kluwer Academic/Plenum Publishers for the smooth co-operation and quick publishing of these proceedings from the first multi-disciplinary conference devoted to the theme of "health hazards and challenges in the new working life".

We have had many requests for a second conference on the same theme and we will be happy to organise such a conference within a few years unless other institutions take the initiative.

Christer Hogstedt   Kerstin Isaksson
President   *Secretary General*
                    National Institute for Working Life
Charli Eriksson   Töres Theorell
Professor   *Professor*
National Institute for   *National Institute for*
Public Health   *Psychosocial Factors and Health*

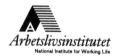 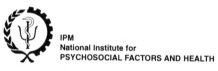

CONTENTS

OPPORTUNITIES AND CONSTRAINTS IN THE LABOUR MARKET

INTRODUCTION

The globalisation of the economies has profound implications for the labour market structures, causes rapid changes, and demands a drastically increased flexibility. The speed of changes is threatening our needs of security and stability as well as the possibilities for collective actions and defence. At the same time there are unique possibilities for personal development, and the human potential for constructive adaptation has many times in history proven to be impressive.

There were three central topics for the conference; Opportunities and Constraints in the Labour Market, Unemployment and Downsizing, Flexibilisation and Stress, all examples of areas where on-going research efforts can already offer new knowledge, but where there are still critical knowledge gaps, which need further exploration. In these proceedings from the conference we have collected a selected number of highly qualified papers with the common purpose of addressing these issues.

The book, as the conference, has three main parts. The first area is that of *Unemployment and downsizing,* where we had the great honour to invite and receive a contribution from a truly distinguished researcher in this domain with more than fifty years experience of unemployment research, Professor Marie Jahoda. Her opening speech to the conference, delivered by video, is also the start of the first book section. The next chapter introduces her impressive career and great contributions to the area of unemployment research. This was done by David Fryer, who also gave a second contribution to the conference by delivering an overview of knowledge about unemployment and health effects. The introduction gives a clear understanding of the negative effects of involuntary unemployment. The effort of this chapter was the same as that of Marie Jahoda, to point out the knowledge gaps and where future research should aim.

After these introductory chapters we have selected six additional papers for this section. All are good examples of research where there is still a lack of knowledge. The following chapter describes an example of efforts from Canada by Allen Kraut and collaborators to deal with the health problems of unemployed people, as they become visible in primary health care. Thereafter, two chapters deal with ways to empower the unemployed, helping them to cope and fight the negative consequences (Westerlund, Levi). A common thread in this section is the critical issue of having a social network and support in a critical situation like this (Arnell-Gustafsson). The last chapter deals with the threat of becoming unemployed, which has become a problem for so many employees during this last decade of the millennium (Isaksson et al.).

The second part of the book, the largest one, consists of ten contributions in the broad area of *Flexibilisation and stress*, here divided into three sub-sections, which cover aspects of the new working life. Organizational change is one, followed by new employment contracts resulting in precarious or contingent employment forms. The subjective contracts, as perceived by employees during organizational change is a critical issue, addressed in a contribution by Schalk and Frese. Other questions concern if the new contracts are for better or for worse, and in what cases they do lead to flexibility for employees as well as companies (Härenstam et al.), or when they seem to cause new hazards such as occupational violence (Mayhew & Quinlan) or increased stress (Sverke et al.). The new contracts and working conditions also impose a challenge to traditional ways of working in the occupational health services (Ertel et al).

A severe effect of long-lasting stress, that of burnout, its definition and measurement, is also addressed. Burnout has become a popular concept in present-day work environment discussions, here it is challenged in a critical discussion and analysis (Söderfeldt). Bejerot presents a theoretical and empirical analysis of the consequences of work redesign based upon Human Resource Management (HRM). Finally, change of working schedules and how this affects employees in terms of their sleeping patters, crucial for well-being forms the last part of this section (Åkerstedt et al., Kecklund et al.).

The last section of the book gives examples of research in the area of *Opportunities and constraints in the labour market*. Five chapters give a wide variety of perspectives, starting with an overview of the polarization of the labour market and the exclusion of vulnerable groups (Gallie). Defining the quality of work only in terms of the content of jobs is insufficient, studies of labour need also to consider the work-family interface (Schouteten & de Witte). A Swedish longitudinal study of work socialization among nurses and engineers illustrates the need for a differentiated perspective on work values and gender issues (Hagström & Kjellberg). A second longitudinal study of early school leavers compares employment rates during the last three decades (Murray). The final chapter in this section gives a truly global perspective by providing an overview of health hazards in the informal sector (Loewenson).

We strongly feel that the conference and the contributions in this book will give a valuable summary of where we stand today. In some of these areas, like labour market change and unemployment, we really know a lot and research has to find new directions, leading among other things to direct action. In other areas such as flexibilisation and stress we are only in the beginning of defining questions for research. Some of these questions are:

Will formal employment contracts be substituted for informal and psychological contracts? Can increased control balance the stress of flexibility? How can you organise occupational safety and health facilities during these new conditions? How will it effect the health equity among men and women and in different professional groups? Which ideologies are formulated by these changes for work and health? What do the unemployed do when they are unemployed; become passive or organise themselves in the so-called "third sector"? Are the trends really global? What is known, guessed and researched?

On the whole we feel that the book constitutes an substantial contribution to this work. It gives a state of the art and we feel that by finishing this book we at least partly achieved one of the ultimate goals of all conferences – to stimulate new ideas and thinking for the future.

Health Effects of
the New Labour Market

UNEMPLOYMENT AND DOWNSIZING

Professor Marie Jahoda

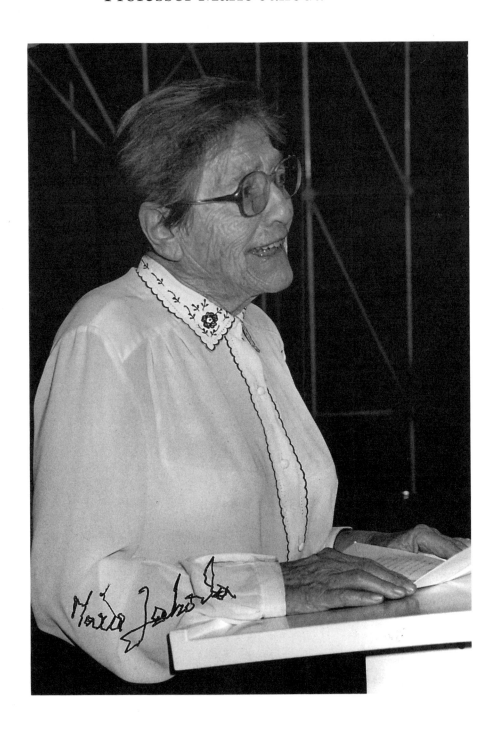

OPENING ADDRESS

Marie Jahoda
Sussex, England

Ladies and Gentlemen, old age prevents me from being with you in person at the opening of this conference but nevertheless modern technology makes it possible to tell you in a few words of all the good wishes I have for the success of your conference.

Over the years I have frequently participated in similar conferences and have learned a lot from them. In addition to learning, I must confess, I have also sometimes had misgivings. This has been when I think of the enormous effort, all the thought and all the research, that goes into such conferences and realise that, despite all this, we have as yet done so little to change the world. Maybe some of you have had similar misgivings? I have taken some comfort from realising that there are some noticeable effects of good thinking and research. It seems, to me at least, that nowadays I hear less often of "the blessings of unemployment" and of "lazy, voluntarily unemployed, people living happy lives of leisure at the expense of the State". I do think that we have at least the possibility of influencing the climate of thought around us.

In addition to this, I have also learned many positive things from the thinking of my colleagues and from discussion at conferences. For me perhaps the most important lesson was the realisation that you cannot look at the experience of people in soul destroying jobs or in unemployment independently from looking at the institutions which have brought them to the state they are in. Individual experiences and institutional arrangements are really inseparable but they are very difficult to combine seriously in research because, you see, people have the inestimable advantage of being countable, leading us to greater precision in our thought. Institutions and their attributes cannot be counted. So we are dealing with two different units, two different essences.

Nonetheless, just because it is difficult to combine the two, there is no excuse for shirking the intellectual task of, all the time, keeping in mind that people create institutions and that institutions shape human experience. In employment and in unemployment the combination of the two thoughts is an essential feature of all the work that we have to do in this area.

In many areas of human endeavour the separation of individual experience from collective arrangements has created havoc in thinking and must be resisted at all costs. You see, for seventy years of this eventful century, the false dichotomy of values between individualism and

Health Effects of the New Labour Market, edited by Isaksson *et al.*
Kluwer Academic / Plenum Publishers, New York, 2000.

collectivism has dominated world political debate. However, if we look at the world in which we live, we must realise that individualism and collectivism - the concern for experience and the concern for the collective group - are complementary and not contrasts to be treated separately.

Thinking about the political events of the century forces us to another realisation. The hated dictatorships of this century have understood, better than the democracies which we cherish, how important it is to deal with the problem of unemployment. However, just because they have done so is no justification for the misery they have spread, no justification for us not trying to think of ways in which justice can be done to basic human values without the horrible means to that end which the dictatorships found.

Unfortunately the social sciences have very often repeated the false dichotomy of values, have specialised either on the one side or the other, have studied institutions or studied individual experience. I do think it possible to do justice to both, to overcome the splits between economics, sociology and psychology and to try to create an image of the world as it is really experienced by people, in which institutions and the human experience condition each other neutrally.

I have often felt that it is almost impossible to do justice to this task in one's thinking and in one's research but this is a failure of intellectual courage. We must continue with the one blind faith that we all need, the blind faith in reason and thought. I am quite convinced that on occasions, here at this conference, you will all face near insurmountable problems and also that you will have the courage to carry on and learn from each other. If so, at some future date, our thinking and our work will translate into a more bearable world for our children and for our children's children. I wish you all success in the learning experience to which you are now open.

A SOCIAL SCIENTIST FOR AND IN THE REAL WORLD: *An introduction to the address by Professor Marie Jahoda*

David Fryer
Department of Psychology, University of Stirling, FK9 4LA Scotland

Professor Marie Jahoda is one of the most distinguished psychologists in the discipline's history and one of the foremost intellectuals of our times. A clue to her profound impact, especially upon psychology, is given by referring to her prodigious publishing output over more than seventy years in mental health, psycho-analysis, prejudice, conformity, anti-semitism, authoritarianism, job-related well-being, education and research methodology. However, this is merely to refer to some of her major themes. Within the last decade, she has also published on time, social psychological perspectives on artificial intelligence and on nationalism and conflict in relation to the former Jugoslavia, for example. This is more than enough work to have filled several very productive academic careers, yet mention has not yet been made of the massive research programme for which Professor Jahoda is probably most well known. From the early 1930s until almost the present day, she has produced a steady stream of influential publications which report her attempts to empirically investigate, describe, explain and widely disseminate information about the psychological consequences of unemployment.

Marie Jahoda read psychology in the 1920s at the University of Vienna. Hers was the scintillating imperial city of Sigmund Freud, of Karl and Charlotte Buhler's legendary Psychological Institute, of the Vienna Circle of positivist philosophers, of a flowering of intellectual and cultural creativity. It was also the Vienna of apparently unlimited progressive political and ideological possibility, at least from the perspective of a young Austro-Marxist social democrat.

The young Marie Jahoda played a full part in each of these spheres. As an 18 year old, she worked with the brilliant and eccentric Gustav Icheiser in the Vocational Guidance Centre of the City of Vienna. She attempted with the philosophers Neurath and Carnap to translate Freud's Massenpsychologie und Ich-Analyse into logical positivist language (the attempt was unsuccessful!) and she also worked with Neurath at the Museum for Social and Economic Affairs. Marie underwent psycho-analysis with Heinz Hartmann as her analyst during 1930 and 1931. Herr Hartmann was one of only two psychoanalysts invited to receive their own training analysis from Sigmund Freud himself. The Freud and Buhler sets moved in very different circles in the Vienna of the time, however Marie recalls meeting Sigmund Freud in person when she was taking tea with Anna Freud. Marie Jahoda also worked intensively with Paul Lazarsfeld, a polymath who would later be known principally as one of the

Health Effects of the New Labour Market, edited by Isaksson *et al.*
Kluwer Academic / Plenum Publishers, New York, 2000.

major sociologists of his time. They were briefly married and had a daughter, Lotte, now Lotte Bailyn, herself now a prominent social scientist in the USA.

Marie was actively involved, all the while, in socialist politics of the Austro Marxist Social Democratic Party, first in the youth movement and later as a mature woman. Indeed at that time Marie, herself, saw her future as in politics rather than in education or social science. As Professor Jahoda herself told me, in an interview published in 1986, "my very active involvement in the social democratic party in Austria ... and my study of Psychology ... were the two great influences. The political activity being overwhelmingly concerned with the impact of the environment on people and the psychological studies being overwhelmingly concerned with the development and functioning of individuals".

Professor Jahoda pioneered the relocation of psychology from the laboratory to the field to tackle pressing social problems. So successful was she that in 1933, still only in her twenties, she was appointed Director of the Industrial Psychology Research Station (Wirtschafts-psychologischen Forschungstelle) in the Institute of Psychology, University of Vienna, by Professor Karl Buhler. This was probably the first occupational psychology research unit, though subsequently much imitated.

In the same year, 1933, she published her collaborative investigation of the disastrous psychological costs of mass unemployment in the Austrian village of Marienthal. Incredibly publication of Marienthal is now more than 65 years ago. It is a mark of the coherence, vision and power of this research that it has effectively dominated the research agenda in the field for the subsequent six and a half decades.

Professor Jahoda's distinguished contribution to social science has been widely recognised. Her distinctions are too many to list exhaustively on this occasion but mention should be made of her Professorial appointments in New York, Brunel and Sussex; her receipt of the Kurt Lewin Memorial and C S Myers Awards; her Honorary Fellowship of the British Psychological Society; her Presidency of the Society for the Psychological Study of Social Issues and her honouring in 1974 with a CBE (Commander of the British Empire). She has also of course received numerous honorary degrees from Universities in Europe (including, I am proud to say, the Highest Honour bestowed by the University of Stirling in Scotland, Doctor of the University).

1.   "SOCIAL PSYCHOLOGY OF THE INVISIBLE"

Initial acquaintance with her work suggests a vast and diverse range of scholarly and research interests. Closer inspection, however, reveals a persistent and unifying concern underlying her work. Whilst she delves systematically below the surface of the obvious to develop what she has called a "social psychology of the invisible", her work is characterised by attention to substantive knowledge - specific problems of actual people in the real world. She aims in her research to understand that `real` world and to contribute to the solution of those problems, rather than, for example, being theory-driven, method-driven or paradigm driven.

Reciprocating, the 'real world' has taken a sometimes sinister interest in her psychological research. We now know that whilst she and her colleagues were observing the unemployed people of Marienthal, the police were clandestinely observing her and her colleagues. The book was published in limited numbers without the researchers' names on the cover. Nevertheless, it fell victim to the Nazi book burnings of 1933, the year of its publication. Because of her work at the Psychological Institute, Marie was imprisoned and subjected to nightly interrogations by the, then Fascist, Austrian State Police in 1937. Only after international appeals at the very highest levels was she released, only to become what she has herself described as a "rootless refugee" living from then on alternately in the UK and the USA. The original book was published on paper made in a, then, new way - based on wood pulp rather than textiles. The acidity content was far too high and the unburned books gradually literally ate themselves away on the shelf. Both main researchers, Marie Jahoda and Paul Lazarsfeld, subsequently distanced themselves from the book and Marie Jahoda actually developed an explanatory account, Latent Functions Deprivation, which is inconsistent with it.

2.   "DIE ARBEIDSLOSEN VON MARIENTHAL"

Professor Jahoda's book, Die Arbeitslosen von Marienthal, written by her at the age of 25 on the basis of research done when she was 24, has a pivotal place in the unemployment and mental health literature. Even in 1938 it was described by the Pilgrim Trust as "the well-known survey of unemployment". Professor P. B. Warr described it as "a classic investigation" and Professor N. T. Feather described it as "a major source of ideas ... unique for its time" which "still stands as an excellent example of what can be achieved". Marie Jahoda was told when she was 26 that she would always be known as the author of Marienthal and this remains true over 65 years and about 150 publications later. How many other social psychological studies have been dramatised as peak hour television viewing? Marienthal has!

At a more prosaic level, Marienthal played a major part in my own life. After completing a conceptual psychology PhD on simulation as a mode of psychological explanation, a Phd which was psychological yet informed by philosophical psychology, the history of science and the sociology of knowledge, I effectively rendered myself unemployable in a modern British psychology department. During nearly two years of unemployment and intermittent low quality employment, I tried to make sense of my own experience - and that of the people I met whilst signing on and working in marginal formal and informal economies - and found the psychology I had been studying for six years almost totally unhelpful. I came across a translation of Marie Jahoda's Marienthal in a public library and read it. My perspective on psychology, and my interpretation of my own experience, was transformed. I saw, applied for and was appointed to a post doctoral position at the Medical Research Council Social & Applied Research Unit (SAPU) in Sheffield where I had the privilege of working on unemployment and mental health with Jean Hartley, Paul Jackson, Stephen McKenna, Roy Payne, Peter Warr and others.

Imagine how I felt when, relatively shortly after I had joined the Unit, the Director, Professor Peter Warr, asked me to go down to a village in Sussex to update a certain Professor Marie Jahoda on SAPU unemployment research. I went and it was the first of, for me, a wonderful series of meetings at which I have had the privilege to talk with Professor Jahoda as fellow unemployment researchers.

Given Professor Jahoda`s eminence and status, it would be impertinent to describe our relationship as one between friends but to me it has been not only a tremendously stimulating but personally important and valued relationship too. I have not always agreed with Professor Jahoda but I have never been anything but inspired by, and in total respect and admiration of, her work and her as a person.

Long after I had first met her, I decided to read the much quoted Marienthal in the original German. I tried in vain to find a copy in the UK and then via the inter-library loan service overseas too. No copy was to be found anywhere. I mentioned this to Marie and soon I found myself opening a parcel containing an infinitely fragile set of decomposing pages. It was Marie Jahoda`s own copy of Marienthal! The University of Stirling Library`s rare books department staff kindly washed, de-acidified and patched it up, created an acid free box for its storage and returned to me what is now one of my most treasured possessions. The reading was full of surprises but that is another story ....

Our meetings over the years have included a series of interviews on audio tape and later video tape, for the American Psychological Association and most recently for the British Psychological Society, the BPS. On one of these occasions, in September 1998, both an interview for BPS archives about Professor Jahoda`s involvement in psychology in the UK and also the video tape a transcription of which you are about to read were recorded. I was the interviewer, the recording itself and subsequent technical editing work was done by Mr Bob Lavery, Senior Technician at the University of Stirling.

At this meeting Professor Jahoda gave me a second, much newer, book which she had written and which was published in 1998 (by Johannes Lang of Munster). It is a translation of 24 sonnets by the woman poet, Louize Labe, originally published in French in 1555, but translated into German by the poet Rainer Maria Rilke and published in 1917 as "Ach, meine Liebe, werft sie mir nicht vor". In her postscript, Marie described Louize Labe (1525-1556) as "an extraordinary woman who lived in .. an extraordinary town, in extraordinary times ... loved and admired by many contemporaries ... as an independent spirit". Marie Jahoda could hardly have described herself better in as few words.

Marie Jahoda was born in January 1907 and is thus 92. She has suffered a number of strokes which have severely damaged her vision. Her conference address, which you are about to read, took place as she recovered from an unpleasant virus-attributed illness. It was delivered from memory without the benefit of notes.

In this, her 9th decade, the social and psychological consequences of unemployment, problems to which Professor Jahoda, has devoted nearly 70 years of inspired and inspiring research, are again at the forefront of our international attention. Whilst it is regrettable that Professor Jahoda was unable to be with us in person, it was surely both appropriate and also a great honour for debate at this major international research conference on Health Hazards and Challenges the New Working Life to be opened by Professor Marie Jahoda.

UNEMPLOYMENT AND MENTAL HEALTH:
Hazards and Challenges of Psychology in the Community

David Fryer
University of Stirling, Scotland

Abstract: There is persuasive evidence for both social causal and individual drift relationships between unemployment and mental health disorders over 80 years of massive social change, differing countries , vastly increasing research method sophistication and differing value assumptions. The number of people at risk of negative psychological effects of unemployment is appalling and usually greatly underestimated. There are also grounds for believing that unemployment negatively affects far more people than just those who are actually unemployed. Given the scale of unemployment and its negative consequences on mental health, interventions to prevent or reduce the psychological costs are clearly important. However many, perhaps most, actual interventions seem problematic regarding their psychological impacts and the dominant psychological account of what it is about being unemployed which causes mental health problems has a number of serious problems at a variety of levels. It is suggested that new ways of conceptualising and investigating the psychological problems of unemployment are needed and that in order to address the conditions which damage the mental health of both employed and unemployed people, it may well be necessary to redesign not only the substandard jobs of many employed people but also the jobs of unemployed people too.

1.   MENTAL HEALTH HAZARDS OF UNEMPLOYMENT

There are powerful grounds for believing that unemployment is central to the social causation of a wide range of mental health problems. Anxiety, depression, dissatisfaction with one's present life, experienced strain, negative self-esteem, hopelessness regarding the future and other negative emotional states, all measured by scales with proven reliability and validity, have again and again been demonstrated by cross-sectional studies to be higher in groups of unemployed people than in matched groups of employed people. Compared with employed people, unemployed people also report greater social isolation and inactivity. There is also growing agreement that the physical, as well as the mental, health of unemployed people is generally

Health Effects of the New Labour Market, edited by Isaksson *et al.*
Kluwer Academic / Plenum Publishers, New York, 2000.

Some of the most persuasive longitudinal quantitative studies, have been done with young people. Typically these studies measure the mental health of large groups of young people in school and follow them out into the labour market - periodically measuring the mental health of those who get jobs and those who do not and comparing group mean scores cross-sectionally and longitudinally. In study after study, groups of unemployed youngsters are demonstrated to have poorer mental health than their employed peers but statistically significant differences are seldom found between the scores of the same groups when at school i.e. poor mental health is overwhelmingly the consequence rather than the cause of the labour market transition.

However, it would be foolish to deny that the individual drift account makes sense at the individual level for some unemployed people. Some pre-existing mental health problems do predispose people to loss of employment and to failure to get a job. Nevertheless, the distinction between social causation and individual drift is less clear cut than some appear to believe.

For example, during economic recession some employers ratchet up their selection criteria to exclude people from employment on mental and physical health grounds who might in other economic circumstances be employed (Catalano and Kennedy, 1998; Catalano, Rook and Dooley, 1986).

On the other hand, if - as it is now beyond reasonable doubt - unemployment is causally responsible for mental health deterioration in the previously mentally healthy, it is likely that unemployment is also pathogenic for those previously mentally unhealthy. Those who become unemployed because of mental health problems (by individual drift) are therefore at risk of having mental health problems compounded - made more severe or new problems added (by social causation).

By the same token, if pre-existing mental health problems disadvantage a person in getting or keeping a paid job, then those who were originally mentally healthy but became unemployed and then suffered deterioration in mental health (social causation) are at risk of remaining unemployed because of the socially caused problems (individual drift).

In brief, it is vital not to make crude static and abstract assumptions about social causation and individual drift accounts. Causation and drift processes will usually be inextricably intertwined as part of dynamic labour market experience and are best seen as in combination rather than as in competition. Other conceptual and methodological concerns arising out of these issues are discussed in Fryer (1997) and Winefield and Fryer (1996).

Many of the above points about the robustness of the findings can be well illustrated by research by Dooley, Catalano & Hough (1992). They interviewed over 10,000 adults in three areas of the United States using a highly structured diagnostic symptom check list developed for use by trained interviewers to reliably assign respondents to specific categories of the American Psychiatric Association diagnostic system. People were categorised as suffering from an alcohol disorder if they were either using alcohol excessively with resulting impairment in work or social functioning as indicated by specified behavioural patterns or if they were physically dependent upon alcohol as indicated by specified behavioural patterns indicating tolerance or withdrawal. Seventy nine per cent of the original sample (over 8,000 people) were re-interviewed one year later. The researchers found that those with a prior history of alcohol disorder were at greater risk of becoming unemployed. However, even more striking was that those people with no prior history of alcohol disorder who had gone from employment at first interview to unemployment at second interview a year later were nine times more likely to have become alcohol disordered in the intervening period than their consistently employed peers. Dooley and colleagues also reanalysed data on "intemperance" which was available from Rowntree's study of York in 1910 (Rowntree and Lasker, 1911) and again found evidence for both a social causation link between unemployment and alcohol disorder as well as evidence for individual drift. This research, then, provides persuasive evidence for both causal and drift relationships between unemployment and a specific serious mental health disorder over 80 years of massive social change, two continents, vastly increasing research method sophistication and differing value assumptions. Many other studies have one the same in relation to other aspects of mental health.

There are also grounds for believing that unemployment negatively affects far more people than those who are unemployed. These include: the babies of unemployed men (Cole, Donnet and Stanfield, 1983); children with unemployed fathers (McLoyd, 1989); the spouses of unemployed people (Pilgrim Trust, 1938; McKee and Bell, 1986; members of the extended family of unemployed people (Binns and Mars, 1984); general medical practitioners working with unemployed people (Smith, 1987; Beale and Nethercott, 1985; Westin et al., 1988); the clergy, probation officers, and police officers (Fineman, 1990); and welfare system employees (Kingfisher, 1996). For further details see Fryer (1995, 1998).

The number of people at risk of negative psychological effects of unemployment is appallingly vast and usually greatly underestimated. Until recently, in the UK, unemployment was officially measured in terms of the seasonally adjusted number of people in receipt of unemployment benefit (the "claimant count"). In March 1999, the announced claimant count was 1,311,000 in the UK. However, very large numbers of changes have been made by UK Governments over the years in the eligibility criteria for receipt of unemployment benefit/ job seekers' allowance. Increasingly strict criteria have excluded many people from state financial support and also had the politically convenient result of reducing the headline number of unemployed people.

For these and other reasons, a survey definition which counts people as unemployed if they have not undertaken any paid work in the survey reference week, have looked for work within the previous four weeks and are available to start work within two weeks, is currently preferred by many. The figure yielded by these criteria, as announced in March 1999, was 1,839,000.

However, given the psychological consequences of unemployment described above, it might be that people who are so discouraged and demoralised that they have not actively looked for employment in the previous four weeks should also be counted as unemployed. The Broad Labour Force Survey includes all those who say they want a job and are available to start within two weeks but have not have been actively looking for a job (because they think there are no jobs to get, that even if they found a job, they would not be offered it etc). The figure yielded for February-April 1998 by using these criteria is over two and a half million.

This is, however, still a very conservative indicator of the number of people competing for jobs. If we also count those on employment and training schemes and the full-time equivalence of involuntary under employed part-time workers, the figure for the same period rises to 4,709,700 – the so-called labour force slack (Unemployment Unit, 1999). The possibility of collateral damage to the babies, children, spouses and extended family members of unemployed people (outlined above), on top of this, suggests a truly appalling number of people at risk of mental health problems due to unemployment.

However so far, I have only referred to the situation in the UK. In February 1998, the EU unemployment rate was 10.3% and in some EU countries the rate was as high as 19.7% (in Spain: source - Eurostat web site). On a wider scale, in 1996 the International Labour Organisation calculated unemployment to stand at 34 million in O.E.C.D. countries and one billion worldwide (Milne and Ryle, 1996).

2.   CHALLENGES FOR MENTAL HEALTH PROMOTION

Given the scale of unemployment and its negative consequences on mental health, interventions to prevent or reduce the psychological costs are clearly very important.

Some favour therapeutic or counselling interventions. However, given the vast numbers of people indicated above, one-to-one treatment on the scale required to dramatically reduce or eliminate the psychological costs of unemployment could arguably never be provided. In any case, research evaluating the outcomes of many forms of individual level one-to-one professional psychiatric treatment, psychotherapy, counselling etc., raises doubts about their effectiveness.

Even if one-to-one treatment were effective, if people who had been successfully "treated" were then sent back into the psychologically toxic conditions of unemployment which caused their mental health problems in the first place, psychological problems would soon result again. Even if the particular people who were successfully treated did not return to the unemployment which originally caused their mental ill health, a constant stream of new cases would arise out of the unemployment conditions which had remained intact and which threatened the mental health of others who found themselves unemployed.

Beyond these considerations, one to one treatment can reinforce victim blaming ideologies: if the mental health problem of the unemployed person is treatable by a therapist, both problem and solution appear to be located at the intra- or inter-personal rather than at the socio-structural level. The victim of pathogenic social arrangements comes to be seen as the cause of those social problems. One to one treatment in these circumstances is offensive, unjust, naive and short sighted.

Others argue that, rather than one to one treatments, social scientists should get involved in the design and implementation of effective interventions which focus on unemployed people individually or in groups in an attempt to make them seek paid employment more assiduously and effectively. Recent examples are Proudfoot et al. (1997:96) who adapted the "principles of cognitive-behavioural therapy ... to create a group-training programme for long term unemployed people" and Caplan, Vinocur and Price (1997:343) who designed, implemented and evaluated the so called JOBS intervention whose "short term goals focus on the enhancement of productive job-seeking skills and on the self confidence to use those skills ... fortifying the job seeker's ability to resist demoralization and to persist in the face of barriers and common setbacks ... inherent in the search for a new job ... the long-term goals focus on providing ... confidence and skills to achieve reemployment in stable settings that maximise economic, social and psychological rewards from re-employment". There are a number of reasons for concern about such interventions. Firstly, such interventions focus on social and job-seeking skills, self-confidence, self-efficacy, perseverance in the face of set-backs, motivational energy, attributional style, negative thinking etc and play down or ignore socio-structural factors.

Secondly, such interventions locate the cause of both the unemployment and of the mental health problem in the unemployed person rather than in social structural factors reflecting the societal distribution of power. They thus blame victims for their own damaging and distressing predicament.

Thirdly, such interventions are insensitive to local variations, such as in the ratio of job seekers to vacancies, the economic cycle, labour market niches etc. Unemployed older unskilled industrial manual workers in recession-bound areas are processed through the same interventions as young unemployed information technology workers in economic-boom areas, even though the chances of the former finding employment are weaker whatever is done and the chances of the latter finding paid work are relatively good even without intervention.

Fourthly, such interventions usually address the problem of unemployment within a strictly limited number of brief sessions, sometimes in group settings. Moreover, they tend to regard employment as the end of the problem, even though the effects of unemployment may run deep and long (Fineman, 1987) and even though many unemployed people move from unemployment into low paid, insecure, casual, part-time, temporary, non-unionised employment of poor psychological quality replete with stressors (Dooley and Catalano, 1999; Fryer and Winefield, 1998; Warr, 1987). The British labour market was for a long time dominated by men employed in permanent full time skilled manual jobs in manufacturing industries. However, currently nearly 50% of the workforce are women, nearly 50% of all workers are in the service sector, short-term and fixed contract employment is growing, over 12% of paid workers are now self-employed and 70% of the jobs which have been created since 1992 are part-time temporary jobs (RSA, 1997).

Fifthly, such interventions may actually increase mental health problems in those remaining unemployed, whilst not substantially decreasing overall unemployment. They usually involve encouraging job seekers to look harder, more often, using more ways, for employment and may disrupt ways which people have found to cope effectively with ongoing unemployment.

Whilst we can urge everyone in a race to run faster, there will still only be one winner, So also with a number of people "competing" for each job vacancy. Given that the number of job vacancies officially notified to government Job centres in February 1999 was less than a quarter of a million (206,574), the mismatch between the number of job seekers and the number of jobs available is stark, whether we regard the number of people in Great Britain competing for jobs at the same time as 1.3 million, 1.8 million, 2.5 million or 4.7 million (see above - all figures courtesy of the independent Unemployment Unit).

Moreover some schemes carry the threat of reduction or stopping of unemployment allowance in case of non-compliance with the letter or the "spirit" of the intervention. Research has shown, however, that unemployed people with higher levels of employment commitment, more financial problems (both objectively and subjectively assessed) and less security are at greater risk of more severe mental health problems than job seekers with lower employment commitment, less financial worries and more security. For further details see: Fryer, 1988; Fryer, 1990; Fryer, 1992; Fryer and Payne, 1986; Fryer and Ullah, 1987. Interventions which combine increasing commitment to paid employment and more vigorous job seeking with the threat of withdrawal of financial support combine stressors, probably multiplicatively, and maximise the likelihood of more negative mental health consequences of unemployment.

Sixthly, such interventions assume that the problem of unemployment lies in the supply side (potential employees) rather than in employers' demand for labour and thus are destined never to make much impact on overall levels of unemployment. Clearly no matter how hard they look, the majority of unemployed people will not find jobs. ·

Although interventions to encourage unemployed people to seek jobs more "diligently" may make a difference regarding which particular individuals are unemployed, they can make no real impression on the overall total of unemployed people, since they create no jobs. They merely reallocate the misery caused by unemployment from one person to another.

Incidentally, a reserve army of unemployed people kept desperate for employment and being seen by employed people to suffer economic, social, health and mental health consequences of unemployment has the additional benefit for some stake holder groups in society of simultaneously acting as an effective incomes policy and disciplining the workforce.

The dominant psychological account of what it is about being unemployed which causes mental health problems (Jahoda's Latent Function deprivation account) is important and ground breaking yet has a number of problems at a variety of levels (see Fryer, 1986). New ways of conceptualising and investigating the psychological problems of unemployment are needed and are being developed. As regards investigative methods, action, intervention and evaluation research methods within a community psychological perspective are particularly promising (Fryer, 1995; Fryer, 1998; Fryer and Fagan, 1993; Fryer and Feather, 1994).

As regards conceptualisation, the problem of unemployment is not merely the problem of the absence of employment. An Agency Restriction account (Fryer and Payne, 1984; Fryer, 1986; Fryer, 1995) takes this into account, arguing that the agency of unemployed people is frequently restricted by future insecurity (Fryer and McKenna, 1988), by information poverty (Cassell, Fitter, Fryer and Smith, 1988) by material poverty (Fryer, 1990; McGhee and Fryer, 1989) and by the very social relationship which is unemployment (Fryer and Winefield, 1998). Looked at this way, "unemployment" sector "employment" by the State in which the "employee's work" involves searching for something virtually extinct in many parts of the world, taking part in humiliating State rituals etc., "working" in poor quality environments (the State unemployment bureaucracy, the streets, impoverished homes etc) with a high risk of "occupational strain" in return for inadequate "pay" delivered in a stigmatising and disempowering fashion with a virtual absence of negotiating rights over "pay" and "working conditions" and with scarcely any scope for collective action. Looked at this way, unemployment has much in common with poor quality, mental health damaging jobs.

In order to address the conditions which damage the mental health of both employed and unemployed people, it may well be necessary to redesign not only the substandard jobs of many employed people but also the jobs of unemployed people too.

REFERENCES

Bakke, E. W. 1933, The Unemployed Man. London: Nisbet.

Barnett, P., Howden-Chapman. P. and Smith, A. 1995, Unemployment, work and health: opportunities for healthy public policy. The New Zealand Medical Journal, 26 April, 108, 998, 138-140.

Bartley, M. 1992, Authorities and Partisans: The Debate on Unemployment and Health. Edinburgh: Edinburgh University Press.

Beale, N. and Nethercott, S, 1985, Job loss and family morbidity: a study of a factory closure. Journal of the Royal College of General Practitioners, 35, 510-14.

Beales, H. L and Lambert, R. S. 1934, Memoirs of the Unemployed. Wakefield: E.P. Publishing.

Binns, D. and Mars, G. 1984, Family, community and unemployment: a study in change. The Sociological Review, 32, 4, 662-695.

Brenner, S-O, Petterson, I-L, Arnetz, B. and Levi, L. 1989, Stress reactions to unemployment among Swedish blue-collar workers. In: B. Starrin, P-G Svensson and Wintersberger, H. (Eds.). Unemployment, Poverty and Quality of Working Life. Berlin: Sigma.

Briscoe, I. 1995, In Whose Service? Making Community Service Work for the Unemployed. London: Demos.

Caplan, R. D., Vinocur, A. D. and Price, R. H. 1997, From job loss to reemployment: field experiments in prevention-focused coping. In Albee, G.W. and Gullotta, T.P. (eds.). Primary Prevention Works. Sage, Thousand Oaks / London: pp 341-379.

Cassell, C., Fitter, M., Fryer, D. and Smith, L. 1988, The development of computer applications by unemployed people in community settings. Journal of Occupational Psychology, 61: 89-102.

Catalano, R. & Kennedy, J. 1998, The effects of unemployment on disability caseloads in California. Journal of Community and Applied Social Psychology, 8, 137-144.

Catalano, R., Rook, K. and Dooley, D, 1986, Labor markets and help seeking: a test of the employment security hypothesis. Journal of Health and Social Behaviour, 27, 277-287.

Claussen, B. and Nygard, J. F. 1994, Unemployed patients in 60 general practices. Tidsskr Nor Laegeforen, 114, 1806-10. (In Norwegian with english summary).

Claussen, B. and Bertran, J. 1999, The International Commission on Occupational Health Working Group 'Unemployment and Health' 25–26 September, 1998. Paris, France. Int Arch Occup Environ Health, 72 (Suppl): 1-48.

Cole, T. J., Donnet, M. L. and Stanfield, J. P. 1983, Unemployment, birth weight and growth in the first year. Archives of Disease in Childhood, 58, 717-722.

Cragg, A. and Dawson, T. 1984, Unemployed Women: A Study of Attitudes and Experiences. Research Paper No. 47. London: Department of Employment.

Daniel, W. W. (1990). The Unemployed Flow. London: PSI.

Dooley, D., and Catalano, R. 1999, Unemployment, disguised unemployment and health: The U.S. case. Int Arch Occup Environ Health, (199)72 (Suppl): 16-19.

Dooley, D., Catalano, R. and Hough, R. 1992, Unemployment and alcohol disorder in 1910 and 1990: drift versus social causation. Journal of Occupational and Organisational Psychology, 65, 4, 277-290.

Eisenberg, P. and Lazarsfeld, P.F, 1938, The psychological effects of unemployment. Psychological Bulletin, 35, 258-390.

Engbersen, G., Schuyt, K., Timmer, J. and Van Waarden, F. 1993, Cultures of Unemployment: A comparative look at long-term unemployment and urban poverty. Oxford: Westview Press.

Feather, N. T. 1992, The Psychological Impact of Unemployment. New York: Springer Verlag.

Fineman, S. 1987, Back to employment. wounds and wisdoms. In D. Fryer & P. Ullah (Eds.): Unemployed People: Social and Psychological Perspectives. Milton Keynes: Open University Press.

Fineman S. 1990, Supporting the Jobless: Doctors, Clergy, Police, Probation Officers. London: Tavistock/Routledge.

Fryer, D. 1986, Employment deprivation and personal agency during unemployment. Social Behaviour, 1, 3-23.

Fryer, D. 1988, The experience of unemployment in social context. In: Fisher, S. and Reason, J. Handbook of Life Stress, Cognition and Health. Chichester: Wiley, pp. 211-238.

Fryer, D. 1990, The mental health costs of unemployment: towards a social psychological concept of poverty. British Journal of Clinical and Social Psychiatry. 7, 4: 164-176.

Fryer, D. 1995, Social and psychological consequences of unemployment: from interviewing to intervening. Journal of Applied Social Behaviour. 2, 1: 25-43.

Fryer, D. 1992, Psychological or material deprivation: why does unemployment have mental health consequences? In E. McLaughlin (Ed.): Understanding Unemployment. London: Routledge.

Fryer, D. 1995, Benefit agency? Labour market disadvantage, deprivation and mental health. The Psychologist, 8, 6, 265-272.

Fryer, D. 1997, International perspectives on youth unemployment and mental health: some central issues. Journal of Adolescence. 20: 333-342.

Fryer, D. (Guest Editor), 1998, Mental Health Consequences of Economic Insecurity, Relative Poverty and Social exclusion: Community Psychology Perspectives on Recession. Special issue of Journal of Community and Applied Social psychology, 8, 2, 75-180.

Fryer, D. and Fagan, R. 1993, Coping with unemployment. International Journal of Political Economy, 23, 3, 95-120.

Fryer, D. and Feather, N. 1994, Intervention research techniques. In: Cassell, C. and Symon, G. (eds). Qualitative Methods in Organizational and Occupational Psychology. London, Sage, pp 230-247.

Fryer, D. and McKenna, S. 1988, Redundant skills: temporary unemployment and mental health. In Patrickson, M. (ed). Readings in Organizational Behaviour. New South Wales: Harper and Row, pp. 44-70.

Fryer, D. and Payne, R. L. 1986, Being unemployed: a review of the literature on the psychological experience of unemployment. In: C. L. Cooper & I. Robertson (Eds.), International Review of Industrial and Organizational Psychology 1986, (pp. 235-278) Chichester: John Wiley & Sons.

Fryer, D. and Ullah, P. 1997, (Eds.): Unemployed People: Social and Psychological Perspectives. Milton Keynes: Open University Press.

Fryer, D. and Winefield, A. H. 1998, Employment stress and unemployment distress as two varieties   of labour market induced psychological strain: an explanatory framework. Australian Journal of Social Research. 5, 1: 3-18.

Gatti, A. 1935, Prima relazione sulla efficienza lavorativa dei disoccupati. Italian Archives of Psychology, xiii, 67-91.

Haworth, J. T. 1997, Work, Leisure and Well Being. London: Routledge.

Jahoda, M. 1938 / 1987, Unemployed Men at Work. In D. Fryer and P. Ullah (Eds.): Unemployed People: Social and Psychological Perspectives. Milton Keynes: Open University Press.

Jahoda, M. 1982, Employment and Unemployment: A Social-Psychological Analysis. Cambridge: Cambridge University Press.

Janlert, U. and Hammarstrom, A. 1992, Alcohol consumption among unemployed youths: results from a prospective study. British Journal of Addiction, 87, 703-714.

Kaufman, H.G. 1982, Professionals in Search of Work: Coping with the Stress of Job Loss and Underemployment. New York: Wiley.

Kingfisher, C. P. 1996, Women in the American Welfare Trap. Philadelphia: University of Pennsylvania Press.

Kirchler, E. 1985, Job loss and mood. Journal of Economic Psychology, 6, 9-25.

Kronauer, M., Vogel, B. and Gerlach, F. 1993, Im Schatten der Arbeitsgesellschaft: Arbeitslose und die Dynamik sozialer Ausgrenzung. Frankfurt & New York: Campus Verlag.

Lahelma, E. and Kangas, R. 1989, Unemployment, re-employment and psychic well being in Finland. In: B. Starrin, P-G Svensson and Wintersberger, H. (Eds.). Unemployment, Poverty and Quality of Working Life. Berlin: Sigma.

Lazarsfeld-Jahoda, M. and Zeisel, H. 1933, Die Arbeitslosen von Marienthal. Psychol. Monographien, 5, 1933. An English language translation appeared in 1971 as Jahoda, M., Lazarsfeld, P. F. and Zeisel, H. 1971, Marienthal: The Sociography of an Unemployed Community. Chicago: Aldine Atherton).

McGhee, J. and Fryer, D. 1989, Unemployment, income and the family: an action research approach. Social Behaviour, 4, 237-252.

McKee, L. and Bell, C. 1986, His unemployment, her problem: the domestic and marital consequences of male unemployment. In S. Allen, S. Waton, K. Purcell and S. Wood (Eds.), 1992, The Experience of Unemployment. Basingstoke: Macmillan.

McLoyd, V. C 1989, Socialisation and development in a changing economy: the effects of paternal job and income loss on children. American Psychologist, 44, 2, 293-302.

Milne, S. and Ryle, S. 1996, World's jobless total 1 billion. The Guardian, Tuesday November 26.

Moylan, S., Millar, J. and Davies, R. 1984, For Richer for Poorer? DHSS Cohort Study of Unemployed Men. DHSS Social Research Branch Research Report 11. London: HMSO.

Murphy, G. C. and Athanasou, J. A. 1999, The effect of unemployment on mental health. Journal of Occupational and Organizational Psychology, 72, 83-100.

O'Brien, G.E. 1986, Psychology of Work and Unemployment, Chichester: Wiley.

Pilgrim Trust 1938, Men Without Work. Cambridge: Cambridge University Press.

Proudfoot, J., Guest, D., Carson, J. Dunn, G. and Gray, J. 1997 Effect of cognitive-behavioural training on job-finding among long-term unemployed people. The Lancet. 350: 96-100.

Pugliese, E. 1993, The Europe of the unemployed. In: M. Kronauer (Guest Editor). Unemployment in Western Europe, Special Issue of the International Journal of Political Economy, 23, 3, 3-120.

Rowntree, B. S. and Lasker, B. 1910, Unemployment: A Social Study. London: Macmillan.

RSA 1997, Key views on the future of work. Redefining Work Discussion Paper, Royal Society of Arts Journal, June, 7-13.

Smith, R. 1987, Unemployment and Health: A Disaster and a Challenge. Oxford: Oxford University Press.

Svensson, P.G. and Wintersberger, H. (Eds.), 1989, Unemployment, Poverty and Quality of Working Life. Berlin: Sigma.

Unemployment Unit 1999, Working Brief, 103, April, 22-24.

van Heeringen, K. and Vanderplasschen, W. 1999, Unemployment and suicidal behaviour in perspective. Int Arch Occup Environ Health, 72 (Suppl), 42-45.

Varela Novo, M. 1999, Unemployment and mental health in Galicia, Spain. Int Arch Occup Environ Health, 72 (Suppl), 14-15.

Verhaar, C. H. A., de Klauer, P. M., de Goede, M. P. M., van Ophem, J. A. C. and de Vries, A. (Eds.), 1996, On the Challenges of Unemployment in a Regional Europe. Aldershot: Avebury.

Warr, P. B. 1987, Work, Unemployment and Mental Health. Oxford: Clarendon Press.

Westin, S. 1990, The structure of a factory closure; individual responses to job-loss and unemployment in a 10-year controlled follow-up study. Social Science and Medicine, 31, 1301-11.

Whelan, C. T. 1992, The role of income, life-style deprivation and financial strain in mediating the impact of unemployment on psychological distress: evidence from the Republic of Ireland, Journal of Occupational and Organisational Psychology, 65, 4, 331-344.

Winefield, A. H. and Fryer, D. 1996, Some emerging threats to the validity of research on unemployment and mental health. The Australian Journal of Social Research, 12, 1, 115-134.

Winefield, A. H., Tiggemann, M, and Winefield, H. R. 1993, Growing Up with Unemployment: A longitudinal study of its psychological impact. London: Routledge.

Ytterdahl, T. 1999, Routine health check-ups of unemployed in Norway. Int Arch Occup Environ Health. 72, (Suppl), 38-39.

Zawadski, B. and Lazarsfeld, P. F. 1935, The psychological consequences of unemployment. Journal of Social Psychology, 6, 224-251.

UNEMPLOYMENT AND HEALTH CARE UTILIZATION

Allen Kraut, MD[1,2], Cam Mustard, ScD[2,3,4,5,6], Randy Walld, BSc[2,3] and Robert Tate, MSc[2,6]

1. Department of Internal Medicine, University of Manitoba, Winnipeg, Canada; 2. Department of Community Health Sciences, University of Manitoba; 3. Manitoba Centre for Health Policy and Evaluation, University of Manitoba; 4. Population Health Program, Canadian Institute for Advanced Research; 5. Institute of Work and Health, Toronto, Canada; 6. Workplace/Workforce Theme HEALNet Network Centre of Excellence

Abstract: OBJECTIVES: To determine if prior use of health services predicts subsequent risk of unemployment and to describe the acute effects of exposure to unemployment on the use of health care services. DESIGN: Prospective population-based study. SETTING/PARTICIPANTS: 18,272 employed and 1,498 unemployed individuals in a Canadian province in 1986. MAIN OUTCOME MEASURE: All cause and cause-specific rates of hospital admission and ambulatory physician contacts over the period 1983-89 were compared between unemployed and employed individuals across four consecutive time periods related to the onset of unemployment. RESULTS: Adjusted rates of hospitalisation admission and physician contacts were higher among the unemployed across all four periods. When persons with a history of mental health treatment were excluded, health care use in the period prior to the onset of unemployment was equivalent among the employed and unemployed. Controlling for mental health treatment history, all-cause and cause-specific health care use was elevated among the unemployed during the unemployment spell. CONCLUSIONS: Unemployed individuals had increased hospitalisation rates before their current spell of unemployment. Much of this difference is due to the subgroup with prior mental health treatment. For individuals without prior mental health care, hospitalisation increased following a period of unemployment.

Key words: Unemployment, Health Care Utilization, Selection, Causation, Mental Health

1. INTRODUCTION

Both cross-sectionally and prospectively, unemployment has been found to be consistently associated with health status deficits across a broad range of health measures, including individual biological and behavioural responses, self-reported or objectively measured health and functional status, and mortality (Moser et al 1987, Linn et al 1985, Martikainen 1990, Morris

Health Effects of the New Labour Market, edited by Isaksson *et al.*
Kluwer Academic / Plenum Publishers, New York, 2000.

et al 1994, D'Arcy & Siddique 1985, Jin et al 1995, Valkonen & Martikainen 1995, Moser et al 1984). This relationship between unemployment and health may potentially be accounted for by three competing explanations: causation, where unemployment precipitates declines in health, perhaps through the combination of effects arising from loss of income, alteration in behaviour, and in some settings, reduced access to medical care (Brenner & Mooney 1983, Brenner 1971); selection, where individuals in poor health experience a higher risk of becoming unemployed (Valkonen and Martikainen 1995); and indirect selection, which refers to the possibility that individual characteristics may place an individual simultaneously at higher risk for both unemployment and poor health (Montgomery et al 1996).

In prospective studies, a number of methodologic issues have limited efforts to estimate the relative contribution of each of these competing explanations in accounting for the observed relationships. Efforts to estimate the direct impact of unemployment on health have been limited by a number of factors, including variations across studies in the definition of 'exposure' to unemployment and whether and how studies adjusted for potential confounding. Similarly, investigation of the hypothesis that the association can be explained primarily by the selection of unhealthy workers into unemployment as been constrained by the relative absence of information on health status prior to the incidence of unemployment.

This prospective study reports on the relationship between unemployment and the use of health care services for a representative sample in one Canadian province. The study was designed to explicitly test two hypotheses: first, that individuals who become unemployed are a random selection of the labour force on measures of health care use prior to unemployment, and second, that the acute effects of unemployment would result in higher use of health care services during unemployment spells.

2.   METHODS

2.1   Study Population and Context, Study Design and Sources of Data

The study population is a sample of labour force participants in the province of Manitoba, Canada. The study design combines comprehensive longitudinal histories of health care utilization over a seven-year period from 1983 to 1989 with cross-sectional information on labour market experiences in the period 1985-86 for a sample of 19,770 individuals 15-64 years of age.

Information on health care utilization was obtained from administrative records of physician services and hospital care maintained by the Manitoba Health Services Insurance Plan (MHSIP), the single payer government funded health care insurance agency in the province. All citizens have equal access to complete medical coverage for both outpatient and in patient insured services. There are no co-payments or deductibles. Payments to either physicians or hospitals are not dependent on diagnosis. Information on labour market experiences, occupation and other socioeconomic attributes of the study sample was obtained from responses provided to the 1986 federal census.

In Manitoba, human rights legislation prevents the indiscriminate laying off of sick individuals, however inability to perform the essential tasks of a job is grounds for dismissal. There is no absolute financial benefit for being unemployed for sickness over other reasons, although sickness may hasten the attainment of unemployment benefits.

2.2   Study Sample

The study sample of labour force participants was drawn from a research database composed of a 5% sample of the 1,050,000 residents of Manitoba, Canada, selected by stratified sampling from respondents to the federal 1986 census.   For each sampled respondent, information on demographic and socioeconomic characteristics was linked to records of health care utilization, migration and vital status for a seven-year period from 1983 to 1989. The method used to link census records to health care utilization records has been described previously (Houle et al 1996, David et al 1992, Mustard et al 1997, Roos & Wajda 1991, Newcombe et al 1959).

A total of 21,483 labour force participants were eligible for inclusion in the study. Individuals not continuously resident in the province over the 7 year observation period (N=1,557) or who reported never working (N=156) were excluded from this sample, leaving a total of 19,770 individuals. Population estimates produced from the sample accurately reflect the sociodemographic profile, mortality experience and health care utilization of Manitoba residents (Houle et al 1996). Figure 1 describes the study sample.

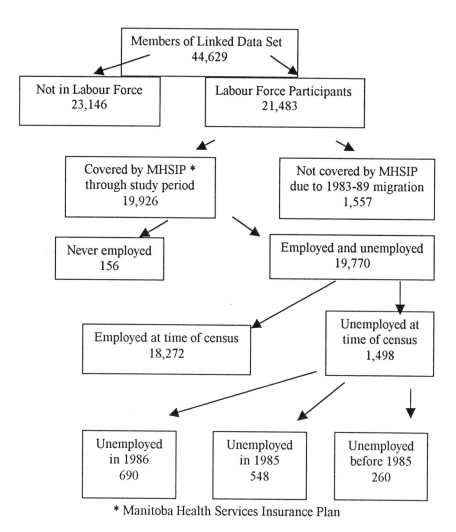

* Manitoba Health Services Insurance Plan

Figure 1. Description of Study Population

2.3   Measures

2.3.1   Outcome Measure

Electronic records of inpatient hospital admissions and ambulatory physician contacts, were the source of the study outcome measures. These records contain unique numeric personal identifiers which can be used to create longitudinal person-based histories of health care utilization (Roos et al 1993). Hospital separation abstracts record up to 16 diagnoses defining patient health status and physician reimbursement claims record a single diagnosis most responsible for the patient encounter. Diagnoses are recorded in the ICD-9-CM standard (International Classification of Disease, 1987). This diagnostic information was used to group health service use into three categories identifying the treatment of: mental health disorders (ICD 290-319), injury and poisoning (ICD 800-999), and cardiovascular disorders (ICD 390-459). Health services associated with pregnancy, labour and delivery (ICD 630-676) were excluded.

2.3.2 Employment Status

Standard Statistics Canada definitions were used to determine the employment status of labour force participants in June 1986. Among unemployed workers, the initiation date of the current unemployment spell was not recorded by the census questionnaire. Approximate information on duration of unemployment was obtained from a question that asked if the unemployed individual last worked in 1986, during 1985 or prior to 1985. No information was available on labour force participation and employment status in the three and one half year observation period following the census. Similarly, no retrospective information on employment status over the period 1983 to June 1986 was available for persons employed on census day. A total of 1,498 individuals were unemployed on census day (weighted estimate 6.3% of labour force), agreeing closely with the official unemployment estimate at the time of the census (6.5%) (Statistics Canada 1997).

For unemployed individuals, health care use was classified into four observation periods: 1) before the current spell of unemployment; 2) a transitional period during which an individual moved from being employed to unemployed; 3) the period of unemployment; and 4) the 36 month period following December 1986. For persons reporting unemployment status in June 1986, the remainder of calendar year 1986 was classified to the 'during unemployment' period. Because the specific date in the transitional period when the individual became unemployed was not measured by the census, this period contains time prior to the individual becoming unemployed and time during a period of unemployment. Since concern about job loss may have adverse health effects (Henry et al 1994, Ferrie et al 1995, Ferrie et al 1998) and the earliest period of unemployment may have acute effects on health and on health care behaviours we separated this period from the 'during unemployment' period. Table 1 describes the temporal organisation of health care use for the unemployed in relation to duration of unemployment.

Table 1. Classification of Health Care Use by Period of Unemployment

Date of Initiation of Unemployment Spell	#	1983	1984	1985	Jan.1 - June 3 1986	June 4 - Dec. 31 1986	1987 - 1989
Prior to 1985	260	B	T	D	D	D	F
In 1985	548	B	B	T	D	D	F
In 1986	690	B	B	B	T	D	F

B = Before; T = Transitional; D = During; F = Follow up

2.4   Demographic and Socioeconomic Characteristics

Measures of age, sex, marital status, Aboriginal heritage (race), attained education, sources and amounts of individual and household income, self-reported occupation and region of residence were obtained from responses to the June 1986 census (Table 2).

2.5   Health Status Prior to Unemployment

Because mental health disorders have negative impacts on labour force participation (Dohrenwend et al 1992), the complete labour force sample was stratified on the basis of a history of treatment for mental health conditions prior to the June 1986 census date. A history of treatment for mental health disorder was defined as one or more hospital admissions or two or more physician contacts for the treatment of mental health conditions (ICD 290-319). Applying this definition, 1,208 respondents (6.1%) had a history of mental health care use.

Table 2. Demographic Characteristics of Labour Force Participants, Manitoba

	Employed	Breakdown of Current Episode of Unemployment		
		Initiation of current episode in 1986	Initiation of current episode in 1985	Initiation of current episode before 1985
Unweighted N	18,272	690	548	260
Weighted N[+]	18,518.0	623.9	435.6	192.3
Mean Age (Years)	38.0	33.2	32.5	36.2
Male (%)	57.6	51.4	53.7	48.0
Residence (%)				
Winnipeg	58.3	62.3	60.6	57.1
Urban non-Winnipeg	14.9	14.6	11.0	13.1
Rural	26.8	23.1	28.4	29.8
Education (%)				
None-Grade 9	17.1	21.0	20.9	24.9
Grade 10-12	36.1	39.1	43.5	38.9
Some university/post secondary	46.9	39.8	35.6	36.2
Married (%)	67.5	51.4	49.0	49.6
Aboriginal race (%)	1.5	5.7	11.1	18.8
Household Income ($)	40,500	35,300	34,200	20,500

[+]All values are derived from weighted sample estimates.

3.   ANALYTIC METHOD

Crude rates of hospital admission and physician service use (1,000 person years) are reported, weighted by respondent sample weights, comparing employed to unemployed cohort members. For the unemployed, rates of health care use are stratified into the four observation periods. Ratios of adjusted rates of health care utilization (and 95% confidence intervals) were computed comparing unemployed to the employed reference group and included adjustment for age, gender, education, race, area of residence, calendar year and household income. Income, although it is an effect of unemployment, was utilized as a measure of socioeconomic status as occupation was not available for individuals who were unemployed for more than 18 months prior to the census. When separate analyses were performed using income and occupation for those individuals for whom both variables were available, similar results were obtained.

Measures of hospital use and physician service use were analysed under assumptions of a Poisson distribution, using the GENMOD procedure in SAS to account for the correlated structure of the repeated measurement of health care use for each person over the seven year period. Interaction terms were included where indicated. Normalised sample weights were incorporated in analyses to adjust effect size estimates arising from the stratified sample design. Because previous work had established that the sampling design had weak effects on variance estimates, analytic tools to adjust variance estimates were not used.

These multivariate analyses were repeated after stratification of the sample by mental health treatment status. Analyses were also conducted for the three subsidiary groupings of health care use: mental health disorders, injuries and poisonings, and cardiovascular disorders. Also included in the reported results are statistical tests for differences in health care utilization for the unemployed group using the before period as a reference for the other observation periods.

4.   RESULTS:

Comparisons of hospital and ambulatory care utilization are reported in Tables 3 and 4. The unemployed had significantly higher rates of hospital admissions than the employed group in all four observation periods, with adjusted relative rate ratios ranging from 1.34 in the period before the current spell of employment to 1.33 in the follow-up period (Table 3). Rates of ambulatory care use were also higher for the unemployed relative to the employed in all four observation periods (Table 4).

Tables 3 and 4 also report results stratified by history of treatment for mental health disorder. For those with no history of mental health treatment, rates of hospital admission and ambulatory care were equivalent between the employed and unemployed groups prior to the current episode of unemployment. In the three subsequent periods, however, rates of both hospital admission and ambulatory care for all disorders combined were significantly elevated in the unemployed group.

Among both the employed and unemployed with a history of treatment for mental health disorder, rates of health care utilization for all disorders combined were consistently 2 to 3 times higher than those without a history of mental health treatment. In the group with a history of mental health treatment, there was no observed difference in the use of ambulatory care between unemployed and employed groups in any of the four observation periods. The unemployed had significantly higher use of hospital care relative to the employed in the before period (adjusted rate ratio (RR) 2.09, 95% confidence interval (CI) 1.46 - 2.99). The hospitalisation rate ratio declined over the subsequent periods.

All cause hospitalisation rates were significantly lower in the follow-up period when compared to the before period for those with a history of prior mental health care. The opposite was true for those without such a history.

Rates of hospital admission for the treatment of mental health disorders were elevated in the unemployed group relative to the employed group in the before and transitional periods (Table 5). Rates of ambulatory care for the treatment of mental health disorders in the unemployed group were elevated in the period during the episode of unemployment and the follow-up period. For both hospital admissions and ambulatory care, these results persisted in analyses excluding labour force participants with a prior history of mental health treatment.

Hospital and ambulatory care utilization rates for the treatment of injury and poisoning were elevated in the unemployed group during the transitional period, the period of unemployment and the follow-up period (Table 6), both for the complete labour force sample, and controlling for prior history of mental health treatment. In the period before the initiation of the current unemployment episode, rates of ambulatory care use for the treatment of injury did not differ between the unemployed and employed. A significant difference in the rate of hospital admission for these conditions in the before period (RR: 1.49, 95% CI: 1.02-2.18) was not sustained when individuals with a history of mental health treatment were excluded from the analysis (RR: 1.38, 95% CI: 0.90-2.11). There were no consistent differences between the employed and unemployed on rates of hospital admission and ambulatory care for the treatment of cardiovascular disorders.

In Table 7, the analytic perspective is reversed. In this table, the relationship between prior health care use and subsequent risk of unemployment is estimated, stratified into three groups; individuals who became unemployed in 1986, in 1985, and prior to 1985. In a consistent finding across all three groups, the approximately 6% of the labour force with a treatment history for mental health conditions had an elevated risk of subsequent unemployment. For example, among the labour force participants employed in 1985 who had two or more ambulatory physician contacts for mental health care in this period (3.5% of the employed cohort in 1985), the risk of 1986 unemployment was 1.57 times greater than those not in treatment in 1985 (95% CI: 1.10-2.25). In contrast, health care utilization for non-mental health disorders prior to unemployment did not consistently predict the risk of becoming unemployed.

Table 3. Comparison of Hospital Admission Rates Between Employed and Unemployed Labour Force Participants, Manitoba 1983-1989*

	EMPLOYED			UNEMPLOYED											
				Before			Transitional			During			Follow-up		
	N#	Rate+	RR^	N	Rate	RR	N	Rate	RR	N	Rate	RR	N	Rate	RR
Entire cohort	9502	72.0	1.0	301	89.8	1.34 (1.12-1.60)	138	102.3	1.45 (1.14-1.86)	158	93.6	1.32 (1.05-1.66)	525	96.6	1.33 (1.13-1.56)
Cohort members with history of MHC**	1289	151.8	1.0	77	331.9	2.09 (1.46-2.99)	17	212.4	1.24 (0.57-2.69)	16	169.4	1.16 (0.57-2.36)	28	84.6	0.71* (0.39-1.27)
Cohort members with no history of MHC	8213	66.1	1.0	224	68.2	1.15 (0.95-1.39)	121	93.1	1.49 (1.15-1.92)	142	87.2	1.36 (1.07-1.72)	497	97.7	1.43* (1.21-1.68)

*Indicates results are significantly different from the **Before** period, for unemployed only.
#Number of hospitalisations.
+Weighted rates per 1,000 person years.
^Rate ratio adjusted for age, gender, education, race, area of residence, calendar year, and household income.
** Mental Health Care

Table 4. Comparison of Ambulatory Care Contact Rates Between Employed and Unemployed Labour Force Participants, Manitoba 1983-1989*

	EMPLOYED			UNEMPLOYED												
				Before			Transitional			During			Follow-up		
	$N^{\#}$	$Rate^{+}$	$RR^{\wedge}$	N	Rate	RR	N	Rate	RR	N	Rate	RR	N	Rate	RR
Entire cohort	485964	4.0	1.0	11395	4.1	1.07 (1.00-1.15)	4351	4.4	1.07 (0.99-1.16)	6247	4.6	1.13 (1.05-1.22)	20717	4.8	1.13 (1.06-1.20)
Cohort members with history of MHC **	74252	9.2	1.0	2080	10.2	1.04 (0.83-1.29)	682	10.7	0.98 (0.73-1.30)	875	10.2	0.94 (0.73-1.23)	2637	9.2	1.02 (0.82-1.27)
Cohort members with no history of MHC	411712	3.6	1.0	9315	3.5	1.06 (0.99-1.13)	3669	3.8	1.09 (1.01-1.17)	5372	4.2	1.15 (1.06-1.24)	18080	4.4	1.14 (1.07-1.22)

*Indicates results are significantly different from the **Before** period, for unemployed only.

#Number of ambulatory contacts.

+Weighted rates per person year.

^Rate ratio adjusted for age, gender, education, race, area of residence, calendar year, and household income.

** Mental Health Care

Table 5. Comparison of Hospital Admission Rates and Ambulatory Care Contact Rates for the Treatment of Mental Health Conditions Between Employed and Unemployed Labour Force Participants, Manitoba 1983-1989*

	EMPLOYED			UNEMPLOYED												
				Before			Transitional			During			Follow-up		
	N#	Rate+	RR^	N	Rate	RR	N	Rate	RR	N	Rate	RR	N	Rate	RR
Entire cohort hospitalisation	420	3.2	1.0	32	11.2	3.60 (2.11-6.14)	17	17.1	4.70 (2.21-9.99)	10	7.4	1.77 (0.72-4.35)	27	5.4	1.21* (0.64-2.30)
Entire cohort ambulatory contacts	34201	296	1.0	788	313	1.37 (0.96-1.95)	430	496	1.40 (0.94-2.07)	620	534	1.61 (1.13-2.30)	1812	468	1.44 (1.08-1.93)
Hospital admissions for cohort members with no history of MHC**	126	1.8	1.0	-	-	-	8	6.8	6.15 (1.50-25.29)	6	3.9	2.79 (0.67-11.74)	18	3.1	1.34 (0.64-2.84)
Ambulatory contacts for cohort members with no history of MHC	11015	168	1.0	-	-	-	166	170	1.42 (0.98-2.05)	311	266	1.87 (1.25-2.80)	1102	295	1.70 (1.21-2.41)

*Indicates those results that are significantly different from the **Before** period when that period was used as the reference.
#Number of events. ^Rate ratio adjusted for age, gender, education, race, area of residence, calendar year, and household income.
+Weighted rates per 1,000 person years. ** Mental Health Care

Table 6. Comparison of Hospital Admission Rates and Ambulatory Care Contact Rates for the Treatment of Injuries and Poisonings Between Employed and Unemployed Labour Force Participants, Manitoba 1983 – 1989

| | EMPLOYED | | | UNEMPLOYED | | | | | | | | | | | |
| | | | | Before | | | Transitional | | | During | | | Follow-up | | |
	N#	Rate+	UR^	N	Rate	RR	N	Rate	RR	N	Rate	RR	N	Rate	RR
Hospital admissions for entire cohort	1052	7.4	1.0	55	14.9	1.49 (1.02-2.18)	32	18.3	1.87 (1.13-3.09)	40	18.6	2.02 (1.27-3.21)	101	15.8	2.00 (1.47-2.73)
Ambulatory contacts for entire cohort	48563	392	1.0	1379	458	1.03 (0.91-1.16)	532	506	1.08 (0.93-1.26)	730	490	1.18 (0.99-1.41)	2360	468	1.13 (1.03-1.25)
Hospital admissions for cohort members with no history of MHC **	942	7.0	1.0	46	13.2	1.38 (0.90-2.11)	32	19.8	2.15 (1.30-3.66)	38	18.1	2.10 (1.29-3.40)	98	16.5	2.25 (1.64-3.09)
Ambulatory contacts for cohort members with no history of MHC	43853	379	1.0	1215	428	1.00 (0.87-1.14)	495	470	1.13 (0.96-1.33)	681	502	1.22 * (1.01-1.47)	2188	482	1.15 (1.04-1.28)

*Indicates results are significantly different from the **Before** period, for unemployed only.
#Number of hospital admissions or ambulatory contacts.
+Weighted rates per 1,000 person years.
^Rate ratio adjusted for age, gender, education, race, area of residence, calendar year, and household income.
** Mental Health Care

Table 7. Risk of Unemployment in Relation to Prior Health Care Use, By Period of Onset of Unemployment, Manitoba Labour Force Participants, 1986

COVARIATE	INITIATION OF CURRENT UNEMPLOYMENT EPISODE		
	In 1986	**In 1985**	**Before 1985**
Healthcare Utilization Variables *			
Mental Health **			
Hospitalisation in 1983	NS	3.17 (1.12-8.98)	NS
Hospitalisation in 1984	NS	5.51 (2.34-12.97)	-
Hospitalisation in 1985	NS	-	-
Hospitalisation in 1986 (pre census)	-	-	-
Ambulatory contacts 1983	NS	NS	2.54 (1.45-4.45)
Ambulatory contacts 1984	NS	NS	-
Ambulatory contacts 1985	1.57 (1.10-2.25)	-	-
Ambulatory contacts 1986 (pre census)	-	-	-
Non Mental Health ^			
Hospitalisation in 1983	NS	NS	NS
Hospitalisation in 1984	NS	NS	-
Hospitalisation in 1985	1.45 (1.07-1.97)	-	-
Hospitalisation in 1986 (pre census)	-	-	-
Ambulatory contacts 1983	1.24 (1.01-1.50)	NS	NS
Ambulatory contacts 1984	NS	NS	-
Ambulatory contacts 1985	NS	-	-
Ambulatory contacts 1986 (pre census)	-	-	-

NS not significant at .05 level.

- not entered.

* Adjusted for age, gender, education, race, area of residence, and marital status.

**Hospitalisations refer to one or more hospitalisations for a mental health diagnosis.

Ambulatory contacts refer to 2 or more physician encounters for a mental health diagnosis.

^Hospitalisations refer to one or more hospitalisations for non-mental health diagnosis.

Ambulatory contacts refer to 5 or more physician contacts for non-mental health diagnosis.

3.   DISCUSSION

This prospective study was designed to test two competing explanations for the frequently observed cross-sectional finding that unemployed labour force participants have evidence of poorer health status compared to the employed: the causal explanation, where unemployment precipitates declines in health and the selection explanation, where individuals in poor health experience a higher risk of becoming unemployed.

To examine these questions, the study has used measures of health care utilization as a proxy for direct measures of health status. In comparisons of the entire cohort of labour force participants, persons who become unemployed were shown not to be a random sample of the labour force on prior health status. In the unemployed group, the use of both hospital care and ambulatory physician services was elevated relative to the employed group in the period prior to the incidence of unemployment. Stratification revealed different patterns in the relationship of health care utilization and unemployment for those who had a history of treatment for mental health care and those that did not. Unemployed individuals with prior mental health care had increased hospitalisation rates before their current period of unemployment. When members of the cohort with a history of mental health treatment were excluded from the analysis, the use of hospital care and ambulatory physician services was comparable between the employed and unemployed in the period prior to the incidence of unemployment. In this group health care utilization increased among the unemployed during the periods of transition to unemployment, the period during unemployment and the follow-up period.

Diagnosis-specific analyses also provided evidence supporting the hypotheses that the experience of unemployment is causally implicated in adverse changes in health status. Among persons with no history of mental health treatment, the incidence of hospital admission for the treatment of injury and poisoning increased among the unemployed during the transitional period, the unemployment period and the follow-up period.

Unemployed individuals with no prior history of treatment for mental health disorders, were more likely to have increased health care utilization for subsequent mental health diagnoses. Our ability to control for education, gender, income, and race and stratify by previous contacts for mental health diagnoses make confounding by these variables less likely. However, administrative data may not correctly identify all individuals who would be considered by clinical criteria to have mental health conditions so confounding by unrecognised mental illness cannot be excluded.

Our study had a number of limitations. An observed increase in healthcare utilization may be due to health care seeking behaviour and not due to a change in health status. Our results showed greater differences in hospitalisations than ambulatory care utilization and in health care treatment for injuries and poisonings than other conditions. This pattern is more in keeping with a change in health status of the unemployed rather than an increase in healthcare seeking behaviour. Misclassification may also have occurred as we were not able to identify employment status at times other than at the census. Generally, misclassification tends to obscure associations (Armstrong 1998), thus our results may have underestimated the true effect of unemployment on healthcare utilization. Another limitation is that the group of unemployed would not include discouraged workers who left the work force prior to the census, or individuals who were selected out of the workforce by poor health status prior. It is highly unlikely that exclusion of these types of individuals would have lead to our findings. A further limitation is that we are not certain of the exact date when unemployment commenced. This limitation was addressed by comparing compare utilization in periods before and during a spell of unemployment that showed changes consistent with an unemployment effect.

Overall our data is consistent with a selection effect of the unwell into unemployment, particularly for those with a history of mental health care utilization. This study is consistent with previous research on labour market experiences indicating that mental health disorders increase the risk of unemployment. However, for the majority of the unemployed in this sample, the elevated use of hospital care and ambulatory physician services during the unemployment experience was not explained by prior histories of health care use, and replicates findings from a limited number of prospective studies which have documented increases in the use of health care during unemployment (Linn et al 1985, Iversen et al 1989, Beale & Nethercott 1988, Platt & Kreitman, 1990).

4.   CONCLUSIONS:

The observed association between increases in healthcare utilisation and unemployment is likely due to combination of selection and causation. Future research that utilises population-based data sets should control for prior mental health care as it may obscure a causal relationship between unemployment and adverse health outcomes

ACKNOWLEDGMENT

Funding for this research was provided in part by the National Health Research Development Program, Health Canada. Dr. Mustard is a recipient of a Medical Research Council of Canada Scientist award. The authors wishes to thank Ms. Lisa Springer for assistance in preparation of the manuscript.

REFERENCES

Armstrong, B., 1998, Effects of measurement error on epidemiological studies of environmental and occupational exposures. *Occup. Environ. Medicine* 55:651-56.

Beale, N., and Nethercott, S., 1988, The nature of unemployment morbidity: 2. description. *Journal of the Royal College of General Practitioners* 38:200-2.

Brenner, M.H., and Mooney, A., 1982, Economic change and sex-specific cardiovascular mortality in Britain 1955-1976. *Soc. Sci. Med.* 16:431-42.

Brenner, M.H., 1971, Economic changes and heart disease mortality. *Am. J. Public Health* 61:606.

D'Arcy, C., and Siddique, C.M., 1985, Unemployment and health: an analysis of "Canada Health Survey" data [published erratum appears in Int. J. Health Services 1987; 17(2):368] *Int. J. Health Services* 15(4):609-35.

David, P., Berthelot, J.M., and Mustard, C., 1992, Linking survey and administrative data to study the determinants of health. *Social and Economic Studies Division.* Statistics Canada.

Dohrenwend, B.P., Levav, I., Shout, P.E., Schwartz, S., Naveh, G., Link, B.G., Skodol, A.E., and Stueve, A., 1992, Socioeconomic status and psychiatric disorders: the causation-selection issue. *Science* 255:946-52.

Ferrie, J.E., Shipley, M.J., Marmot, M.G., Stansfeld, S., and Smith, G.D., 1995, Health effects of anticipation of job change and non-employment: longitudinal data from the Whitehall II study. *B.M.J.* 311(7015):1264-9.

Ferrie, J.E., Shipley, M.J., Marmot, M.G., Stansfeld, S., and Smith, G.D., 1998, An uncertain future: the health effects of threats to employment security in white-collar men and women. *Am. J. Public Health* 88:1030-36.

International Classification of Disease, 1987, Clinical Modification DHEW.

Heaney, C.A., Israel, B.A., and House, J.S., 1994, Chronic job insecurity among automobile workers: effects on job satisfaction and health. *Soc. Sci. Med.* 38(10):1431-7.

Houle, C., Berthelot, J.M., David, P., Mustard, C.A., Roos, L.L., and Wolfson, M.C., 1996, Project on matching census 1986 database and Manitoba health care files: private households component. Research Papers Series No91, Analytic Studies Branch, Statistics Canada, Ottawa.

Iversen, L., Sabroe, S., and Damsgaard, M.T., 1989, Hospital admissions before and after shipyard closure. *B.M.J.* 299(6707):1073-6.

Jin, R.L., Shah, C.P., and Svoboda, T.J., 1995, The impact of unemployment on health: a review of the evidence. *Can. Med. Assoc. J.* 153(5):529-40.

Lavis, J.N., An inquiry into the links between labour-market experiences and health (unpublished dissertation). Cambridge MA: Harvard University.

Linn, M.W., Sandifer, R., and Stein, S., 1985, Effects of unemployment of mental and physical health. *Am. J. Public Health* 75(5):502-6.

Martikainen, P.T., 1990, Unemployment and mortality among Finnish men, 1981-5. *B.M.J.* 301: 407-11.

Morris, J.K., Cook, D.G., and Shaper, A.G., 1994, Loss of employment and mortality. *B.M.J.* 308:1135-9.

Montgomery, S.M., Bartley, M.J., Cook, D.G., and Wadsworth, M.E., 1996, Health and social precursors of unemployment in young men in Great Britain. *J. Epidemiol. Comm. Hlth.* 50(4):415-22.

Moser, K.A., Fox, A.J., and Jones, D.R., 1984, Unemployment and mortality in the OPCS longitudinal study. *The Lancet* 1324-28.

Moser, K.A., Goldblatt, P.O., Fox, A.J., and Jones, D.R., 1987, Unemployment and mortality: comparison of the 1971 and 1981 longitudinal study census samples. *B.M.J. (Clin. Res. Ed.)* 294(6564):86-90.

Mustard, C.A., Derksen, S., Berthelot, J.M., Wolfson, M., and Roos, L.L., 1997, Age-specific education and income gradients in morbidity and mortality in a Canadian province. *Soc. Sci. Med.* 45:383-97.

Newcombe, H.B., Kennedy, J.M., Axford, S.J., and James, A., 1959, Automatic linkage of vital records. *Science* 130:954-59.

Platt, S., and Kreitman, N., 1990, Long term trends in parasuicide and unemployment in Edinburgh, 1968-87. *Social Psychiatry and Psychiatric Epidemiology* 25:56-61.

Roos, L.L., and Wajda, A., 1991, Record linkage strategies part I: estimating information and evaluation approaches. *Methods Inf. Med.* 30:117-23.

Roos, L.L., Mustard, C.A., Nicol, P., McLerran, D.F., Malenka, D.J., Young, T.K., and Cohen, M.M., 1993, Registries and administrative data: organization and accuracy. *Med. Care* 31:201-12.

Statistics Canada, 1997, *Historical Labour Force Statistics*. Catalogue no. 71-201-xpb. Ottawa, Canada.

Valkonen, T., and Martikainen, P., 1995, *The association between unemployment and mortality: causation or selection? Adult mortality in developed countries: from description to explanation.* (Lopez, A.D., Caselli, G., and Valkonen, T., eds.) Clarendon Press, Oxford , pp.201-22.

UNEMPLOYMENT AND SOCIAL NETWORKS AMONG YOUNG PERSONS IN SWEDEN

Ulla Arnell Gustafsson
National Institute for Working Life, 171 84 Solna, Sweden

Abstract   A concentration of unemployment in social networks has been found in a number of European countries, including the United Kingdom and the Netherlands. These are countries that have had high unemployment rates for a number of years. The phenomenon can be seen as an indicator of a process of marginalisation of the unemployed, via which they become isolated from people at work. This is likely to be a major threat to solidarity and integration in society. What is the situation like in Sweden? The country has enjoyed a long period of low unemployment, but the situation has changed dramatically during the 90s. The study describes unemployment concentration among young people, and their parents, siblings and friends, over the first eight months after leaving school (in June 1996). Results indicate a tendency to concentration even after controlling for a number of structural factors (education, sex, ethnicity, parents' socio-economic status, and local unemployment rate).

1.   INTRODUCTION

For a long time the level of unemployment in Sweden was lower than that of other countries. However, during the 1990s there was a qualitative change in the pattern of unemployment growth. Unemployment grew dramatically. For example, in 1997 - one of the relevant years in the present study - about 8 percent of people were unemployed, not including people in government work programs. For young people the rate was even higher. The figure for the 20-24 age range was 16 percent, while in 1990 the corresponding figure had been 3 percent. In addition, many young people participated in government work programs. Many young people did not join the labour force; for example, instead of starting work they continued their studies. In 1990, 82 percent of young people aged 20-24 belonged to the labour force (annual average). In 1997, the corresponding figure was 63 percent (Statistics Sweden 1990 and 1997).

When unemployment increases as dramatically as it has in Sweden, there is reason to expect various other social changes to occur (e.g. Arnell Gustafsson, 1996, Åberg et al 1997). One consequence could be a sharpened distinction or segregation between the unemployed and people with jobs.

Health Effects of the New Labour Market, edited by Isaksson *et al.*
Kluwer Academic / Plenum Publishers, New York, 2000.

Populations of unemployed people could become concentrated in particular housing areas, in particular families or other networks. Unemployment per se – irrespective of education, social class, ethnicity and sex – might become a segregating factor in society. This segregation would in turn lead to a great risk of marginalisation as unemployment often means withdrawal from important societal functions.

2.   AIM OF THE STUDY

The main aim of the present study is to describe the concentration of unemployment in young people's social networks, with the networks defined as their parents, siblings and friends. Are young people who have experienced unemployment more likely to come from families with unemployed parents and siblings than young people who have never experienced unemployment? And are they more likely to have unemployed friends? The structural factors of education, sex, ethnicity, the parents' socio-economic status and the local unemployment rate are controlled for in this study, allowing the specific contribution of unemployment as a segregating factor to be isolated.

A secondary aim of this paper is to discuss different explanations for the demonstrated tendencies for concentration of unemployment in social networks. These explanations are summarily tested on the material. However, more research is needed to explore the validity of these explanations.

3.   CONCENTRATION OF UNEMPLOYMENT

Research on the concentration of unemployment in social networks has primarily been conducted in the United Kingdom and the Netherlands, countries that have had high unemployment rates for a number of years. The studies have mainly focused on unemployment in families. Several studies have found relationships between spouses' unemployment (e.g. Davies, Elias & Penn 1994, Henkens, Kraykamp & Siegers 1993, Morris 1995, Murphy 1995, Pahl 1988). In addition, relationships between unemployment in young people and their family members have been found. Thus, for example, Payne (1988) found that unemployed young persons lived in households with other unemployed persons more often than employed young persons. She found clearly significant differences - 35 percent of the unemployed young people (age 16-19) lived in families with at least one other member unemployed, whilst the corresponding figure for young people who were working was 12 percent. In addition, only 78 percent of the unemployed young people lived in families with at least one working person, while the figure was 94 percent for young people who were working. Thus, having family members who are not active in working life seems to have a negative effect on the likelihood of young people being employed themselves. The relationship between the young person's unemployment and unemployment or economic inactivity in the family remained after controlling for education, age, sex, ethnicity, illness or disability, unemployment rate in the region and socio-economic status of the head of the household. In particular, there was a strong relationship between an individual's unemployment and that of other household members aged 16-24, who were presumably most likely to be siblings. One reason for this could be the special features of the youth labour market, and the impact this currently has on the young members in a household. In Sweden studies such as those of Nordenmark (1999) and Soidre (1999) have looked at the relationship between young people's unemployment and their parents' unemployment. The preliminary results show that, even in Sweden, there are tendencies to unemployment concentration. However, there have not been many studies in Sweden on unemployment concentration which also look at siblings' unemployment.

In addition to these studies on concentration of unemployment in households and families, there have also been some studies looking at the phenomenon among other relatives and among friends (Allatt & Yeandle, 1992; Gallie, Gershuny & Vogler, 1994; Morris, 1995; Morris & Irwin, 1992). In Sweden, Nordenmark (1999) found that the longer a person had been unemployed, the greater the number of his friends who were unemployed. For example, 10 percent of those who had been unemployed for less than one year had more than 50 percent of their friends unemployed compared with 28 percent of those who had been unemployed more than 3 years. This relationship was significant at the 0.01 level even when age, class and local unemployment rate were controlled for.

4. SOME EXPLANATIONS FOR THE CONCENTRATION OF UNEMPLOYMENT

Several theories about the concentration of unemployment in social networks have been discussed in the literature. However, most of these theories lack empirical evidence. The structural explanations, however, are almost self-evident. As it is well known - and empirically well supported - that the risk of unemployment differs between geographical regions, between educational, socio-economic and ethnic groups etc., the concentration of unemployment in families and other networks will vary between these structures as well. A high unemployment rate in a municipality will, for example, not only hit a son but also his father and mother. Studying the concentration of unemployment without controlling for these structural variables is next to meaningless. Yet there is a lack of high-quality studies, which control for the relevant structural variables, probably because such studies would demand a considerable amount of quite specific data. In Sweden this is a rather new area of research and the aim of this article is to study the concentration of unemployment, whilst controlling for the most relevant structural variables.

Another important explanation for the concentration of unemployment in families and other networks is the importance of informal or personal contacts in getting a job. Korpi (1998) studied this in Sweden, using longitudinal data from the years 1992 and 1993. He showed that the chance of getting a job for an unemployed person was higher the larger their social network. This finding remained even after controlling for a great number of background factors. Korpi's data covered about 600 individuals, aged 20-54. These findings would probably be even more marked in young people, as they, more often than adults, get their jobs through informal contacts (Holzer 1988). In addition, getting a job through informal contacts is probably even more important in a situation of high unemployment (e.g. Allatt & Yeandle 1992; Jenkins et al 1983). This may also explain why the results from Payne (1987), referred to above, showed that not only the unemployment of parents but also their absence from the labour market for other reasons had effects on the risk of young person's unemployment. It might not first and foremost be the stigmatizing effects of a parent's unemployment that is important, but that the parent's absence from the labour market in general reduces the informal inroads to the labour market for young people. In this study we examine separately the effect unemployment of parents, compared with work activity of parents, has on the risk of unemployment for young people.

A third explanation for the concentration of unemployment in families or networks is the development of particular norms, values and attitudes among unemployed people. These types of values and attitudes could be spread within groups of unemployed people and affect search behaviour and activity on the labour market. We know rather well that, on the individual level, unemployment causes many problems. Several studies show that unemployed people suffer more health problems and reduced self-confidence (e.g. Burchell 1994, Colbjörnsen et al 1992, Janlert 1992, Lahelma 1989, Warr & Jackson 1985, Warr et al 1988, Starrin & Jönsson 1998). But are these attitudes spread in the unemployed person's social network and do they influence their behaviour on the labour market? Another explanation emphasises a so-called "unemployment culture"- that is, attitudes that decrease commitment to work and encourage a more tolerant attitude towards social welfare, which also might influence behaviour on the labour market. However, it is not easy to find empirical evidence for the hypothesis that "commitment to work" is lower among unemployed people than among others. There is no evidence of this from studies looking at environments with a high proportion of unemployed people (Nordenmark 1999, Gallie & Vogler 1994).

For the present study we do not have data on work commitment or attitudes to social welfare. We do, however, have one variable measuring the young person's assessment of his/her future possibilities in terms of the labour market, which is related to the findings discussed above on self-confidence and mental health. We use this variable in the analysis in an exploratory manner to see how much an attitudinal variable of this kind might improve our model of the unemployment experience of young people.

5.   METHOD

5.1   Data

A representative, stratified sample of 6388 young people responded to a questionnaire, three years and ten months after having left compulsory school in 1993. The data were collected in May 1997, and are part of the set of standard follow-up studies conducted by Statistics Sweden. As most young people (over 90 percent) continue to three-year upper-secondary school this means that most of the questionnaires were answered ten months after students finally left school. The sample was stratified in terms of what type of educational program the students had followed in upper-secondary school and in terms of sex; this produced 44 different strata. The weighted non-response rate was 20.2 percent. In the analysis six strata were excluded: Youths who were still in upper secondary school (men and women), youths who had never begun in upper secondary school (men and women) and dropouts (men and women). After this 38 strata, with totally 5617 individuals, remained.

5.2   Variables and strategy of the analysis

In the questionnaires the young people were asked about their activities in terms of education or on the labour market, month by month, during the first eight months after having left upper secondary school. Thereafter the number of months in unemployment or in government work programs was counted and a dichotomous variable was created: those who during their first eight months after school had ever been unemployed/in government work programs, and those who had not. The former category contained 41 percent and the latter 59 percent respectively.

The first part of the analysis consists of simple cross-tabulations, which indicate the principal focus of the study. These illustrate the relationship between the young person's experience of unemployment and:

- unemployment of the father, mother and sibling(s);
- unemployment of best friends;
- index of unemployment concentration;
- father's and mother's work activity.

Later, these relationships were controlled for in terms of the following structural variables:

- sex and education (the stratification variable);
- socio-economic status of the parents;
- ethnicity;
- unemployment rate in the municipality where the young person lived at the time of the data collection.

And, added to one of the initial models, the attitudinal variable:

- the young person's assessment of their opportunities on the labour market.

The statistical method employed was logistic regression. The results are shown as odds ratios, which are interpreted as follows. For every variable used in the analyses, there is a reference group with a value of 1. A figure higher than 1 means that the impact on the dependent variable is increased, a figure of lower than 1 indicates that the impact is decreased. Roughly speaking, an odds ratio of 2 means that the impact is doubled, and an odds ratio of 1.5 that the impact is about one and a half times as great as for the reference group. A confidence interval (95%) is also given for every odds ratio as a measure of the certainty of the estimation. As a measure of how well the chosen model fits the data, R^2 (Nagelkerke) is given.

5.3   Operationalisation of the variables

Unemployment of the father, mother and siblings was based on answers to the following question: "Has anyone in your family (mother, father or siblings) been unemployed or in government work programs during the last year?" The possible responses were: Yes, father; Yes, mother; Yes, siblings; and, No.

Friend's unemployment was based on the following question: "Have any of your best friends been unemployed or in government work programs during the last year?" The possible responses were Yes and No.

Index of unemployment was the sum of unemployed people in various categories in the individual's social network. It runs from 0 (none unemployed) to 4 (father, mother, siblings and friends unemployed).

Parents' work activity was based on the following questions: "Is your mother working?" Possible responses for this were: Working full time; Working part time; Other (e g studying, unemployed/in government work programs, retired, not alive). The same question was asked about the person's father.

What is termed *the stratum* is the stratification variable, and was determined by a combination of the education and the sex of the individual. Education was categorised in terms of the program taken in upper - secondary school. In most cases boys and girls were separated and formed different strata. Those programs which were strongly dominated by one sex, however, were not divided. This variable is divided into 44 different categories and is, compared with other studies, well defined and specified.

Socio-economic status of parents was determined by their occupations. The categorisation is the standard system used in official Swedish statistics. The categories are: - non-skilled workers, - semi-skilled workers and lower-level white-collar workers, - middle-level white-collar workers, - upper-level white-collar workers, - self-employed people and farmers. The socio-economic status of the parents where their occupations fell into different categories was determined as in official Swedish statistics. The rule is that the highest socio-economic status is chosen as the family characteristic. For further details, see Statistics Sweden 1995.

Ethnicity was categorised in terms of whether the individual was born in Sweden or not. This is, of course, a crude categorisation but the relatively few individuals in the sample who had been born outside Sweden would have made any finer categorisation problematic. – Another measure of ethnicity, was if the young person had *any parent* born outside Sweden or not should have been preferable in this context. However, data on this were not available in the study.

Unemployment rate in the municipality where the person lived at the time of the interview consisted of five categories, as follows: Municipalities with 0-4.99%, 5.00-7.49%, 7.50-9.99%, 10.00-12.49%, and 12.50% or more unemployed or in government work programs. These figures relate to the population in the age range 16-64, and not to the labour force as a whole, which means that the numbers are somewhat lower than the numbers given in Sweden's official statistics.

Assessment of one's own opportunities in terms of the labour market was assessed by the response to the following question: "What do you consider the likelihood of you having a permanent position in the labour market within the next four to five years?" Possible responses were: Very likely, Quite likely, Not very likely, Not likely at all.

Data were weighted according to the stratification procedure. The percentages shown in table 1 are based on weighted data. The absolute frequencies in the table, however, are based on the unweighted sample. In the logistic regression no data were weighted. Instead the stratifying variable was controlled for.

6.   RESULTS

6.1   Concentration of Unemployment

Table 1 shows simple cross-tabulations for the most relevant variables in the analysis. Of young people coming from families where the father had been unemployed during the previous year, 50 percent had themselves been unemployed during the same period, compared with 40 percent of the young people coming from families where the father had not been unemployed. If the mother had been unemployed the corresponding figure was 51 percent compared with 40 percent. Both differences were highly significant. In terms of siblings, the association with unemployment seemed to be more pronounced than was the case for parents; 54 percent of young people coming from families with unemployed siblings had been unemployed themselves compared with 38 percent coming from families with no unemployed siblings. Still greater differences were seen concerning friends; nearly 20 percent more of the young people with unemployed friends had themselves been unemployed compared with those with no unemployed friends. However, unemployment among friends seems to have a somewhat different meaning to unemployment in the family. The norm for young people in Sweden in the 90s is to have unemployed friends; about 80 percent reported that they had at least one unemployed friend. It was unusual to report having no unemployed friends, and doing so meant that the risk of being unemployed oneself was substantially decreased; only 25 percent of this group reported that they had themselves been unemployed during the first eight months after school compared with 41 percent of the total sample.

Table 1. Youths being unemployed during their first eight months after school in relation to unemployment and work activity in the social network.

Having experienced unemployment during the first eight months after school	Yes %	No %	Sum(n) %	Missing cases	Sign.(chi square)
Father unemployed	50	50	100(531)	41	***
Father not unemployed	40	60	100(5045)		
Mother unemployed	51	49	100(688)	41	***
Mother not unemployed	40	60	100(4888)		
Some sibling unemployed	54	46	100(1033)	41	***
Siblings not unemployed	38	62	100(4543)		
Some friend unemployed	45	55	100(4566)	63	***
Friends not unemployed	25	75	100(988)		
Index of unemployment concentration					
0	22	78	100(772)	114	***
1	41	59	100(3005)		
2	51	49	100(1451)		
3	59	41	100(244)		
4	75	25	100(31)		
Father not on the labor market	51	49	100(863)	160	***
Father working part time	53	47	100(174)		
Father working full time	39	61	100(4420)		
Mother not on the labor market	51	49	100(947)	120	***
Mother working part time	40	60	100(1336)		
Mother working full time	39	61	100(3214)		

*** p< 0,001

As mentioned above, an index had been constructed, where the father's, mother's, siblings' and friends' unemployment were summed. Using this index, the concentration of unemployment in social networks can be seen even more clearly. Of those in networks with no-one unemployed only 22 percent had experience of being unemployed themselves whilst amongst those in networks with an unemployment concentration index of 3, 59 percent had been unemployed. The figure rises to 75 percent in networks where father, mother, siblings and friends (concentration index = 4) had been unemployed. However, it should be noted that only 0.6 percent of the sample belonged to this kind of network.

A methodological problem with the study is that the data do not give information on size or composition of household. Thus, we do not know whether the father or mother is living in the household or not. One or both could, for example, have died or moved away. Nor do we know if the interviewee has any siblings. This means that the categories "father/mother/sibling not employed" contain cases where there is no father/mother/sibling in the household as well as those where the father/mother/sibling is actually unemployed. Therefore, what is measured is the absolute presence/absence of unemployed members in the network.

This also means that the additive index measures the absolute number of unemployed members in the young person's network. Thus a value of "2" on the index might indicate various different network make-ups; either, for example, the mother and best friends are unemployed and there is no father and siblings in the household, or the mother and best friends are unemployed and the father and siblings are working. The index does not therefore discriminate so much between varying amounts of contact with the world of work as between different amounts of contact with the world of unemployment.

The variable "parents' work activity", which measures the extent to which parents are in direct contact with the labour market - and could be an indicator of possible, informal contacts with a potential employer, also shows a significant relationship with young person's unemployment. Of those young people not having a father who is active on the labour market, 51 percent had experienced unemployment. The corresponding figure for those having a father working full-time is 39 percent. The effect of having a mother who is not active in the labour market against having a mother who is working full-time seems to be about the same as for the father. One difference in terms of the impact of the father's as opposed to the mother's labour-market status can be seen in terms of part-time work. The effect of having a father who works part-time seems to be the same as having a father who is not working at all, whereas having a mother who works part-time appears to have the same effect as having a mother who works full-time. The father who works part-time is probably as deviant a case as the father who does not work at all, whereas the mother who works part-time is as acceptable as a mother who works full-time. In this analysis as well, however, missing information about household size is a problem. A household containing no father/mother who is active in the labour market, may mean a household with an unemployed, sick, studying or dead father/mother. Thus, it is the presence or absence of a working father/mother that is focused on here, whatever the reason might be for their absence.

Lack of information on the composition of the household is, of course, unfortunate. However, its impact on the results concerning unemployment concentration will probably lead to an under-estimation of the tendencies investigated. This type of error is to be preferred to an error in the opposite direction.

Our hypothesis was that general absence from the labour market, as measured by work activity, might yield different results from simply looking at whether the parents were unemployed. However, neither the results in table 1 nor the results of the logistic regression (not shown here) offer information interpretable in terms of our hypothesis. The data on parents' work activity was therefore not analysed further.

6.2   Concentration of Unemployment and Structural Factors.

As mentioned above, unemployment concentration is likely to be highly dependent on various structural factors. Table 2 shows unemployment concentration when the structural variables, that is, stratum (sex/education), ethnicity, parents' socio-economic status and unemployment rate in the municipality, are controlled for. Three different models are presented. In the first, the association between the young person's experience of unemployment and the unemployment of his/her father, mother, siblings and friends is focused upon. In the second this model is extended, and also contains the variable "assessment of one's own opportunities in the labour market". In the third model the number of unemployed members of the close social network – the additive index described earlier – is utilised.

Nearly all the structural variables (sex, education, country of birth, parents' socio-economic status, unemployment rate in the municipality) show effects in terms of the young person's unemployment. However, these effects must be interpreted with great caution, since the sample contains various kinds of young people – studying, working, and doing compulsory military service. The latter, for example, means that sex differences are difficult to interpret. As military service is done almost entirely by young men – and since during this time they do not belong to the labour force and

Table 2. Unemployment during the first eight months after school and unemployment in the family, parent's work activity, unemployment among friends, index of unemployment concentration and assessment of the future chances on the labour market. Controlled for sex, education, parent's socio-economic status, birth country and municipal unemployment rate. Odds ratio and confidence interval (95%).

	Model 1	Model 2	Model 3
Father unemployed(n=475)	1,21 (*) 0.99-1.48	ns (1.18; 0.96-1.45)	
Father not unemployed(n=4739)	1.00	1.00	
Mother unemployed(n=592)	1.31** 1.09-1.58	1.25*1.04-1.51	
Mother not unemployed(n=4622)	1.00	1.00	
Some sibling unemployed(n=957)	1.42*** 1.23-1.65	1.38***1.18-1.60	
Siblings not unemployed(n=4257)	1.00	1.00	
Some friend unemployed(n=4279)	1.95*** 1.66-2.30	1.96***1.66-2.32	
Friends not unemployed(n=935)	1.00	1.00	
Chances to have a permanent position on the labor market in about 4-5 years			
Very great(n= 1082)		1.00	
Rather great(n=2426)		1.53***1.30-1.79	
Rather small(n=1304)		2.44***2.03-2.93	
Very small(n=330)		2.54***1.94-3.32	
Index of unemployment concentration			
0 (n=737)			1.00
1(n=2851)			1.96*** 1.62-2.37
2(n=1352)			2.62***2.13-3.23
3(n=207)			3.55***2.52-5.01
4(n=20)			4.37**1.62-11.8
Stratum (education and sex; 38 strata; not specified here)	***	***	***

Table 2 (continuing)

Parents' socio-economic status			
Non-skilled workers (n=791)	1.76*** 1.40-2.28	1.76***1.39-2.23	1.75***1.39-2.20
Skilled workers and lower-level white-collar workers (n=1630)	1.51***1.23-1.85	1.51***1.23-1.87	1.50***1.22-1.84
Middle-level white-collar workers(n=1222)	ns (1.19; 0.96-1.48)	ns (1.22; 0.98-1.52)	ns(1.20; 0.97-1.49)
Upper-level white-collar workers (n=992)	ns(0.97; 0.77-1.21)	ns (1.09; 0.80-1.28	ns (0.98; 0.78-1.23)
Self-employed and farmers (n=579)	1.00	1.00	1.00
Birth country			
Outside Sweden (n=193)	ns (1.31; 0.97-1.79)	ns (1.27; 0.93-1.74)	ns(1.29; 0.95-1.76)
Sweden (n=5021)	1.00	1.00	1.00
Unemployment rate in the municipality			
- 4,99% (n=193)	1.00	1.00	1.00
5-7,49% (n=1511)	1.45*1.04-2.03	1.45*1.03-2.04	1.46*1.05-2.05
7,5 - 9,99% (n=1576)	1.67**1.20-2.34	1.60*1.13-2.25	1.66 **1.19-2.31
10,0 - 12,49%(n=1582)	1.86***1.34-2.60	1.76**1.25-2.49	1.86***1.33-2.59
12,5 - % (n=352)	1.96***1.33-2.88	1.83**1.23-2.72	1.93***1.31-2.84
Nagelkerke R ^{2}	0.094	0.115	0.093

* = p< 0.05   **= p<0.01   ***=p<0.001

"cannot" be unemployed – there is a bias in the data. Accordingly, the structural variables in this respect function solely as control variables for the relationship focused upon in this study, namely how young people's unemployment is associated with the unemployment of their family and friends. This also explains why we show the stratum variable in the form of a mixture of education and sex. Separation of the two variables is not very useful in this context.

Model 1 shows that the earlier relationship found between the young person's experience of unemployment and father's and mother's unemployment is weakened when the structural variables are controlled for. The relationship with father's unemployment becomes insignificant, while the relationship with the mother's unemployment is still significant but at a lower level (p<0.01). This may, however, be due to the methodological problem discussed above, that is, the fact that we do not know whether the father/mother/sibling is living in the household or not. Since it is more common for the father rather than the mother to be missing from a household, the father's labour status may therefore have less impact on the labour status of the young person.

The relationship between a person's own experience of unemployment and unemployment among their siblings and friends remains strongly significant. Unemployment among friends in particular shows a relatively high odds ratio. This could be explained in at least two ways. The first explanation is that the effect is due to selection; whereas you cannot choose your siblings or parents you can choose your friends. Unemployment gives a person a different structure to their day; they are free when other people work, and this might confine their circle of friends to those with the same structure to their day as they have. The second is that the effect is due to peer influence. For young people friends are very important; the growth of a "youth culture" has been focused in more classical as well as in more recent sociological literature (e g Coleman 1961, Fornäs and others 1984). This may also be the case in terms of attitudes and behaviour related to unemployment.

An illustration to this is given in model 2. There the attitude variable "assessment of one's own chances on the labour market" is added to the structural variables. This rises the power of explanation with more than two percent and the risks of unemployment differs significantly between young people with an optimistic contra a pessimistic view of their chances on the labour market. Certainly, it is difficult to make any statements based on the data from our study regarding the casual direction here. The logistic regression assumes the variable as independent, which means that the assessment of the future chances on the labour market should influence the risk of being unemployed. This is worth considering: the assessment of one's own chances on the labour market is an indicator of self-confidence, which in turn can influence the behavior, for example the way to apply for jobs and for the behavior in an interview situation. However, also the other casual direction is possible: experience of unemployment may influence the assessment of one's own assessment on the labour market. Most likely both the processes are going on: in our model, however, it is the first direction which is tested and found significant.

Even if the variable "assessment of one's own chances on the labour market" seems to be very important for the *individual risk of unemployment*, the importance for the *unemployment concentration* is more difficult to answer. Adding the variable "assessment of one's own chances on the labour market" in model 2 doesn't change the odds ratios of the relationships between own unemployment and unemployment of neither the father, the mother, the siblings nor the friends in comparison with model 1. The hypothesis that the unemployment concentration is due to the diffusion of an "unemployment culture" in the network is not supported from the data. However, the analysis, and the operationalization of "unemployment culture" is very crude and explorative; more research as well as better data is needed to test the hypothesis.

Model 3 shows that the relationship between the young person's unemployment and the index of unemployment concentration remains strong after controlling for the structural variables. The index yields strongly significant differences for all values. The greater the number of unemployed people in the close social network, the greater is the odds ratio for the person having been unemployed during the first year after school. The odds ratio or the risk of unemployment is more than four times as great when a person has four unemployed people in his/her network as opposed to having none.

7. CONCLUSION

The study demonstrates that there is a significant relationship between being unemployed during the first eight months after school and having unemployed parents, siblings and friends. To some extent this relationship is explained by structural factors; unemployed young people and their parents, siblings and friends are located in the same kind of structures in terms of risks of unemployment. This is particularly the case with regard to the relationship between the unemployment of young people and that of their parents, although this relationship is weakened when the structural variables education, sex, socio-economic status, ethnicity and the municipality's rate of unemployment are controlled for. By contrast, the association with unemployment of siblings and friends remains highly significant even after controlling for structural variables.

In relation to previous research in Sweden, this study produced some new findings, and also some that replicate the results of earlier investigations. This is the first study in Sweden where unemployment concentration among siblings is considered. Some results are particularly noteworthy. The finding that young people belonging to the same family are more affected by unemployment than others is an indicator that unemployment "runs in families". Also, the findings with regard to unemployment concentration among friends are new in a Swedish context. Although Nordenmark (1999) found concentration tendencies among friends, his data could not distinguish between employed and unemployed people, only between unemployed people with different lengths of periods of unemployment. It should be noted that his sample consisted of people of all ages, rather than concentrating on young people.

Swedish research on unemployment concentration has previously focused on the relationship between parents' and the young people's unemployment, and in this respect the results of the present study are in line with those of earlier studies. There is a tendency for the unemployment-concentration effect to weaken when structural variables are controlled for. This has also been shown by Nordenmark (1999) and Soidre (1999).

However, both these previous studies used different sorts of data to those used in the present study, meaning that the results are not directly comparable. For example, Nordenmark and Soidre both used fairly heterogeneous registry data. On the other hand, it could be argued that registry information on labour-market status is more valid than the self-report data used in the present study. The different kinds of studies therefore have their own advantages and disadvantages. However, as there have been few studies concerning unemployment concentration in Sweden, the need for alternative approaches is considerable. Large quantities of specific data are probably required to illuminate the subject matter in detail.

REFERENCES

Allatt, P & Yeandle, S., 1992, Young Person Employment and the Family. Routledge, London.

Arnell Gustafsson, U., 1996, När arbetslösheten stiger. Om sociala konsekvenser och forskningsbehov (When Unemployment Rises. On Social Consequences and the Needs for Research). Arbetsmarknad & Arbetsliv, 1996:2, pp 99-115.

Burchell, B., 1994, The Psychological Consequences of Unemployment: An Assessment of the Jahoda Thesis. In Gallie D, Marsh C & Vogler C (ed) Social Change and the Experience of Unemployment, Oxford University Press, Oxford, pp 188-213.

Colbjörnsen T, Dahl S. and Hansen H., 1992, Langtidsarbeidslöshet. Årsaker, konsekvenser og mestring (Long Term Unemployment. Reasons, Consequences and Coping). Stiftelsen for samfunns-og näringslivsforskning. Bergen.

Coleman, J S., 1961, The Adolescent Society. The Social Life of the Teenager and Its Impact on Education, New York.

Davis R B, Elias P and Penn R., 1994, The Relationship between a Husband's and his Wife's Participation in the Labour Force. In Gallie D, Marsh C and Vogler C (ed) Social Change and the Experience of Unemployment. Oxford University Press, Oxford, pp 154-188.

Janlert, U., 1992, Arbetslöshet som folkhälsoproblem (Unemployment as a Public-Health Problem). Allmänna förlaget, Stockholm.

Fornäs J, Lindberg U and Sernhede O., (red), 1984, Ungdomskultur: Identitet - Motstånd (Youth Culture: Identity - Resistence) Stockholm.

Gallie D, Marsh C and Vogler C (ed), 1994, Social Change and the Experience of Unemployment. Oxford University Press, Oxford.

Gallie D, Gershuny J and Vogler C., 1994, Unemployment, the Household, and Social Networks in Gallie D, Marsh C and Vogler C (ed) Social Change and the Experience of Unemployment. Oxford University Press, Oxford, pp 231-264.

Gallie D & Vogler C., 1994, Unemployment and Attitudes to Work in Gallie D, Marsh C and Vogler C (ed) Social Change and the Experience of Unemployment. Oxford University Press, Oxford, pp 115-153.

Henkens, K , Kraaykramp, G and Siegers, J., 1993, Married Couples and Their Labour Market Status. A Study of the Relationship between the Labour Market Status of Partners. European Sociological Review, No 9, pp 67-78.

Holzer, H., 1988, Search Method Use by Unemployed Young Person. Journal of Labour Economics, Vol 6, No 1, pp 1-20.

Jenkins R, Bryman A, Ford J, and Keil T., 1983, Information in the Labour Market: The Impact of Recession. Sociology 17, pp 260-267.

Korpi,T., 1998, The Unemployment Process: Studies in Search, Selection and Social Mobility in the Labour Market, Department of Sociology, Stockholm University.

Lahelma E., 1989, Unemployment, Re-employment and Mental Well-Being. A Panel Survey of Industrial Job-Seekers in Finland. Scandinavian Journal of Social Medicine, Suppl 43.

Morris, L., 1995, Social Divisions. Economic Decline and Social Structural Change. London. UCL Press Limited.

Morris, L and Irwin, S., 1992., Unemployment and Informal Support: Dependancy, Exclusion, or Participation? Work, Employment and Society. Vol 6, No 2 pp 185-207.

Murphy, A., 1995, Female Labour Force Participation and Unemployment in Northern Ireland: Religion and Family Effects. The Economic and Social Review, No 27, pp 67-84.

Nordenmark, M., 1999, The Concentration of Unemployment within Families and Social Networks. European Sociological Review 1999:1

Pahl, R E., 1988, Some Remarks on Informal Work, Social Polarization and the Social Structure. International Journal of Urban and Regional Research 13, 709-20

Payne,J., 1987, Does Unemployment Run in Families? Some Findings from the General Household Survey. Sociology, Vol 21, No 2, pp 199-214.

Soidre T., 1999, Arbetslöshet och generation - unga kvinnor och män och deras föräldrar (Unemployment and Generation - Young Women and Men and their Parents). Department of Sociology, University of Gothenburg.

Starrin B and Jönsson L., 1998, Ekonomisk påfrestning, skamgörande erfarenheter och ohälsa under arbetslöshet. En prövning av ekonomi-skam modellen (Economic Stress, Experience of Shame and Ill-Health during Unemployment). Arbetsmarknad & Arbetsliv vol 4, No 2 pp 91-108.

Statistics Sweden, 1995, Occupations in Population and Housing Census (FoB 85) According to Nordic Standard Occupational Classification (NYK) and Swedish Socio-Economic Classification (SEI). Örebro, Statistics Sweden.

Statistics Sweden, 1990, Arbetskraftsundersökningarna. Årsmedeltal (Labour Force Statistics, Sweden).

Statistics Sweden 1997, Arbetskraftsundersökningarna. Årsmedeltal (Labour Force Statistics, Sweden).

Warr P and Jackson P., 1985, Factors influencing the psychological impact of prolonged unemployment and re-employment. Psychological Medicine 15, pp 795-807.

Warr P, Jackson P and Banks M., 1988, Unemployment and Mental Health: Some British Studies, Journal of Social Issues 1988, Vol 44, pp 47-68.

Åberg. R, Strand M, Nordenmark M and Bolinder M., 1997, Arbetslöshet i goda och dåliga tider (Unemployment in Good and Bad Times). Working Paper No 7, Department of Sociology, Umeå University.

ON EMPOWERMENT AND HEALTH EFFECTS OF TEMPORARY ALTERNATIVE EMPLOYMENT

Some reflections on the general implications of the experiences from an experimental labour market project in West Sweden

Hugo Westerlund
National Institute for Psychosocial Factors and Health

Abstract: Comparatively very high unemployment figures in the wake of the economic crisis in the 1990's have prompted new initiatives in Swedish labour market policy. One such initiative, aimed at creating alternative employment in the third sector, is discussed in terms of empowerment and health effects. The project, called Use for Everyone (UfE), is open to all people who are involuntarily excluded from the active labour force, mainly long-term unemployed and disabled persons, plus immigrants. UfE advocates a bottom-up perspective based on solidarity to stimulate empowerment, and is implemented through two associations representing authorities and participants respectively. The evaluation of UfE, which has been conducted with a combination of quantitative and qualitative methods, including a longitudinal biopsychosocial study, shows significant gains in self-rated health and quality of life, but also physiological indications of adaptation to a situation characterised by powerlessness. It is argued that the projects has been hampered by lacking resources and restrictive rules and regulations pertaining to the unemployment insurance system, but also that the experimental nature of the project highlights a number of important questions about activation and labour market policy.

Key words: unemployment, empowerment, health, psychophysiology, third sector

1. BACKGROUND

For many years, Sweden was known for its successful implementation of an active labour market policy. Despite internationally very high employment rates, comparatively equally distributed between men and women, the government maintained large-scale vocational training programmes, thus effectively ensuring a good match between labour demand and supply. A large and growing public sector in combination with markedly

Health Effects of the New Labour Market, edited by Isaksson *et al.*
Kluwer Academic / Plenum Publishers, New York, 2000.

Keynesian economic policy also contributed to keeping unemployment at bay, even in the wake of the 1973 oil crisis. Long-term unemployment did exist for especially vulnerable groups and in certain geographical areas, but its consequences were mitigated by generous unemployment benefits, various activating schemes and public relief work for the most disadvantaged.

The situation changed drastically in the beginning of the 1990's. Unemployment rose steeply as Sweden entered its worst economic crisis since the thirties. Although efforts were made to counteract unemployment, largely with the same instruments that had been successful before, the government's freedom of action was severely restricted by large budget deficits and earlier market deregulations. In fact, cuts in the public sector significantly contributed to unemployment.

Although still active in scope, the labour market policy was by necessity becoming increasingly concerned with alleviating the social consequences of long-term unemployment—which was rapidly growing into a major problem—rather than focusing on labour market demands. Cheaper activating schemes were radically scaled up to accommodate more people and keep them from demoralising passivity, leaving less resources for specialised vocational training. Consequently, the policy lost some of its effectiveness, among other things leading to visible bottleneck problems despite high open unemployment.

For the individual unemployed person, however, these changes had other consequences. Due to the severe shortage of job openings, many people did not find a job despite participating in various activating schemes and training programmes. Indeed, because periodic activation was required for continued unemployment benefit, these measures tended to become little more than formalities to ensure survival for many people. The fact that hopes were raised and repeatedly frustrated could for some individuals even make the activating schemes counterproductive, in effect reinforcing learned helplessness and passivity.

Another result of rising mass unemployment was that the employment offices had less time and resources to spend on each individual, leading to a decrease in guidance and placement quality. A major problem seems to have been that action plans, although formally required, were often not properly implemented. Since unemployment among other things is characterised by a state of financial and psychological dependence, however, these inadequacies might have had ramifications that are even more serious. Not infrequently, people felt disempowered and subjected to the decisions of the employment office rather than actively involved in their own processes, which in turn may lead to further resignation and passivity (Westerlund, 1999; cf. Fryer, 1999).

The latter problem can be construed as one of lacking communication between the employment offices and individual unemployed persons. There is, however, a real power imbalance between the two parties, exacerbated by the fact that the placement officers, in addition to being counsellors, are also expected to check that the unemployed fulfil their duties in relation to the unemployment insurance system.

Experiences of disempowerment can be very humiliating, giving rise to feelings of shame, which is also in itself a common concomitant of unemployment. Especially in combination with financial hardship, shame has been shown to be related to psychosomatic symptoms and mental health problems among the unemployed (Starrin *et al.*, 1997). It can be argued that unemployment becomes less of a stigma when it affects a comparatively large proportion of the population. However, mass unemployment has also lead to lowered unemployment benefit and calls for a more stringent application of rules pertaining to the unemployment insurance, thus making unemployment more difficult to bear economically.

Disempowerment, shame and economic hardship are parts of the wider issue of ill-health among the unemployed (Hallsten *et al*, 1999). It is fairly well established that unemployment can lead to mental health problems, psychosomatic complaints and social isolation, possibly also indirectly to increased mortality and incidence of severe somatic illness. Health problems, in turn, negatively influence the chances of finding or keeping a job, thus creating a vicious circle that can lead to more or less permanent exclusion from the labour market. Since both unemployment and ill-health are unequally distributed in the population, these mechanisms have the strongest effect on more vulnerable groups, exacerbating pre-existent inequalities in health.

Unemployment has thus also become a major public health problem. As discussed earlier, this has warranted a greater emphasis on the social aspects of labour market programmes, although placement and job creation are still the main goals of Swedish labour market policy. Although it can be argued that no activation scheme can fully replace regular employment, some of the vital factors or 'vitamins' as described by Warr (1987) may to some extent be provided by alternative employment, namely:
- Opportunity for control
- Opportunity for skill use
- Externally generated goals
- Variety
- Environmental clarity
- Availability of money
- Physical security
- Opportunity for interpersonal contact

– Valued social position

Furthermore, some authors, notably Rifkin (1995) and Martin & Schumann (1997), argue that only a portion of the available workforce will be needed in regular jobs in the future due to technical and economic development. As an alternative to massive unemployment and possible social unrest, Rifkin (ibid.) suggests employment within the third sector or social economy (*économie sociale*), which mainly comprises small, community-based enterprises, co-operatives and voluntary organisation. A large multinational study does indeed show that the non-profit sector is growing much faster than other sectors in terms of employment (Salamon & Anheier, 1996).

Two additional aspects that are ideally characteristic of the social economy are of importance here. Firstly, because of the social and not-for-profit nature of the activities, it can be easier for people with weak health or other limitations to take part in them than it is in ordinary worklife. Secondly, in contrast to traditional labour market activating schemes, a bottom-up perspective is often presupposed, opening for both collective and individual empowerment of groups that otherwise tend to be disempowered and clientised.

In this paper, some results and experiences from a combined labour market and public health project involving third sector activities will be discussed. After a brief outline of the programme itself, some data from the evaluation are presented, followed by a more speculative discussion about how the results can be generalised.

2.   USE FOR EVERYONE – A PRESENTATION

During the first years of the 1990's, rising unemployment and pending lay-offs within the public health services prompted the County Council of Skaraborg, West Sweden, to look for new ways of counteracting the negative effects of unemployment, especially on public health. Denmark, with its much longer experience of mass unemployment in modern times, was in focus for this work and provided some ideas that were up to then foreign to Sweden.

Danish labour market policy at the time may—in contrast to Swedish—be characterised by a partial acceptance of, and adaptation to, more or less permanently high unemployment figures. As a result, alternative ways of activating, mobilising and 'employing' the unemployed were encouraged. Apart from this basic Danish attitude towards unemployment, there seem to have been two particular aspects that impressed the Swedish working group: the use of unemployed people to mobilise other unemployed, plus creative ways of exploring new 'jobs' within the social economy. Adult pedagogy was also used more extensively and consciously in Danish labour market measures than it was in Sweden.

Two politically active county directors of finance—who after retirement were free to operate more independently than before, while still retaining their old professional networks—were instrumental in the development of a local Swedish initiative. Based on the Danish ideas and on their own experiences, e.g. from mental health care reorganisation, they developed an 'ideology' or 'attitude' centred on solidarity and belief in the positive potential of each individual, even the most disadvantaged and socially excluded.

As a result, a non-profit association was formed in 1994 by local authorities and politicians from all major political parties to implement a programme called *Use for Everyone* (UfE; Swedish: "Det finns bruk för alla") in four municipalities in West Sweden. The basic idea was to stimulate—and provide opportunities for—people outside the active workforce to start activities within the third sector. The main goal of the project was formulated in terms of increased health, defined as "how much influence people have over their own lives."

As a first step, unemployed and people on temporary disability pension were offered a ten week course to become so called process leaders in the programme. Of the applicants, 24 were selected because of their apparent interest in the social aspects of the project rather than on formal merits. The group comprised 12 men and 12 women aged 22 to 56 and with a varied background, both blue and white collar. Three were on sick-leave, the rest unemployed.

In January 1995, the newly educated leaders started to recruit participants to the project (or "process" as it is preferably called by the initiators to distinguish it from short-term and top-down "projects"). The leaders, individually or in pairs, formed working groups around activities such as recycling, handicraft or voluntary social service. The activities were generally based on the leaders' own interests, but participants were also encouraged to come up with their own ideas, some of which might lead to independent businesses or co-operatives. Because there is no formal hierarchy or codified methodology apart from the ideological principles, the different process leaders tend to work according to their personal preferences, making UfE a heterogeneous phenomenon. For a more detailed description, see Westerlund & Bergström (1997).

During the period 1995-98, around 1,000 people took part in the programme (Westerlund & Bergström, 1998). A good two third lived mainly off unemployment benefit, 12% had temporary or permanent disability pension, while the rest were mainly on welfare or special refugee allowance.

Two thirds were women and the mean age 39 years. For the majority, participation was in the form of a six month Work Experience Scheme ('ALU') entitling to renewed unemployment benefit—*not* as an entirely voluntary activity as originally envisioned. Infrequently, ALU participation has been extended for another six months, and a few people on occupational rehabilitation have been allowed to stay in the project for up to several years. More common, however, is that people return for a new period after some months of open unemployment.

UfE, however, is intended to be more than a labour market project. Since unemployment by the founders is considered to be a more or less permanent aspect of the future, UfE advocates the development of a new, alternative labour market where allowances are transformed into wages in return for activities of advantage to the community. In order both to create opinion regarding this goal and to mobilise unemployed people, a participants' union has been formed with the intention that it spread across the country as a democratic, bottom-up movement. So far, this has happened only to a limited extent, largely because of the above mentioned restrictions. UfE in practice can therefore to some degree be compared to other labour market and rehabilitation projects and has largely been evaluated as such.

3.   EVALUATION

Use for Everyone has been evaluated by Forskningsstation Mösseberg, a local research station associated with the National Institute for Psychosocial Factors and Health in Stockholm. Several approaches have been used. The project itself has been studied qualitatively, mainly focusing on methodological aspects (Westerlund & Bergström, 1997; Westerlund & Bergström, 1998) and how the project ideology is reflected in the organisational culture of UfE (Mårtensson, 1997). In addition, all participants are followed up by a short telephone interview one year after entering the project. A sample selected to be representative of the participants has also been followed longitudinally with extensive psychosocial questionnaires and psychophysiological data (blood pressure and analyses of blood samples).

One year follow-up shows that a majority of the participants were satisfied or very satisfied: 80% and 76% for those starting in 1995 and 1996 respectively (Westerlund & Bergström, 1998). Around 10% were dissatisfied and the rest neutral. Among those on occupational rehabilitation, the satisfaction rate was even higher, 93% in 1995. Although very positive, these figures are not exceptional when compared with other evaluations of labour market programmes. In response to the question whether they had gained in self-confidence, 43% said that it had improved while only 3% had experienced a deterioration. 33% believed that the project had increased their chances on the labour market to at least some degree. When asked to name the best aspects of UfE, two answers were by far the most common: social interaction and generally having something to do. The results may have been affected by the fact that younger participants had a higher drop-out rate along with those who had higher education and/or only participated for a short period of time.

One year after entering the programme, 13% of the originally unemployed participants of 1995 had sufficient regular employment (i.e. full time or the desired percentage of this), which is comparative to (or slightly higher than) other Work Experience Schemes in the region during the same period (Westerlund & Bergström, 1997). While the general pattern was that re-employment was more common among men (13% vs. 8%), however, the reverse was true in UfE, where women had the best success rate (15% vs. 7%). This could indicate that UfE offers something that is lacking in other projects, while the low percentage of men who had been re-employed could be explained by a relatively high mean age and low educational level among the male participants.

A preliminary study indicated that the participants' self-rated health was better than among openly unemployed, but that there also was a significant reversal during the two last months of participation (Westerlund & Bergström, 1997). A first analysis of the longitudinal data, however, failed to replicate these findings and indicated significant improvements in self-rated health and quality of life during participation that were retained also at six month follow-up (Westerlund & Bergström, 1998). Especially encouraging was the fact that the mean value of a 100 millimetre visual-analogue scale intended to measure individual control—the main goal of the project—rose significantly from 65 at baseline to 75 at follow-up.

The hypothesis that physiological data would show corresponding improvements was, however, not confirmed (Westerlund *et al.*, 1999). Serum prolactin, which has been shown to increase in situations characterised by powerlessness and passive coping (Theorell, 1992) and decrease when working conditions improve (Grossi *et al.*, 1999), rose from a mean level of 5.9 to 9.0 µg/l during participation and remained at that level at six month follow-up. DHEA-s (dehydroepiandrosterone sulphate), a hormone that is related to anabolism and can be hypothesised to be positively correlated with psychosocial working conditions (Theorell, 1993), decreased significantly during participation. There were also tendencies towards increased systolic blood pressure and ALAT (possibly reflecting increased use of alcoholic beverages) at follow-up. Although not significant, the changes in the other measured physiological variables also appear to indicate a deterioration of psychosocial conditions rather than the opposite.

Moreover, the subjects in the longitudinal study are not fully representative due to skewed drop-out, especially regarding blood tests. Women and people with only primary education are over-represented in the analysed longitudinal sample, which could have affected the results. Recent unpublished analyses of short questionnaires that were administered to all participants every two months during a period of a couple of years do indeed suggest that UfE does not have the same positive influence on self-rated health for all categories of participants. Although the relatively low quality of these data makes inferences uncertain, it seems as if youth, low education and a history of disablement pension or social welfare were independently related to improvements in self-rated data, while the majority actually rated their psychosocial health as somewhat worse at the end of the participation period than in the beginning – in line with the first published study.

The finding that UfE has had the most palpable effects on people with a weak position on the labour market is partly corroborated by case histories and data of a more anecdotal nature. Participants who have full working capacity and are mainly looking for a job opening not infrequently complain that the project is disorganised or irrelevant in relation to their needs. In contrast, quite a few people who initially had very low self-confidence, were socially isolated or had given up worklife altogether because of illness, have obviously developed new hope and found the environment congenial to psychological growth. There also seems to be a tendency that immigrants and people who have only recently moved to the area are particularly positive in their evaluations, which to a large extent could be because they gain a social network through the project.

In its present form, UfE thus seems most fit for participants with a weak connection to the labour market, while it may be less suited for some other groups. The findings must, however, also be understood in the context of how the project has been implemented. From its inception, UfE has been met by considerable resistance, not the least from representatives of labour market authorities who have been challenged by the somewhat provocative project ideology, for instance by the insistence that unemployment is here to stay and only can be effectively met by the creation of an alternative labour market.

The financial situation has been problematic throughout the history of UfE. The process leaders have generally been appointed for very short periods at a time, down to a few days, and the threat of a close-down has been strongly felt. The work has also been hampered by rules and regulations pertaining to the unemployment insurance system. As in other Work Experience Schemes, most participants enter UfE because they need a renewed benefit period and have to leave after six months. In addition to creating an unproductive psychological set among the participants, this makes it difficult both for the leaders to pass on responsibility to the ever-changing group of participants with varying motivation, and to develop the activities into well-functioning third sector enterprises. All forms of market competition are prohibited and unemployed participants are not allowed to handle money, which further complicates an economically sound development within the project. Even more troublesome is that these problems seem to have contributed to difficulties to develop the organisation itself and especially the methods to achieve empowerment among the participants (Westerlund & Bergström, 1998).

4. DISCUSSION

Use for Everyone is difficult both to describe and to assess due to its heterogeneous nature and the complex interplay between internal and external factors. It must also be remembered that the somewhat mixed results reflect the difficulties that UfE has had, rather than its potential, which still largely remains a matter of speculation. However, studying the difficulties and struggles may in fact be more rewarding than simply measuring the 'success' or 'failure' of a more straightforward project.

In a study of several more experimental programmes for the unemployed in Sweden and Denmark, Westerlund (1999) found similar problems in many of the projects. A particularly difficult question seems to be how to design an activating measure that does not in fact take the active personal initiative from the participants by forcing activity upon them by external means. When people take initiatives on their own accord, the solution can simply be to allow and support their initiatives (which is by no means always easy in practice), but when no spontaneous initiative is forthcoming, there are two basic alternatives: to wait, or to take an initiative on behalf of the 'passivated' participant. The latter can be both counterproductive and humiliating, as described earlier. UfE, whose process leaders in many cases have had own experiences of humiliating treatment, has thus to a large extent chosen a cautious approach, waiting for development to occur spontaneously. This is also a result of an ideological emphasis on the positive aspects of human nature—people are expected to be responsible and active in themselves unless directly hindered by the environment.

For some people, especially those who have severe difficulties and need a long rehabilitation process, this careful approach seems to have worked quite well. Part of the explanation for this could be that the environment itself offers sufficient challenges to promote development (basic time structure, social contacts, simple tasks etc.) and that the process leaders successfully protect the participants against environmental overload. Mårtensson (1997) describes how the strong value—as opposed to goal—orientation in the project can help participants in finding new hope and self-confidence despite sometimes pronounced objective difficulties.

The latter improvements are often relatively easily seen by the process leaders in their daily contacts with the participants, but are difficult to quantify and measure—especially when self-rated and physiological data are seemingly contradictory as in this case. Since the gains appear to be most pronounced among the weakest participants, re-employment is not a good measure of success, nor can the medical or psychiatric conditions of many of these people be expected to be completely cured. Percentages and measures of central tendency can also be misleading if the major gains are found in a relatively small group of especially difficult cases.

Anecdotes and case histories describing quite spectacular improvements in subjective health and quality of life are indeed partly backed up by more objective data, such as decreased consumption of (especially psychiatric) health care and medication. For those participants who have no such initial difficulties, however, UfE may be somewhat lacking in challenges, leading to a less pronounced overall result. Indeed, a significant part of the latter group may not even need any improvements except in employment status, which UfE cannot offer.

It is, however, questionable whether UfE has resulted in any significant *collective* mobilisation within the project. Although quite a few individuals have broken their personal passivity and isolation and become part of a social network, there are few signs of a growing grass roots movement in a political sense. The participants' union acts almost solely through the board, which is made up of process leaders and a few participants who are generally regarded as future leaders, and the dependence on the founders is still fairly strong. The average participant, although generally positive towards UfE, does not get involved in the common cause as formulated in the ideological framework.

There has, however, been an extensive series of political activities arranged by UfE as an organisation and involving mainly a core of highly dedicated process leaders, politicians and civil servants along with the founders. These activities have included local workshops and study visits with participants form different parts of Sweden, participation in public debates in different media as well as two seminars in the Parliament for members of the Parliament. Partly as a result of this, a number of projects and organisations have been started in other parts of Sweden based on the ideology of UfE. In some cases, these have been original grass roots initiatives resulting in significant collective mobilisation. In most cases, however, the latter projects have been fraught with other problems and have not had the longevity of UfE with its stronger support on a political and administrative level.

The physiological results that apparently gainsay the more positive self-rated data also put into question whether there is any real empowerment on an individual level. Indeed, rising prolactin seems to indicate quite the opposite—growing passivity and powerlessness. However, the increase in prolactin could also be viewed as an adaptive response to a situation that the subject, rightly or not, feels unable to alter. Studies on both animals and humans indicate that prolactin can have a protective effect against stress by inducing emotional and behavioural changes (somewhat similar to maternal 'cocooning', in which prolactin plays a part) that shield off adverse external stimuli and narrow the emotional field of vision, as it were (cf. Sobrinho, 1998). This could also explain the improved subjective ratings of individual control and quality of life. Ambitions are lowered, leading to less discrepancy between expectations and actual life situation.

If there is an element of resignation, this need not, however, be an effect of UfE *per se*. Between baseline and follow-up, average time outside regular employment increases from one and a half to two and a half years, which could in itself warrant adaptation to more or less permanent unemployment. Although acceptance of an unemployment role seems to be contrary to empowerment from a labour market perspective, it is not altogether irreconcilable with the objectives of UfE. If unemployment is regarded as a permanent aspect of the future, there is a need for a re-evaluation of work, something which UfE actively encourages. For people with a higher level of employability, such adaptation might have considerable detrimental effects. Especially for people with small chances on the labour market, however, the negative effects of possible impediments in motivation to find a job may be outweighed by the protective effects.

The longitudinal sample analysed so far consists of a higher percentage of women and people with only primary education than the total population of participants due to skewed drop-out. Both these subgroups tend to have a weaker position on the labour market, and might therefore benefit more from refocusing. This could explain the finding that these groups tend to express more (relative) improvements in self-rated health and quality of life, while still being severely restricted or 'powerless' in relation to their work situation, which could be responsible for the apparent deterioration in physiological data. This need not, however, be true for the whole group and the results may therefore be distorted as a result of the drop-out pattern.

The question of adaptation to a permanent shortage of jobs is also problematic on a societal level. As long as work in the third sector is either voluntary (often carried out by people with high status) or paid in the same manner as in the private and public sectors, which is generally the case today, there is no stigma attached to it. If, however, this sector is extensively used as an alternative for people who are not needed on the open market, stigmatisation clearly becomes an issue. Massive alternative employment—which to a certain extent already exists in the form of large scale activating schemes—may also decrease the incentives of the workforce to adapt to the demands of the (open) labour market, thus creating bottle-neck effects. Instead of closing the gaps between employed and unemployed, alternative labour markets could thus perpetuate the social exclusion of large groups of people.

Indeed, people in labour market programmes already play a considerable role both in the third sector, often as administrative aids in small clubs and voluntary organisations, and in the public sector, especially the municipalities where they perform many simpler tasks such as weeding and archive work. Not infrequently, these 'extra workers' feel exploited while the unions at the same time worry that their members are being replaced by free labour. This *de facto* division of the work force into 'real' jobs, with relatively good pay and considerable security, and various forms low-paid labour market measures lacking in basic workers' rights, is likely to have significant negative effects for the latter group (Fryer, 1999).

Sheltered employment could also be regarded as a species of alternative employment. But since the target group is people with obvious handicaps, whose only realistic alternative would be early retirement, such employment is probably more de-stigmatising than the other way around. Thus, it seems to be a question not so much of the content of the work or the organisational mode, as of the fit between work and worker. A job that for one person in a certain situation is challenging, empowering and uplifting, can for another be boring, disempowering and humiliating. A major problem arises when people are forced to perform low status, low priority tasks far below their capacity due to a shortage of 'real' jobs.

UfE has developed aspects of both sheltered employment and ordinary labour market projects focusing on occupation (rather than education). It has, however, so far failed to create convincing alternatives to regular employment. Because programmes of a mainly activating nature have proved to be largely ineffective from a labour market perspective, the government has recently removed the volume goals and given higher priority to more targeted efforts that are likely to have better effects on matching and job creation. As a result, a large number of projects–some of which by many people have been regarded as fairly pointless–are likely to be terminated.

For so called vulnerable groups, however, there is a danger that this new policy will lead to fewer opportunities to daily social contacts and meaningful occupation. Since alternative employment for these groups is unlikely to contribute to bottleneck effects or perpetuated social exclusion, it seems reasonable to retain some of the better projects that exist today and develop their social aspects even further. UfE is one such project that could offer viable alternatives for people with small chances on the labour market and for those who need a gentle settling-in period at the beginning of a rehabilitation programme. The fact that there seem to be some adaptation effects can in fact be an advantage for these groups. For the individual, it may lead to better health and quality of life in the face of a difficult situation and on a societal level counteract widening health gaps. In the long run, protective resignation may indeed uphold employability, even if the short-term effect is decreased job seeking behaviour.

When the results of UfE are evaluated, it must also be kept in mind that the 'process' has not been provided with the opportunities to develop in the direction that was first envisioned. It is still an open question how much of the original ambitions could be achieved under more congenial circumstances. Although it seems unlikely that UfE could become a general solution to the problem of unemployment, collective mobilisation, empowerment and grass roots initiatives will probably play an important role in developing the third sector as an alternative to a shrinking public sector and a private sector characterised by jobless growth. Not the least importantly, an experimental process like UfE also creates many new experiences that can be utilised in other programmes.

REFERENCES

Fryer, D. For better or for worse? Interventions and mental health consequences of unemployment. *International Archives of Occupational and Environmental Health* 1999;**72**(Suppl.1):S34-37.

Grossi, G., Theorell, T., Jürisoo, M. & Setterlind, S. Psychophysiological correlates of organizational change and threat of unemployment among police inspectors. *Integrative Physiological and Behavioral Science* 1999;(1):30-42.

Hallsten, L., Grossi, G. & Westerlund, H. Unemployment, labour market policy and health in Sweden during the 1990's – some tendencies and experiences. *International Archives of Occupational and Environmental Health* 1999;**72**(Suppl.1):S28-30.

Martin, H.P. & Schumann, H. The Global Trap: *Globalization and the Assault on Prosperity and Democracy*. London: Zed, 1997.

Mårtensson, F. [To Live or Just to Survive.] *Leva eller bara överleva*. Stress Research Reports 277. Stockholm: National Institute for Psychosocial Factors and Health, 1997. (English summary, Swedish text.)

Rifkin, J. *The End of Work. The Decline of the Global Labor Force and the Dawn of the Post-Market Era*. New York: Putnam Books, 1995.

Salamon, L.M. & Anheier, H.K. *The emerging nonprofit sector. An overview*. Manchester: Manchester University Press, 1996.

Sobrinho, L.G. Emotional aspects of hyperprolactinemia. *Psychotherapy and Psychosomatics* 1998;**67**(3):133-9.

Starrin, B., Rantakeisu, U. & Hagquist, C. In the wake of recession – economic hardship, shame and social disintegration. *Scandinavian Journal of Work, Environment and Health* 1997;**23**(Suppl.4):47-54.

Theorell, T. Prolactin–a Hormone that Mirrors Passiveness in Crisis Situations. *Integrative Physiological and Behavioural Science* 1992;**27**(1):32-38.

Theorell, T. Psychosocial aspects of work in the health care professions. On the psychosocial environment in care. **In:** Hagberg, M., Hoffmann, F., Stössel, U., Westlander, G. (eds.). *Occupational Health for Health Care Workers.* Landsberg: Lech, Ecomed, 1993.

Warr, P. *Work, Unemployment and Mental Health.* Oxford: Claredon Press, 1987.

Westerlund, H. [Activating measures and active initiatives – two opposites in Swedish labour market policy practice?] *Aktiverande åtgärder och aktiva initiativ – två motpoler i svensk arbetsmarknadspolitisk praktik?* Manuscript, 1999. (English summary, Swedish text.)

Westerlund, H. & Bergström, A. [Use for Everyone – a method under development.] *Det finns bruk för alla – en metod i utveckling.* Stress Research Reports, no. 276. Stockholm: National Institute for Psychosocial Factors and Health, 1997. (English summary, Swedish text.)

Westerlund, H. & Bergström, A. ["Use for Everyone" – Empowerment in Practice?] *Det finns bruk för alla – empowerment i praktiken?* Work Life Report 1998:16. Solna: National Institute for Working Life, 1998. (English summary, Swedish text.)

Westerlund, H., Theorell, T. & Bergström, A. Psychophysiological effects of temporary alternative employment. *Manuscript,* 1999.

EMPOWERMENT, LEARNING AND SOCIAL ACTION DURING UNEMPLOYMENT

Lennart Levi
Department of Public Health Sciences, Division of Psychosocial Factors and Health,
Karolinska institutet, P.O. Box 220, SE-171 77, Stockholm, Sweden

Abstract: A good job helps to give life purpose and meaning. It provides the day, week,
year and lifetime with structure and content. The worker gains identity and
self-respect and is able to give, and receive, social support in social networks.
In addition, a job provides material advantages and a reasonable living. A
person *excluded* from the labour market risks losing or perhaps never
accessing, all of these benefits and also runs an increased risk of physical and
mental ill health. To prevent this, the European Council's Summit on
Employment advocated developing entrepreneurship, improving
employability, encouraging the adaptability of business and their employees,
and strengthening the policies for equal opportunities as a co-ordinated EU
strategy. This approach is based on a necessary but probably insufficient *top-
down* strategy. A necessary complement to this is a *bottom-up* approach, an
attempt to empower, train, and mobilise the 16 millions of European
unemployed for mutual help and self-help (social economy), and to remove
obstacles to their initiatives to do so. Both approaches need to be applied
across societal sectors and academic disciplines, and at all societal levels, in a
systems approach.

Eurostat (1998) estimates that some 16 million men and women were
jobless in the 15 European Union (EU) Member States. The official
unemployment rate of the EU 15 was 9.8% in October 1998, same as in
September when it fell to under 10% for the first time in six years.

Lowest unemployment rates were Luxembourg's 2.2% and the
Netherlands' 3.7% (both September 1998). Next came Denmark (4.2%),
Austria (4.4%) and Portugal (4.5%). Spain's 18.2% was still by far the EU's
highest rate, but down more than two percentage points on the same month a
year ago (20.3%). Big falls over the year were also recorded in Portugal
(6.5% to 4-5%) and Sweden (9.5 to 7.5).

However, these *official* figures do not reflect the *actual* magnitude of the
problem. Out of Sweden's working age population (18-64 years, 5.3
million), only 4.0 million (75%) are employed. Accordingly, 25% are
unemployed (cf. Berg, 1997).

Out of the latter, at least 500 000 are *fully* fit for work; and approximately
another 500 000 are *conditionally* fit for work.

As the unemployed pay little or no tax, this leads to a strong decrease in
total revenue basis and a corresponding increase in governmental

Health Effects of the New Labour Market, edited by Isaksson *et al.*
Kluwer Academic / Plenum Publishers, New York, 2000.

belttightening. The *total fiscal costs* of unemployment in Sweden annually have been estimated to staggering SEK 153 billion = EURO 17.2 billion (Behrenz and Delander, 1997).

At the same time, 59% of those still at work report "far too much to do" (Statistics Sweden, 1998), indicating not "lean" but "anorectic" production. There is also a *widespread fear* of: quitting; reporting industrial injury; or registering and/or asking economic compensation for overtime worked. In addition, a type of *captivity in unsuitable jobs* is created - employees do not dare to quit jobs they do not like or are unsuited for, because it seems better to have a bad job with tenure than a better one that one may loose at any time due to the practice - last hired, first fired.

All of these situations can be detrimental to health and well being. Overemployment, unemployment and unsatisfactory conditions of work, all cause stress, and stress can lead to ill-health as well as reduced physical, mental and social well-being (Levi, 1972, 1981, 1984; Kompier and Levi, 1994; Levi and Lunde-Jensen 1996; Dooley et al., 1996; Wilkinson and Marmot, 1998). This is where we are heading. The question is whether we have already reached this point. And there are no signs of any real improvement.

Even the most optimistic of the Swedish Government's and Opposition's various scenarios would still mean that at least one fifth of Sweden's population of working age would be permanently excluded from the labour market at the turn of the millennium.

The above example concerning some important social determinants of health (cf. Wilkinson and Marmot, 1998) illustrates the changes taking place in one of our most important social environments and the effects that these changes might have on the health and well-being of the population and subsequently on its welfare (Levi, 1999).

1.   WHY WORK IS IMPORTANT

But why is work so important for health, well being and a good life?

According to Jahoda (1979), a good job helps to give life purpose and meaning. It provides the day, week, year and lifetime with structure and content. The worker gains identity and self-esteem and is able to give and receive social support in social networks. In addition, a job provides material advantages and a reasonable living.

A person *excluded* from the labour market risks losing or perhaps never even accessing all of these benefits.

The EU's Social Commissioner, Mr. P. Flynn, has bluntly pointed out that the European unemployment figures are 'intolerable'. Part of their intolerability lies in the fact that unemployment within the EU costs as much as EURO 200 billion (= SEK 1,780 billion) annually. This is much more than the entire Swedish national debt and as much as the total gross national product of Belgium. It is indeed intolerable - from both public health, welfare and financial perspectives.

The fact that it is also financially intolerable perhaps gives us cause for hope that the labour market's three social parties - the employers, the employees and the Governments - will eventually realise that it is in their common interest to increase both employment and productivity without increasing wear. If wear is also increased, the longer term results are both lower productivity and higher social and health costs - which of course is beneficial to no-one (cf. Cooper et al, 1996; Levi and Lunde-Jensen, 1996).

2.   GUIDELINES FOR EMPLOYMENT

Developing entrepreneurship, improving employability, encouraging the adaptability of business and their employees, and strengthening the policies for equal opportunities were the core conclusions of the extraordinary European Council meeting on employment (Eur-Op News, No.4, 1997). This summit launched a corresponding, co-ordinated strategy for national employment policies defining a number of guidelines for employment at EU level. The approaches advocated by the Summit are based on a necessary but probably insufficient *top-down* strategy. What seems to be forgotten is the necessary complement to this of a *bottom-up* approach, an attempt to empower, train, and mobilise the 16 millions of European unemployed for mutual help and self-help, and to remove obstacles to their initiatives to do so. And both approaches must be applied across societal sectors and academic disciplines, and at all societal levels, in a *systems* approach.

According to a common dictionary, a "system" can be seen as "a group of interacting, interrelated, or interdependent elements forming a complex whole". A systems analysis accordingly implies "the study of an activity or a procedure to determine the desired end and the most efficient method(s) of obtaining this end". The term is derived from late Latin "systema", from Greek "sustema" - to combine.

A most interesting initiative not specifically geared to, but easily applicable to the problem area of "unemployment and health", has been made recently by the British Government, in its Green Paper on "Our Healthier Nation - A Contract For Health" presented to the British Parliament in February 1998. In essence, this paper spells out five types of factors affecting health. The first category is referred to as "fixed". It includes genes, sex and ageing, and is accordingly difficult to influence in a disease preventing and/or health promoting manner. In contrast, the other four categories could and should be approached (British Government, 1998):

- *social and economic* (such as unemployment, poverty, social exclusion)
- *environment* (such as air and water quality, housing, and social environment)
- *lifestyle* (such as physical activity, diet, smoking, alcohol, sexual behaviour, drugs) and
- *access to services* (such as education, health and social services, transport, and leisure).

3.   A CONTRACT FOR HEALTH

All these and related factors can be dealt with in a co-ordinated, systems approach, *across sectors and societal levels*, in a Contract for Health. The three groups of *partners* in such a contract are

- central government and national players
- local players and communities, and
- all citizens.

On a central level, the governments should lead the way, establishing broad *cross-ministerial Cupertino* with directives and objectives to set up a corresponding Cupertino at central and local authority and administrative levels. It is also a matter of breaking down structural barriers and implementing joint solutions to problems - with regard to planning, and allocation of funds and personnel. A corresponding system of *'communicating vessels'* should be set up between local authorities with Cupertino between employment offices, social insurance offices, social services, primary health care, the educational establishments, companies, trade unions, voluntary organisations and the unemployed themselves.

An important step in this direction has been made recently in Sweden (Swedish Government Bill 1996/97:63), dealing with collaboration across sectors and societal levels. This bill has its focus on concerted action in the field of *rehabilitation* - of bringing unemployed people with physical, mental and/or social handicaps back to gainful employment. One may hope that the principles spelt out in this bill will be applied to the general problem of unemployment and to many other societal problem areas as well.

Briefly, then, the two bills emphasise the need for collaboration both across *sectors* (such as health care, labour exchange, social welfare, and social insurance) and across public sector *levels* (central government, counties, municipalities). Still lacking is the integration also of education and training policies regarding elementary and secondary schools but also colleges and universities into such a *systems* approach. It is further likely that such integrative initiatives will have to overcome very considerable amounts of intrasectoral "territoriality" thinking and bureaucratic inertia.

Kickbusch (1997) considers *health promotion* to be "a theory based process of social change contributing to the goal of human development, building on many disciplines and applying interdisciplinary knowledge in a professional, methodical and creative way". In her view, "health promotion outcome" can be determined by an organised, partnership-based community effort contributing to health, quality of life and social capital of a society.

Thus, there is a growing awareness - nationally and internationally - of the problems that people are experiencing both with regard to various aspects of their social situation as determinants of their health, well-being and quality of life as well as of ways to prevent ill health and promote health and well-being (Wilkinson and Marmot, 1998). However, there still seems to be a long way to go before effective measures are taken to deal with existing problems, to prevent other ones from occurring, and to the promotion of positive health. There is a wide *science-policy gap*. The high unemployment in Sweden and in most of the other 14 EU Member States serves as an example of this inability.

4.   ACTION FOR FULL EMPLOYMENT

Briefly, then, national governments, local authorities, and "grassroots" should *co-ordinate* their efforts to achieve six major goals: (1) to save and/or develop good jobs, and to abolish obsolete ones; (2) to find those vacant jobs that already exist; (3) to create new jobs; (4) to develop individual professional and social competence (life skills), and to empower the "grassroots"; (5) to improve community climate, in terms of awareness, involvement, and social support, (i.e. social capital); and (6) to protect and/or promote health, well-being and functional ability of the individual to enable him or her to fill a new position once it has been offered, found, or created (IPM et al., 1994).

Action to promote the achievement of these six goals is possible on eight levels, namely: (1) *supranationally*, e.g. through the United Nations and its specialised agencies, the European Union etc; (2) *nationally*, through governmental bills and parliamentary acts concerning laws and regulations, taxes and allowances, administered through various ministries and branches of civil service; (3) *regionally*, through County Councils, County Administrative Boards, County Labour Market Boards etc; (4) *municipally*, through Local Social Insurance Offices, Employment Exchange Offices, Social Welfare Offices, the school system, and units for adult education; (5) through *the parties on the labour market* and their collective bargaining and agreements; (6) through *voluntary organisations*, including self-help groups, religious and charity organisations etc; (7) through local *co-operative* approaches (social economy); and (8) *individually*, through initiatives and actions from each individual in conjunction with his or her close network, and their mutual help and self-help.

The challenge here is to design and implement a *co-ordinated* approach of many concerted actions across sectors and societal levels, in such a way, that the various actions facilitate and reinforce rather than counteract or obstruct each other.

4.1   Life-long education and training

A sizeable proportion of all Swedes is 'functionally illiterate' at the end of his/her compulsory 9-year schooling (cf. National Agency for Education, 1995, 1997, 1999). He or she is unable, or barely able to read, write and do simple arithmetic *sufficiently for everyday occupational purposes*. Not surprisingly, these young persons have considerable and increasing difficulties entering the labour market and managing to stay in it. The routine jobs in mass production industries which the generation of their parents had access to have been increasingly rationalised or made redundant as a result of technical development (computerisation and robotisation) and global competition.

Even those educated to upper secondary level but with incomplete, poor or mediocre grades can be faced with these kinds of difficulties.

The problems are intensified by the fact that many upper secondary and post upper secondary education programs fail in their task to train the pupil's capacity for abstract thinking - to detect patterns and purpose, to think analogously, in models, pictures and categories. Nor is the education system effective in teaching the pupils to think in systems, to view things holistically, to discover cross-disciplinary and cross-sectoral causes and relationships, to work experimentally and to work together with others to solve problems (cf. Reich, 1993).

Bert-Olof Svanholm, the late MD, of the ASEA Brown Bovery Group (ABB), maintained that his company could not promise its employees life-long employment - but it could offer *life-long employability*, by offering them continuous professional development, thereby maintaining and increasing their attractiveness on the labour market.

The Swedish government has realised the importance of developing professional skills both as a measure against unemployment and in order to maintain and increase the international competitiveness of the Swedish workforce, by offering continued education for more than 100,000 adults considered to be in need of it.

However, skills mean more than just professional expertise. Life skills are just as important - the ability to manage one's life both in prosperity and adversity.

4.2   Skills for life

Nowadays, many unemployed are so downhearted, helpless and have such low self-confidence that they give up, feel defeated, stop looking for new solutions. In such situations, vocational education and training, however ambitious and necessary, is not going to be sufficient. A person with low self-confidence will find it hard to profit from such options. Furthermore, the person will subsequently find it hard to apply for and to get, or create a good job.

WHO, in good Cupertino with the European Commission and the Council of Europe, has attracted attention to this problem, based on a broader health perspective. One of WHO's ideas is to improve school-age children's 'introduction to life' by teaching them how to live in a way which promotes health and well-being. 500 schools in 40 countries in Europe have entered the "European Network of Health promoting Schools" (WHO, European Commission, Council of Europe, 1997). These schools are fully committed to:
- create socio-educational settings which support health;
- strengthen collaboration between schools and their communities;
- develop and sustain the school as a healthy physical environment;
- build personal health skills among pupils, teachers and parents.

The health-promoting schools' complementary curriculum includes increasing the pupils' knowledge and understanding of a number of lifestyles known to be hazardous - smoking, drinking, drugs, unhealthy diets, lack of exercise etc., in order to promote healthy life-styles. In addition, and equally important, the programme attempts to promote 'social skills' or 'skills for life'. The pupils have learning opportunities, for example, to:
- communicate effectively
- make decisions
- solve problems
- think critically
- hold their own
- resist peer pressure
- manage their own worry, depression and stress
- adapt to new environmental demands, and
- get to know themselves

Anybody possessing such 'skills for life' - related to but not identical with *emotional intelligence* (cf. Stone and Dillehunt, 1978; Grant Consortium,

1992; Goleman, 1995) - will not remain unemployed for long. Nor will they remain in a bad job. They will improve their job or find another.

The notion of 'skills for life' is very similar to the notion of *'self-power'* which was introduced by Karl-Petter Thorwaldsson, former president of the Social-Democratic Youth of Sweden. 'Self-power' is having power and influence over your own everyday life. This can be gained partly through life skills and partly by society not hindering individual and co-operative bottom-up efforts to solve problems but rather promoting and encouraging such efforts (Levi, 1998), as a complement to society's own central and regional top-down resolution of problems. In this way we could get popular movements against unemployment and other large-scale social and health problems.

These "skills for life" are also very much in line with what Antonovsky referred to as *salutogenesis* (Antonovsky, 1987) which could be defined as *"the development of a condition of health"*. To have an idea of where you are heading and how and why - to have a salutogenic 'sense of coherence' (Antonovsky, 1987). This consists of three components: *Understandability* - people want to understand what is happening to them, *Manageability* - people want to be able to manage their current situation, to adjust it, to cope with it, and *Meaningfulness*.

4.3   Social support

Sweden has a long and honourable tradition of solidarity between people - a solidarity not only expressed in readiness to pay progressive taxes, but also in a will to 'carry each other's burdens', a mutual consideration for other people, not only those within a given circle of family and friends (Putnam, 1993).

Alone is not strong. It is crucial for our welfare and our health that we have someone to 'hold our hand' in the storm. Someone who cares. Who gives us support and appreciation, helps us to orientate ourselves in our life conditions and to interpret them, to encourage, to listen, to comfort, even to lend us a practical hand. It may be a close relative or a good friend. It may be a colleague at work. Or a neighbour. We feel better and can tolerate more if we have somebody to stand up for us. But also when we ourselves have somebody to stand up for. When we do not only receive - but also give - social support. (Putnam, 1993; Wilkinson, 1996).

This support can be applied to both our own and other's self-esteem, for example, through receiving and giving appreciation and praise. We can get help to interpret a social situation correctly - to realise that what is causing us problems is perhaps an annoyance rather than a catastrophe. We can get, and give, a feeling of solidarity. Or practical advice.

A person who has access to all of this and can take advantage of it will feel better and will become more resistant to life's various trials (cf. Johnson, 1986). Welfare will be improved along with health. It is, in fact, another option for "investment for health".

All of this cannot be achieved overnight. It must be based on arduous, long-term efforts. It will not be possible to achieve without clear-cut political signals from all relevant levels, complementing a popular movement both centrally and locally.

Isn't this all very difficult? Of course it is, it's *very* difficult, complicated and hard to master.

But do we really have any alternative?

REFERENCES

Antonovsky, A. 1987, Unravelling the Mystery of Health: How People Manage Stress and Stay Well. Jossey-Bass, San Francisco.

Behrenz, L and Delander, L. 1997, The Total Fiscal Costs of Unemployment - an Estimation for Sweden. Report to the European Commission. Växjö.

Berg, J.O. 1997, Förnyare, frustrerade och fria agenter (Renewers, Frustrated, and Free Agents). City University Press, Stockholm.

British Government. 1998, Our Healthier Nation. A Contract for Health. Green Paper. London.

Cooper, CL, Liukkonen, P, and Cartwright, S. 1996, Assessing the Benefits of Stress Prevention at Company Level. European Foundation for the Improvement of Living and Working Conditions, Dublin.

Dooley, D, Fielding, J. and Levi, L. 1996, Health and Unemployment. Annu. Rev. Public Health, 17:449-65.

Eurostat: News Release No. 94/98. 1998, Luxembourg, Statistical Office of the European Communities.

Goleman, D. 1995, Emotional Intelligence. Bantam, New York.

Grant Consortium, 1992, School-Based Promotion of Social Competence, in: Hawkins, JD et al. (eds.). Communities that Care. Jossey-Bass, San Francisco.

IPM, FHI & AMFO, 1994, Från idé till handling. (From Idea to Action). Arbetsmiljöfonden, Stocholm.

Jahoda, M. 1979, The Impact of Unemployment in the 1930's and the 1970's. Bulletin of the British Psychological Society, 32, 309-314.

Johnson, JV. 1986, The Impact of Workplace Social Support, Job Demands and Work Control Upon Cardiovascular Disease in Sweden. PhD Dissertation, Department of Psychology, Stockholm University.

Kickbusch, I. 1997, Think Health. What Makes the Difference? Key Speech at the 4th International Conference on Health Promotion. World Health Organization, Geneva. WHO/HPR/HEP/41CHP/SP/97.1.

Kompier, M and Levi, L. 1994, Stress At Work: Causes, Effects, and Prevention. A Guide for Small and Medium Sized Enterprises. European Foundation, Dublin.

Levi, L. 1972, Stress and Distress in Response to Psychosocial Stimuli.Pergamon Press, New York.

Levi, L. (ed.), 1981, Society, Stress and Disease. Vol. 4: Working Life. Oxford Univ. Press, Oxford.

Levi, L. 1984, Stress in Industry - Causes, Effects and Prevention. International Labour Office, Geneva.

Levi, L and Lunde-Jensen, P. 1996, Socio-Economic Costs of Work Stress in Two EU Member States. A Model for Assessing the Costs of Stressors At National Level. European Foundation, Dublin.

Levi L: 1998, Folkhälsa, makt, demokrati (Public Health, Power, Democracy). Stockholm, Landsorganisationen.

Levi L: 1998, The Welfare of the Future - A Swedish Case Study. In: European Macro-Trends and Implications for Investing for Health. Report from the First Verona Meeting 14-17 October. Copenhagen: WHO/Euro, 1999 (in press).

National Agency for Education, 1995, Hur i all världen läser svenska elever? (How in the World do Swedish Pupils Read?) Skolverket, Stockholm, (Report 95:164).

National Agency for Education, 1997, Svenska. Läsning, skrivning, muntlig framställning (Swedish. Reading, Writing, Expression). Skolverket, Stockholm, (Report   97:268)

National Agency for Education, 1999, Barnomsorg & skola i siffror 1999 (Child Care and School in Figures 1999). Skolverket, Stockholm.

Putnam RD, 1993, Making Democracy Work. Civic Traditions in Modern Italy. Princeton University Press, Princeton.

Reich, RB. 1993, The Work of Nations. A Blueprint for the Future. Simon & Schuster, London.

Statistics Sweden, 1988, The Working Environment 1997. Statistical Bulletin SM9801. Stockholm: SCB.

Stone, KF and Dillehunt, HQ, 1978, Self Science. The Subject is Me. Goodyear, Santa Monica.

Wilkinson RG, 1996, Unhealthy Societies. The Affliction of Inequality. Routledge, London and New York.

Wilkinson R and Marmot M, 1998, The Solid Facts. Social Determinants of Health.   World Health Organization, Copenhagen.

WHO/Euro, European Commission, Council of Europe, 1997, The Health Promoting School An Investment in Education, Health and Democracy. Conference Report.   1st Conference of the European Network of Health Promoting Schools, Greece, 1-5 May.

REPEATED DOWNSIZING: *Attitudes and well-being for surviving personnel in a Swedish retail company*

Isaksson, K. [1], Hellgren, J. [2] & Pettersson, P. [2]

[1]*National Institute for Working Life, Sweden,* [2]*Department of Psychology, Stockholm University, Sweden*

Abstract: The study evaluates consequences of the major restructuring and downsizing of a large Swedish retail company. Efforts were made to investigate the impacts of perceived job insecurity, influence over the restructuring process, and perceived fairness of the process on well-being of remaining personnel, "survivors" of the process. A second aim was to investigate effects of repeated downsizing on work perceptions, attitudes and health of "survivors". Data were collected by means of a questionnaire on two occasions with a 12-month interval. The response rate was 71% for survivors at Time 1 (n=555), and 71% again for survivors at Time 2 (n=395). Results indicated that the most important predictors of distress at Time 1 was perceived job insecurity and perceived participation in the process. Furthermore, that a new wave of organizational change between measurement occasions was associated with higher personal ratings of workload and lower ratings of job satisfaction, whereas mean distress scores remained unchanged. At Time 2 perceived insecurity together with experience from repeated downsizing were critical factors predicting distress symptoms.

1.   BACKGROUND

The general aim of this paper was to investigate the health and work-related consequences for surviving of the reorganization and downsizing of the administration of KF, a major wholesale and retail supplier of foodstuffs and other merchandise in Sweden. 1993 saw the initiation of a wide-ranging process of rationalization and restructuring within KF, which impacted on both work organization and job content.

1.1   Changes to the central administration

The process of change was initiated during the autumn of 1992 when details of the design of a new administrative organization were first presented. The proposed restructuring was to entail substantial lay-offs among the 1,570 white-collar workers within the administration. In total,

Health Effects of the New Labour Market, edited by Isaksson *et al.*
Kluwer Academic / Plenum Publishers, New York, 2000.

85

there would be room for 880 new positions within what was to become KF/KD AB (a corporate organization). This also entailed that many current employees would be surplus to requirements, and would be laid off. All 1,570 employees were given notice, and had to apply for one of the 880 positions in the new company. The first stage - in what proved to be a series of changes in the new KF/KD AB - was completed on March 31, 1993 and all excess personnel were given notice. A total of 660 persons were regarded as surplus to requirements, of whom 200 were granted a negotiated early-retirement pension for the turn of the year.

In this context, it is important to point out that there had been a traditional conception within KF that co-operation should enable the interests of its employees to be safeguarded and that social responsibilities would be met. There was major confidence in the organization's commitment to job security, and redundancies on this scale had never previously been contemplated throughout its history. This may have contributed to personnel being relatively late to realize that this thorough-going change, with the personnel cutbacks it would entail, was in fact to be effected. Accordingly, the statement on over-manning and the scale of the forthcoming lay-offs came as a shock. Everyone had known that something would happen, but not that the staffing consequences would be so severe.

1.2   Theoretical background

Two perspectives have predominated in research into downsizing and personnel cutbacks. The first is a purely *organizational* perspective, including consideration of, for example, decision-making, strategic choice, and efficiency (Kozlowski, Chao, Smith & Hedlund, 1993). Personnel cutbacks may be either proactive (with long-term development in mind) or reactive (simply reacting to changes in the environment). The two approaches focus on different basic conditions that might determine frames for what opportunities are available and what sequences of events might be. It has proved that choice of method for the effecting of downsizing is governed largely by legal and ethical considerations, but also to some extent by weighing costs against skills (Mabon & Westling, 1997). And other factors, such as how quickly cutbacks have to be made and the need to exert control over who is going to leave are also important. In KF's case, restructuring entailed a largely proactive process of change, which was designed – in the long term – to secure the profitability of the new company. At the same time, the fact that profitability had been poor meant that there was an element of reactivity.

With regard to efficiency, organization researchers – at least in recent years – have adopted an increasingly critical stance towards the extent to which downsizing achieves the goals intended for it by management (Kets de Vries & Balazs, 1997; Cascio, 1998). It has been pointed out that negative impacts on the the so-called survivors have been underestimated, and that far too little attention has been paid to their reactions when retroactive evaluations are made of how successful rationalization has been. In extreme cases, downsizing can be a highly destructive process that sets off a downward spiral. It can have negative effects on profitability, which may then trigger off new cutbacks.

The second principal approach in this research arena has been to adopt an *individual perspective,* i.e. to take employees themselves as the point of departure. For long, there was a concentration on individuals leaving the organization, i.e. the persons made redundant and about to be unemployed. Above all, studies of corporate closures were conducted. The negative effects of unemployment, primarily with regard to psychological health, have been made familiar by previous research. But research into unemployment has also shown that the period when employees have to wait for information on whether or not they are to be laid off is the most stressful (Joelsson & Wahlqvist, 1987). Survivors of downsizing often find themselves in such a situation. It is common for them to be informed that one phase of downsizing has been completed, but that further cutbacks will be needed.

In an earlier study of downsizing of a large Swedish insurance company (Isaksson & Johansson, 1997) the persons on early retirement who made a voluntary departure were found as the most satisfied following personnel cutbacks. Persons who had been compelled to take early retirement, however, expressed very negative experiences – ones that had affected their well-being for several years. The study clearly showed that the way in which downsizing is effected is of decisive importance for the well-being of surviving personnel, in particular that the process takes place in collaboration with the workforce.

1.2.1   Effects on survivors

A number of studies of downsizing, primarily from the USA, have examined impacts on remaining personnel. Kets de Vries and Balazs (1997) drew the conclusion that it is the manner in which the process is effected that has decisive consequences.

Brockner and colleagues (Brockner, 1988; Brockner, Grover, O'Mally, Reed & Glynn, 1993) have dominated this research niche. Above all, they have examined the attitudes of survivors to their work and to the company. Downsizing seems to have impacts on job contentment and motivation (see also Kets de Vries & Balazs, 1997). The findings of these and other studies clearly point to cutbacks reducing levels of job satisfaction and commitment at work, and often increasing desire to leave the company (see, e.g., Ashford, Lee & Bobko, 1989; Rosenblatt & Ruvio, 1996). Impacts vary, in part according to the degree of social support available inside and outside the workplace (Lim, 1996), and also to previous level of personal work commitment within the company (Begley & Czajka, 1993).

In previous research, the factors in the change-and-downsizing process that have been shown to be most significant in terms of the reaction of survivors are:

1. The degree of residual insecurity and extent of the threat of unemployment (Greenhalgh & Rosenblatt, 1984; Kozlowski et al., 1993);

2. Whether or not employees regard the downsizing process as fair (Brockner, 1988; Davy, Kinicki, & Scheck, 1991)

3. The extent of the opportunities available to personnel to influence and participate in the process of change (Covin, 1993; Davy, Kinicki, & Scheck, 1991).

1.2.2   Studies of insecurity and personnel stress/ill-health following downsizing

Worry and stress during periods of reorganization and downsizing have been shown to be strongly associated with inherent situational uncertainty, in particular in that job security is threatened by imminent personnel cutbacks. Job insecurity can be regarded as involving a discrepancy between desired and actual employment security (Jacobson, 1991). Attitudes to the company and to the work are affected by downsizing, often followed by reduced well-being (Van Vuuren, Klandermans, Jacobson & Hartley, 1991), and also by a tendency to leave the organization.

Perceived insecurity in any given situation varies between individuals, not only due to personality factors but also as a product of a variety of factors, such as the degree of social support offered inside and outside work (Lim, 1996). Acute insecurity and long-term insecurity also seem to differ in their effects. Most studies of the impacts of insecurity have shown negative short-term effects with regard to health and well-being. But a study by Heaney, Israel and House (1994) has also shown long-term negative health effects in cases of chronic and long-term insecurity.

A study recently presented by Parker, Chmiel and Wall (1997) found that the negative effects of personnel cutbacks might be prevented by strategic planning and the taking of special measures on behalf of personnel. The study, however, was performed in a situation where the personnel concerned had a relatively secure future.

In sum, while it is clear that research has certainly expanded in this arena in recent years, it still has its limitations, in particular with regard to long-term effects. In the short term, it is clear that personnel cutbacks have a major impact, even on persons who remain in employment. The pleasure they take in work is reduced, and their attitude to the company deteriorates. Many also seem to experience worry and anguish, and display mild symptoms of psychological ill-health. Insecurity and the threat of unemployment seem to be perceived as the factor giving rise to the greatest strain. This study has its focus on whether such effects last, at least in the medium term, and on the impact on survivors of repeated changes and feelings of enclosure.

1.3 Aim and questions posed

The aim of this paper was to examine the effects on affected personnel within KF/KD AB of the major restructuring and downsizing effected since 1992. The impacts of repeated change are investigated primarily in terms of perceptions of work characteristics, such as workload, attitudes to the work and the company, and well-being and health. Predictors of distress symptoms were also investigated.

1.3.1 Questions:

1. What importance did repeated downsizing between times 1 and 2 have for survivors' perceptions of their situation at Time 2?
2. What predictive value do various elements in the process of change have in relation to distress of personnel during various phases of the process?

2. METHOD

The investigation was designed to follow up the reorganizing and downsizing that took place in conjunction with the transformation of the KF cooperative society into KF/KD AB (a corporate organization). Following the major structural change made to the organization, a number of further reorganizations were effected to work processes and work content within its central administration, each of which entailed further rationalization and personnel cutbacks. When our first questionnaire was about to be administered in December 1995, management had just announced that a reorganization of buying operations would be implemented during 1996. By the time of administration of the second questionnaire in November 1996, this change had already been effected. Remaining parts of the administration and the service units were to be rationalized during 1997. This means that everyone who took part in the survey had witnessed the restructuring that had taken place prior to the formation of the company, KD AB. A large group of personnel had experienced a second wave of downsizing between the initial survey and the follow-up. Others were awaiting new changes, which had still not been completed by the time of writing of this paper.

2.1   Data collection

In December 1995 (Time 1), a questionnaire was administered to all remaining personnel within KF/KD AB (786 in total). The questionnaires were sent by post to respondents together with a post-addressed envelope to the research team at the Department of Psychology, Stockholm University. Each questionnaire was accompanied by a letter explaining the purpose of the study and guaranteeing full anonymity and also by a letter from company management encouraging participation. A reminder to persons not returning their questionnaire was sent three weeks later.

On the second occasion of investigation in November 1996 (Time 2), the questionnaire was distributed solely to those who had responded to the first questionnaire and who were still employed in the company (555). Otherwise, the data-collection procedure was precisely the same as at Time 1.

2.2   Respondents and non-respondents

Of the 786 survivors at Time 1, there was a total of 555 (71%) who returned their questionnaire to the research team. The average age of survivors was 49 (SD=8.85). Average length of previous employment was 22 years, and 69% of respondents in this group were women.

Representativeness: Registry data from the company showed that the mean age of all employees at time of administration of the first questionnaire was 47.2 years, that the average period of previous employment was 17.6 years, and that 53% of employees were women. This indicates that older persons with relative long periods of prior employment at KF had a higher questionnaire-response rate, and also that women are somewhat over-represented in the material.

At Time 2, 395 of the 555 survivors who had responded at Time 1 also responded to the second questionnaire (72%). Their mean age was 49 (SD=8.35), and their average period of previous employment at KF was 22.5 years. On the second occasion of administration, 54% of respondents were women. Of the original group of 786 survivors at Time 1, 62 had left KF by

Time 2. These individuals were not sent a questionnaire at Time 2, meaning that the sample constituted 55% of the original survivor group.

Given that 160 individuals did not respond to the second questionnaire, a MANOVA was performed to control for possible differences between persons who responded on the first occasion and those responding on both. No main effect between the two groups was found ($\underline{F}$ [14,507]=0.958, $\underline{p}$<.495). This means that non-respondents did not differ from respondents with regard to perceptions, attitudes or health at time of first investigation.

2.3   Measuring instruments

All but two of the variables encompassed by the study were measured on the same five-point scale (ranging from 1=do not agree at all, 5=agree entirely). The exceptions were well-being (GHQ symptoms), which was measured on a 0-3 scale, and presence of health complaints, where 1 refers to "never or almost never" and 3 to "always or almost always". The analyses are based on mean values on indexes, constructed for each scale following recoding of negative statements. With a few exceptions, the reliability estimates show a value in excess of 0.70, indicating that most of the measuring instruments have satisfactory properties (see, e.g., Nunnaly, 1978). Table 1 below shows correlation coefficients, descriptive statistics, and reliability estimates (as measured by Cronbach's α) for survivors at Time 1.

Table 1. Descriptive statistics for measures used (n = 368)

Variables	M	SD	1	2	3	4	5	6	7	8	9
1. Age	48.2	8.7	-								
2. Sex	1.4	0.5	.04	-							
3. Neg. affectivity	1.4	0.5	-.06	.07	-						
4. Influence	2.2	1.1	.03	.17	.03	-					
5. Perc. justice	2.8	0.9	.22	.02	-.01	.30	-				
6. Perc. insecurity	3.0	1.2	-.07	.05	.27	.23	.01	-			
7. New downsizing	1.5	0.5	-.13	.07	.09	-.07	-.01	-.23	-		
8. Distress T 1	9.6	5.0	.09	-.14	.50	-.26	-.07	-.34	.19	-	
9. Distress T 2	9.3	5.0	.11	-.08	.31	-.19	-.06	-.36	.25	.59	-

.09 =p<.05

2.3.1.1   Change-related variables

Participation in the process of change was measured (only at Time 1) by means of responses to three statements concerning what information was regarded as having being obtainable and influence exertable (e.g. "I had the opportunity to be involved and decide at the time my work situation was changing") in the course of the organizational change (α=0.77). The authors developed the scale specifically for the purposes of the study.

Three statements were employed to measure *fairness in the process of change,* reflecting the individual's perception of fairness with regard to the lay-offs, the offers of early-retirement pensions, and appointments to the new positions (e.g. "I think that the decisions over who could keep their jobs and who had to leave were fair"). The index was developed by the authors specifically for the purposes of the study (α=0.79).

Perceived job insecurity was measured on the basis of three statements (e.g. "I am worried about having to leave my job before I would like to") concerning the individual's perception of employment security and continuity (α=0.79 for both Time 1 and Time 2). The index is based on questionnaire items in English developed by Ashford, Lee and Bobko (1989), which were translated into Swedish and then modified by the authors.

2.3.2   Work situation

Quantitative workload was measured on the basis of responses to three statements (e.g. "It happens quite often that I have to work under severe time pressure") focusing on whether work was perceived as time-pressurized and stressful (α for Time 1=0.81; for Time 2=0.84). The three statements are taken from Nystedt's (1992) four-affirmation scale.

Qualitative workload was examined using three statements (e.g. "Unreasonable demands are imposed upon me at work") reflecting whether the individual feels his/her responsibilities are too great and the scale of job demands (α for Time 1=0.65; for Time 2=0.64). The scale for measuring qualitative load was developed by Sjöberg (1990).

A scale developed by Hovmark and Thomsson (1995) was employed to measure *social support in the workplace.* Three support dimensions are utilized: evaluative, instrumental and emotional. Each dimension is measured on the basis of three statements. For this study, an aggregated measure of social support was employed (α for Time 1=0.87; for Time 2=0.88) that encompassed all three dimensions. Accordingly, nine statements were employed to measure social support (e.g. "When you take the initiative in the workplace do you seek out what others think of your efforts").

Work group climate is concerned with support and community in the work group. It was measured on the basis of four statements (e.g. "Relations between members of my work group are open and straight"), taken directly from Nystedt (1992).

Learning and skills development were measured on the basis of four statements (e.g. "I am always learning something new at work") developed by Hellgren, Sjöberg and Sverke (1997). The index illuminates the individual's perception of job variability and the opportunities for personal development offered at work (α for Time 1=0.85; for Time 2=0.86).

2.3.3 Attitudinal variables

Three attitudinal variables were included in the study. One represented perception of work situation (job satisfaction), while another focused on identification with the organization (organizational commitment). The third reflects an intention to act in a specific manner, namely to give notice and leave.

Job satisfaction was measured using three statements modified by Hellgren and colleagues (1997) from a scale originally developed by Brayfield and Roth (1951). Responses to the statements (e.g. "I feel that I enjoy my work") reflect the individual's overall perception of his/her work (α for Time 1=0.88; for Time 2=0.86).

Organizational commitment was examined on the basis of four statements (e.g. "It often feels that the company's problems are the same as my own") developed by Allen and Meyer (1990). The purpose of the scale is to shed light on the individual's psychological identification with the organization (α for Time 1=0.74; for Time 2=0.70).

To measure *intention to quit,* three questions, developed by Sjöberg and Sverke (1996) were employed (e.g. "I feel like giving up my current job"). The scale reflects the strength of the individual's intention voluntarily to give notice of termination of employment (α for Time 1=0.79; for Time 2=0.75).

Repeated downsizing Responses to the second questionnaire revealed that 200 survivors (51%) perceived their work situation to have changed while 192 (49%) saw no difference with regard to either the nature of the work or its content.

Negative affectivity was measured using the NA part of the PANAS scale (Watson, Clark & Tellegen, 1984), in which the construct is assessed using 10 item mood scales.

2.3.4 Health

Two separate indexes were employed to obtain an idea of how the health states of individuals were affected by the reorganization and personnel cutbacks. The one reflects the individual's perception of psychological well-being, the other the frequency of experienced physical complaints.

Distress (GHQ symptoms) was measured on the basis of twelve statements illuminating various aspects of well-being (e.g. In the light of current circumstances have you been feeling more or less alright in recent times?). The scale was developed by Goldberg (1979). See also Goldberg & Williams (1988). The reliability estimate for both Time 1 and Time 2 was 0.84.

Health complaints were measured on the basis of seven statements, forming a scale originally developed by Andersson (1986). For this study, a later version, modified and previously used by Isaksson and Johansson (1997), was employed. The scale is based on assertions with regard to the appearance of various kinds of somatic health complaints, such as aching of muscles and joints, and so on (α for Time 1=0.67; for Time 2=0.73).

3.   RESULTS

The consequences of the reorganization for personnel are described from both a short-term (Time 1) and a somewhat longer-term (Time 2) perspective. The impacts of the new set of changes between the two occasions of measurement are also tested.

Two multiple regression analyses were performed to see what change-related and health variables (at Time 1) were associated with the level of distress of survivors. The first analysis represented an attempt to predict well-being at Time 1. Results of the first analysis are presented in Table 2.

Table 2. Effects of change-related factors on distress symptoms (GHQ-12) of survivors at Time 1

	Distress Time 1	
Predictor	Step 1	Step 2
Age	.11**	.10**
Sex	-.19***	-.14***
Negative affectivity	.52	.50***
Influence		-.21***
Perc. justice		-.04
Perc. insecurity		.14***
R^2 Adjusted	.30***	.38***
	n=519	n=516

$* p < .05$ $** p < .01$ $*** p < .001$

From the table it emerges that participation in the process and job insecurity are the change-related variables that predict level of distress symptoms at Time 1. Lower senses of influence and high job insecurity gives a higher degree of distress symptoms. There was also a significant age effect indicating that older persons tend to feel more distressed. These relations remain significant even after introducing negative affectivity as a control.

3.1   Changes over time and long-term effects of subsequent changes

The next analytic step was to investigate how perspectives on and attitudes to work of remaining personnel, and also their health, changed over the period of one year between the occasions of data collection. To examine whether there were any differences between those who had obtained new work tasks by Time 2 and survived a second wave of downsizing and those who had not, a MANOVA was performed in which individual Time 2 data was used for the dependent variable. In order to control for Time 1 differences, individual values for Time 1 were treated as covariates, while change in work tasks or not was regarded as an independent variable.

Table 3. Mean value changes over time and test of differences between persons who survived repeated downsizing and those reporting no change at Time 2.

Variable	Mean Working cond.	Time 1	Time 2	T^a	F^b
Perc. job insecurity	Changed	2.72	3.14	-4.87***	
	Unchanged	3.26	2.95	3.33***	17.76***
Workload (Quantitative)	Changed	3.63	3.73	n s	
	Unchanged	3.32	3.26	n s	9.19**
Workload (Qualitative)	Changed	2.06	2.27	-3.42***	
	Unchanged	1.83	1.77	n s	14.74***
Work group climate	Changed	3.82	3.82	n s	
	Unchanged	3.78	3.73	n s	1.00
Participation	Changed	3.70	3.55	2.65**	
	Unchanged	3.89	3.79	2.10*	1.66
Learning, skills develop.	Changed	3.42	3.41	n s	
	Unchanged	3.57	3.46	2.22*	0.48
Social support	Changed	3.32	3.22	2.10*	
	Unchanged	3.39	3.32	n s	1.08
Job satisfaction	Changed	3.48	3.24	2.87**	
	Unchanged	3.65	3.68	n s	9.76**
Work involvement	Changed	2.99	2.87	2.08*	
	Unchanged	3.08	3.00	n s	1.84
Intention to quit	Changed	2.13	2.29	- 2.15*	
	Unchanged	2.03	2.00	n s	3.62
Phys. health complaints	Changed	2.10	2.01	2.53*	
	Unchanged	1.93	1.81	2.83**	2.48
Distress (GHQ-12)	Changed	0.87	0.87	n s	
	Unchanged	0.71	0.65	2.19*	5.22*

[a] Paired t-test for mean differences withtin each group over time

[b] Univariat F-test for Time 2 differences between groups, controlling for Time 1 values (df = 1,357). *p<.05; **p<.01; ***p<.001.

Table 3 shows mean values for both groups at Time 1 and Time 2. The t-values indicate the significance of changes between Time 1 and Time 2, and the F-values that of the effects of change/no change.

Differences between the two groups were detected even at Time 1. These were probably the result of the "Change Group" having received information about the imminent transformations that were to be effected during the one-year period between the occasions of data collection. For example, the Change Group had lower perceived job security and higher workload, and reported higher distress levels at Time 1 than the other group. At Time 2 significantly lower values of perceived influence and health complaints were found for *both* groups compared to the Time 1 levels.

MANOVA results show a significant main effect of new changes made after Time 1 (for changed/unchanged work situation $F[12,346]=4.54$, $p<.001$). This means that there is a significant difference between the Change/No Change groups at Time 2 in terms of some of the investigated factors after controlling for individuals' Time 1 scores on the same variables.

Differences between the groups proved to be significant on five factors. There was an effect with regard to *perceived job security* ($F [1,357]=17.76$, $p\leq.001$) in that the group that had experienced changes had a significantly greater sense of job security at Time 2. Values for both groups changed between Time 1 and Time 2. But sense of job security increased for the group obtaining changed work tasks ($t [196]=-4.87$, $p<.001$), while it fell among those who had the same tasks but had received information about the changes due to be implemented during the forthcoming year ($t [183]=3.33$, $p<.001$).

Significant effects of change/no change were found for two of the work-related variables. The results reveal significant univariate effects on both *quantitative workload* ($F [1,357]=9.19$, $p\leq.01$) and *qualitative workload* ($F[1,357]=14.74$, $p\leq.001$). In both cases, the group experiencing changes had the higher value. In the case of quantitative load, no within-group changes were detected over time, indicating that persons who had changed work tasks by Time 2 were already perceiving higher quantitative load than others were at Time 1. Qualitative load, however, was found to increase for the group with changed work tasks ($t[197]=-3.42$, $p<.001$), but to remain stable for the other group.

Among the attitudinal variables only one effect was found, that on *job satisfaction* ($F[1,357]=9.76$, $p\leq.002$). Job satisfaction was found to be lower at Time 1 among those who had obtained changed tasks, and was also observed to fall over time ($t[196]=2.87$, $p<.01$). By contrast, it remained unchanged for the other group.

Turning finally to the health variables, a significant univariate effect on *distress symptoms,* as measured by GHQ-12, was found ($F[1,357]=5.22$, p≤.05). The group with changed work tasks shows a higher mean value and does not display any change over time, whereas the group with unchanged tasks displays a somewhat lower average symptom level at Time 2 (t[188]=2.83, p<.01).

3.2   Distress at Time 2: effects of repeated downsizing

From looking at predictors of distress levels as measured by GHQ-12 at Time 2, it emerges that job insecurity is again a significant predictor (B=.24, p<.001). And the effect remains significant even when Time 1 scores are entered into the analysis. The relationship is positive, which entails that high job insecurity is independently related to high distress scores one year later. Perceived influence over the change process at Time 1 was also related to well-being at Time 2.

Table 4. Effects of change-related factors and repeated downsizing on distress symptoms at Time 2

| Predictors | Distress symptoms Time 2 | | | |
	Step 1	Step2	Step 3	Step 4
1.Age	.14**	.13**	.16***	.08
2.Sex	-.11*	-.07	-.09*	-.02
3.Negative affectivity	.33***	.27***	.27***	.02
4.Perc. influence		-.12*	-.11**	-.01
5. Perc. justice		-.04	-.05	-.03
6. Perc. insecurity		.24***	.19***	.14**
7. New downsizing			.20***	.13**
8. GHQ-Time 1				.50***
R^2 Adjusted	.12***	.21***	.25***	.40***
	n=365	n=362	n=361	n=360

The factor introduced in the analysis of distress at Time 2, repeated downsizing was clearly associated with higher distress scores. Finally, there is also an age effect with older persons reporting higher levels of distress.

4.   DISCUSSION

The most important explanatory factor with regard to well-being (at both Time 1 and Time 2) was found to be perceived job insecurity. This factor was clearly the most important in terms of explaining variation in distress. Participation in the process of change was influential at Time 1 but not at Time 2 after the second wave of downsizing. Perceived fairness proved to have no significant explanatory value. In several studies (e.g. Brockner, 1988; Davy, Kinicki & Scheck, 1991) effects in the form of changed attitudes have been detected. It is possible that perceived job insecurity is of more fundamental importance, and has a clearer impact on distress. In the case of KF/KD AB, attitudes do not seem to have been affected to the extent that earlier findings suggest. Despite repeated reorganizations and generally critical attitudes, there were still fairly high degrees of job satisfaction and personal identification with the company (at about 3 on a five-point scale).

By Time 2, half of our respondents had experienced further changes. Following the structural transformation of 1993, the organization and content of work underwent further radical changes between 1995 and 1996, including the introduction of the so-called "flow organization". Those who had experienced new changes during the year between our occasions of investigation showed higher values on quantitative and qualitative work load and lower job satisfaction than those who had not, and also a continuing high level of GHQ symptoms. Perceived job insecurity, however, had decreased significantly in this subgroup by Time 2.

The time scale of the study is too restricted to say anything about long-term durability of reactions. But, for the group that had experienced further changes, GHQ symptoms remained at the same fairly high level despite the fact that perceived insecurity had diminished. This means that the negative impact of reorganization was still apparent, although it is impossible to say whether this was a case of delayed effect or lasting deterioration. Taking measurements after a longer period of time has elapsed might provide answers to these questions.

The effort to identify predictors of distress at Time 2 clearly indicated that repeated change and downsizing was related to a higher distress level. The results support the assumption that a major part of the distress reported after downsizing is caused by a sense of powerlessness among survivors. Threats of losing the job and a feeling of not being able to influence the process appeared to lead to very high levels of distress. The consistent age effect is also an interesting result. Older employees appear to be especially vulnerable in the process of downsizing probably due to the fact that age barriers in the labour market makes it difficult to obtain new employment for older persons.

On the whole, our results are very much in line with what has been reported from other studies. The longitudinal nature of this study and the possibility to secure results after repeated downsizing confirm that the changes in perceptions and attitudes are indeed related to change processes in the company.

Our findings might reasonably be supposed to be of interest to companies and other organizations about to embark on major reorganizations and personnel cutbacks. Perhaps the most important of these is that perceptions of job insecurity (in that employees feel the threat of redundancy) have on symptoms of ill-health and well-being. Since the scale of physical complaints seemed to decline during the follow-up period in both groups, it seems that it is psychological health, which is primarily affected. Quite clearly, organizational change is a source of stress for personnel. It means that work is perceived as a greater strain, in terms of both quantitative and qualitative load. Repeated changes also seem to have a negative impact on job satisfaction.

The study provides reason critically to examine the results presented by Parker, Chmiel and Wall (1997), who suggest that the negative effects of downsizing can be prevented by means of strategic planning. It should be pointed out, that their study was performed under circumstances of relative security in that no further lay-offs were planned. But, our findings tend to suggest that in so far as any reorganization entails further personnel cutbacks, negative health effects cannot be avoided.

ACKNOWLEDGEMENTS

The research on which this paper is based was supported by grants from the Swedish Council for Work Life Research, The KF group. the Salaried Employees' Union and the Cooperative Employers Association.

REFERENCES

Allen, N. J., and Meyer, J. P., 1990, The measurement and antecedents of affective, continuance and normative commitment to the organization. *Journal of Occupational Psychology, 63*, 1-18.

Andersson, K., 1986,. *Utveckling och prövning av ett frågeformulärstystem rörande arbetsmiljö och hälsotillstånd* (Development and test of a questionnaire on work environment and health). Örebro: Yrkesmedicinska kliniken, Report No. 5.

Ashford, S., Lee, C., and Bobko, P., 1989, Content, causes and consequences of job insecurity: a theory-based measure and substantive test. *Academy of Management Journal, 32*(4), 803-829.

Begley, T., and Czajka, J., 1993, Panel analysis of the moderating effects of commitment on job satisfaction, intent to quit and health following organizational change. *Journal of Applied Psychology, 78*(4), 552-556.

Brayfield, R., and Roth, H. F., 1951, An index of job satisfaction. Journal of Applied Psychology, 35, 307-311.

Brockner, J., 1988, Scope of justice in the workplace: How survivors react to co-worker layoffs. *Journal of Social Issues, 46*, 95-106.

Brockner, J., Grover, S., O'Mally, M. N., Reed, T. F., and Glynn, M. A., 1993, Threat of future layoffs, self-esteem and survivors' reactions: Evidence from the laboratory and the field. *Strategic Management Journal, 14*, 153-166.

Cascio, W., 1998, Learning from Outcomes: Financial experience of 311 firms that have downsized. In M. Gowing, et al (Eds.). *The New Organizational Reality*. (pp. 55-70). Washington DC: APA.

Covin, T., 1993, Managing workforce reduction: a survey of employee reactions & implications for management consultants. Organiszation Development Journal, 11(Spring), 67-76.

Davy, J. A., Kinicki, A. J., and Scheck, C. l., 1991, Developing and testing a model of survivors responses to layoffs. Journal of Vocational Behavior, 38, 302-317.

Goldberg, D., 1979, *Manual of the General Health Questionnaire*. London: NFER Nelson.

Goldberg, D., and Williams, P., 1988, *A User's guide to the General Health Questionnaire*. London: NFER Nelson.

Greenhalgh, L., and Rosenblatt, Z., 1984, Job insecurity: Towards conceptual clarity. *Academy of Management Review, 9*(3), 438-448.

Heaney, C., Israel, B., and House, J., 1994, Chronic job insecurity among automobile workers: effects on job satisfaction and health. Social Science and Medicine, 38, 1431-1437.

Hellgren, J., Sjöberg, A., and Sverke, M., 1997, *Intention to quit: Effects of job satisfaction and job perceptions*. Paper presented at the EAWOP, Verona.

Hovmark, S., and Thomsson, H., 1995, *ASK - ett frågeformulär för att mäta arbetsbelastning, socialt stöd, kontroll och kompetens i arbetslivet* (Rapport nr 86). Stockholm: Psykologiska institutionen, Stockholms universitet.

Isaksson, K., and Johansson, G., 1997, *Avtalspension med vinst och förlust*. (Gains and Losses of Early Retirement) Stockholm: Folksam.

Jacobson, D., 1991, The conceptual approach to job insecurity. In J. Hartley, D. Jacobson, B. Klandermans, and T. Van Vuuren (Eds.), *Job insecurity* (pp. 23-39). London: Sage.

Joelsson, l., and Wahlqvist, L., 1987, The psychological meaning of job insecurity and job loss. *Social Science and Medicine, 25,* 179-182.

Kets de Vries, M., and Balazs, K., 1997, The downside of downsizing. Human Relations, 50(1), 11-50.

Kozlowski, S., Chao, G., Smith, E., and Hedlund, J. (Eds.), 1993, Organizational downsizing: strategies, interventions and research. In C. L. Cooper and I. T. Robertson *International Review of Industrial and Organizational Psychology*. (Vol. 8). Chichester: Wiley.

Lim, V., 1996, Job insecurity and its outcomes: moderating effects of work-based and non vork-based social support. *Human Relations, 49*, 171-193.

Mabon, H., and Westling, G., 1997, Personalekonomiska aspekter. In K. Isaksson and G. Johansson (Eds.), *Avtalspension med vinst och förlust* (pp. 177-186). Stockholm: Folksam.

Nunnaly, J. C., 1978, *Psychometric Theory*. New York: McGraw Hill.

Nystedt, L., 1992, *Yrkesofficerares arbetsmiljö i armén* (FOA rapport nr C 50093-5.3). Stockholm: Försvarets Forskningsanstalt.

Parker, S. K., Chmiel, N., and Wall, T., 1997, Work characteristics and employee well-being within a context of strategic downsizing. *Journal of Occupational Health Psychology, 3*(4), 289-303.

Rosenblatt, Z., and Ruvio, A., 1996, A test of a multidimensional model of job insecurity: the case of Israeli teachers. *Journal of Organizational Behavior, 17*, 587-605.

Sjöberg, A., 1990, *Arbetstrivsel, lojalitet och frivillig avgång bland byggnadsarbetare.* (C-uppsats). Stockholm: Psykologiska institutionen.

Sjöberg, A., and Sverke, M., 1996, Predicting turnover intention among nurses: The role of work values. In V.V. Baba (Ed.), *Work Values and Behavior: Research and Applications* (pp.213-223), Montreal: International Society for the Study of Work and Organizational Values.

Van Vuuren, T., Klandermans, B., Jacobson, D., and Hartley, J., 1991, Employees' reactions to job insecurity. In J. Hartley, D. Jacobson, B. Klandermans, and T. Van Vuuren (Eds.), *Job insecurity* (pp. 79-103). London: Sage.

Watson, D., Clark, L. A. and Tellegen, A., 1988, Development and validation of brief measures of positive and negative affect: The PANAS scales. *Journal of Personality and Social Psychology, 6,* 1063-1070.

FLEXIBILIZATION AND STRESS

WORK LIFE AND ORGANIZATIONAL CHANGES AND HOW THEY ARE PERCEIVED BY THE EMPLOYEES

Annika Härenstam[1], Anna Rydbeck[2], Kerstin Johansson[1], Monica Karlqvist[1], and Per Wiklund[1].

[1]*Division of Occupational Health, Department of Public Health Sciences, Karolinska Institute, Stockholm, Sweden,* [2]*Department of Occupational and Environmental Medicine, Medical Center Hospital, Örebro, Sweden.*

Abstract: The aim is to investigate the association between different kinds of organizational changes during the last years and how the working conditions have been affected. In a study of working conditions for women and men in Swedish work life of today (the MOA-study[1]), data were collected on the organizational as well as on the individual level. Characteristics of 72 private and public work sites were assessed by using interviews with managers and written documents about the organizations. More changes were identified in the public compared to the private sector. Five different patterns of organizational changes were identified by means of a cluster analysis. 104 women and 104 men were selected for the investigation of working conditions by using open personal interviews and questionnaires regarding perceived consequences of the changes. The results of logistic regressions showed that the pattern of organizational changes was significantly associated with self-reported work load, development and control possibilities, job security and salary in relation to effort. Organizational changes directed at lean production systems seem to have a great impact on psychosocial working conditions, particularly for women.

1. INTRODUCTION

Work life is undergoing major changes as are many organizations[i]. The organization of work has changed as a consequence of the hardening economic reality and new management trends[ii]. The question is if the organizational context has an important, and perhaps increasing relevance for studies of working conditions and health. However, few studies in work life research combine the organizational and the individual levels in spite of

---

[1] Modern work and living conditions for women and men.

Health Effects of the New Labour Market, edited by Isaksson *et al.*
Kluwer Academic / Plenum Publishers, New York, 2000.

the theoretical presumptions on the association between the organizational context, working conditions, and health as proposed by many researchers, for example, Robert Karasek and Töres Theorell (1990), Tage Kristensen (1995), Jeffrey Johnson and Ellen Hall (1996), Björn Söderfeldt et al (1997). The most common associations investigated are between psychosocial factors and ill-health indicators, excluding the organizational level. However, it would be very useful for health promotion in work life if we knew more about early indicators of changes in risk factors. Data on changes in work organizations would offer that kind of information. An ultimate model aiming at describing a chain of mechanisms would also include the society level, e.g. unemployment data, and link all the levels together, preferably by multilevel analyses.

Changes in society ➡ *in work organizations* ➡ *of working conditions* ➡ *health*

Results of a study performed in USA by Fenwick and Tausig (1994) indicated that structural changes on the macro level had an impact on job stress; however, mainly indirectly through changes of the working conditions. There are a few examples from Sweden combining the organizational and the individual levels. One is a study of more than a thousand work places (by interviewing managers) and associations with working conditions, on the individual level, using data from the Swedish survey of level of living conditions (Le Grand, Szulkin & Thålin, 1993). In another study human service organizations are investigated on both levels (Söderfeldt et al 1997). In a study of working conditions for professionals data from both levels are analyzed; however, assessed only on the individual level (Härenstam & Bejerot 1995, Bejerot et al 1998).

2.   AIM, METHOD AND STUDY GROUP

The aim of the present study is to investigate the associations between different kinds of organizational changes during the late 1990's and how the consequences are perceived by the workers themselves. The data was collected within an interdisciplinary Swedish study, (the MOA-study[iii]) performed between late 1994 until the end of 1997. Work sites and a sample of the employees at each work site were successively chosen by means of a strategical selection process with the support of current statistics and reports on different branches of the Swedish labor market and of working conditions for different occupations.

Based on criteria defined in advance regarding gender, distribution of age, type of work, and socioeconomic position, male and female employees were selected. The whole study group consists of approximately 1/3 respectively working with *'people', 'things'* and *'symbols'* (according to the classification by Kohn & Schooler, 1983). Seventy-five percent of the sample were pair-wise matched by gender, type of work, and socioeconomic position. Statistical methods were used as a support and a test of the sample in relation to the criteria. Variation, rather than representativity, characterizes the study group comprising of 104 women and 104 men, long term as well as temporarily employed, with varying age and educational level at seventy-two work sites in public (36%) and private enterprises (64%) in five counties in Sweden. The sample includes typical work sites as well as work sites where new forms of organization and production were implemented. Drop out rate of work sites and individuals were 30% and 1% respectively. The data collection started with structured interviews with managers at the work sites and personal interviews and a public health questionnaire including items on work for the selected employees. Subsequent data collection lasted about two months for each study person. Both quantitative and qualitative methods such as expert assessments, observations, field measure-ments, interviews, and questionnaires were used.

3.   QUALITATIVE ANALYSIS OF INTERVIEWS WITH EMPLOYEES

In the personal open interviews, the study persons were requested to tell us about their work and the interface between work and private life. The interviews were tape-recorded and transcribed word by word. The analysis started with searching for and identifying recurring themes within each interview and also between interviews.

We found that most of the interviewees talked about how their work had changed and continued to change. Quite often the high unemployment rate was referred to as a cause of negative consequences. What happens in today's work life appears to be so central for the individual that the main thread running through the interviews can be designated as *"struggling for human worth and dignity and a position in a changing work life"*. Both negative and positive aspects came up. According to the results of the qualitative analysis changes are perceived either as threatening or enhancing important personal life values (Härenstam et al 1997). Common changes in work life seem to enhance values which are of an individual nature and threaten values that are more collective and social. The results indicate that organizational changes have great importance – both as health promoters and health hazards and should be an important aspect in studies of work and health. Two typical citations illustrate different perceptions of the consequences of the changes. Both the man and the woman work in organizations with so called lean production systems.

Female supermarket assistant: " We hadn't worked that way before. Then, they turned it all around with this flow scheme .... Partly to save hours. And then it was like this. We shall take care of the product – follow it 'from quay to cash-point' as it's called ... They said there shouldn't be any dead time, but it's there automatically – because it's hard to pick up exactly from where you left off. So, there's all those little stress stages, and even if you try, they're in your hands, whatever you do."

Male industrial worker: "All I did was to pick pumps. I picked them up from a truck and handed them to someone else, who put them down on a pallet. That was my job. In the old days, when you had done your thing, you didn't care if the pallet was fully loaded or not. Now, we do everything from beginning to end. It's like there should be a seamless flow, no demarcation lines between departments. Everyone should be able to work in any department, that's the goal, isn't it?"

4. PROCEDURE, METHODS AND RESULTS OF THE QUANTITATIVE DATA

4.1 The Organizational level

Characteristics of the included seventy-two private and public work sites were assessed by five behavioral scientists in the MOA-research group using interviews with managers and written material about the organizations. The interviews were loosely structured and covered several areas such as:
– Ownership
– Power structure, hierarchical levels
– Control and management systems
– Characteristics of the organization and the production process
– Integration/fragmentation of the work content for the workers
– Use of technology, including IT
– The context regarding market, competition and customers
– Staff size, structure and policy
– Reward systems

- Changes in all aspects above

In all more than sixty variables were assessed and classified according to
the same criteria for all work sites and finally reduced into several indices.
Of all assessed characteristics of changes in the organizations during the last
two years, the most common were: structural changes of the work
organization (in 60 % of the work sites), changes of the production process
and technology (38%), increased demands of competence (56%), decreased
size of staff (28%), increased use of result monitoring (22%), increased use
of soft control systems (14%), increased vertical and horizontal integration
of the work process (15%) and decreased hierarchical levels (15%). More
changes were identified in work sites in the public compared to the private
sector (figure 1).

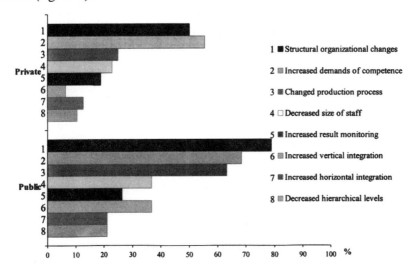

Figure 1 Proportion of work sites (n=72) in the public and private sectors
where the different aspects of changes were identified.

As we wanted to investigate what kind of changes are found in Swedish
work life of today, an empirically based strategy by means of cluster analysis
(Ward's hierarchical method, SPSS procedure) was chosen for the
categorization of the seventy-two work sites. This means that within each
cluster there are some differences between the work sites. However, when all
dimensions are considered together, work sites having most in common are
clustered together. The variables included in the cluster analysis are
theoretically based and consist of all dimensions on changes listed in figure
1 except 'changes of staff size' as 'decreased staff' was not classified as to
differentiate between 'downsizing', 'outsourcing', and 'divisionalization'.

Furthermore, an index of number of aspects that had been changed at each work site was included (range 0-11) as well as three variables regarding "levels"; 'degree of vertical and horizontal integration of work process', 'degree of centralized structure of power', 'degree of competition on the market'. Five different patterns of changes were identified as a result of the cluster analysis. In table 1 the most evident characteristics for each cluster are listed. Furthermore, the five clusters of work sites were compared regarding changes in staff size. Significantly more of the *'lean production'* as well as the *'centralizing'* work sites were classified as having decreased size of staff during the past two years compared to the others.

Table 1. Characteristics of the five different patterns of changes.

Patterns of changes (keywords)	Number of work sites	Most important characteristics
Lean Production	11	Extensive structural changes Increased integration of work process Increased demands of competence Decreased hierarchical levels. Decreased staff size (not included in cluster analysis)
Result Monitoring	10	Increased use of result monitoring Few/small other changes
Market Adjusting	24	High market adjustment and competition No other changes
Centralizing	7	Centralized power structure Increased centralization Extensive structural changes Decreased staff size (not included in cluster analysis)
Stable	20	No extensive changes

In the cluster named *'lean production'*, there are mainly large work sites: a hospital, three schools, a large passenger traffic company, a supermarket, large industrial production plants, and a company working with IT, and computer systems. In the cluster called *'result monitoring',* we found a food process plant, a hotel, hospitals, as well as, transport and cleaning enterprises. What is called "result monitoring" here, the most evident and almost only characteristic of this cluster, had many names when talking to managers and reading the written documents for these work sites. For example; total quality management, bench-marking, economic-administrative routines necessary when introducing buy-and sell models in the public sector. Those who are called *'market adjusting'* are mainly small and medium sized private work sites within service, trade, finance, construction, and transport. Work sites called *'centralizing'* are mainly large within industrial production, juridical and financial work. The *'stable'* are mainly medium sized and large work sites within public administration, schools, child and elderly care, and consulting firms within marketing and IT. Both the private and public sector and work sites with gender mixed, male dominated and female dominated staff, are represented in all clusters.

4.2   The individual level

For the investigation of perceived consequences of the changes for one's own working conditions, a specially designed questionnaire was used. Thirteen questionnaire items covered several aspects such as the individual's own development possibilities, work control, participation, support, team-work, work load, job security, salary in relation to effort, possibilities to adjust work and family interface, gender equality, and co-determination. The respondents were asked to evaluate if their working conditions had been affected as a consequence of changes in their work sites in the aspects described above. The answer alternatives were 'increased', 'decreased', or 'unchanged'. Most of the items were constructed for a previous study of working conditions for professionals in Sweden (Härenstam & Bejerot 1994). The levels of job demands, skill discretion and control according to the job strain model by Karasek and Theorell (1990), as well as the demand/control ratio, were also tested in relation to the patterns of changes and the consequences for working conditions.

The largest changes in working conditions reported in the questionnaires were both negative and positive. The negative, for example, consisted of increased work load, decreased job security, decreased possibilities to adjust work and family interface and decreased salary in relation to effort. Increased possibilities for development and control are examples of positive consequences. Men and women generally reported similar consequences.

4.3   Results of analyses of data on both levels

The employees were grouped by the five "patterns of changes" at the work sites according to the results of the cluster analysis. The study group on the individual level consists of 25 women and 27 men in "lean production" work sites, 26 women and 16 men in "result monitoring", 21 women and 28 men in "market adjusting", 12 women and 12 men in the "centralizing" work site group and finally, 20 women and 21 men in the group of "stable" work sites. Some differences between the five groups of employees regarding the distribution of age, education level, and type of work were found. For example, the proportion of employees with a high educational level was higher in the "centralizing" and "stable" work sites compared to the others. Also, the youngest age group was over represented in the "market adjusting" work sites.

Response frequencies regarding increased work load and job control from employees in the different patterns of changes according to the cluster analysis are shown in figure 2. Almost eighty percent of those working in an organization called *'lean production'* reported increased work load compared to less than forty percent in the cluster called *'centralized'*. Furthermore, of those working in the *'lean production'* work sites just over forty percent reported increased control and just over ten percent among the *'centralized'*. Thus, there are clear differences between the clusters. The question now is if this can be explained by other factors, such as differences in type of work, age, educational level etc. among the study persons within each group of work sites. The standard logistic regression models applied so far might not be the most optimal ones for our data and further analyses by some kind of multi-level method will be performed.

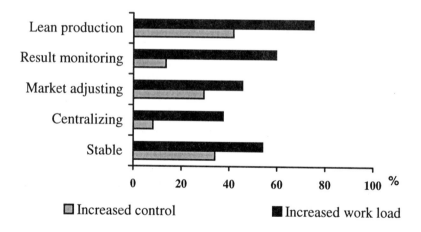

Figure 2. Proportion of employees in the five patterns of changes reporting increased work load and control. (N= 104 women and 104 men).

The strategy for the modeling of the regressions aimed at investigating if patterns of changes contributed independently to explain the variation in the working conditions when other possible explaining factors were adjusted for. The five patterns of changes were included in the analyses as categorical independent variables. Two more work site characteristics were investigated: employer (public, public owned company and private) and proportion of women in the staff (male and female dominated, and gender mixed). Three more individually related characteristics -all with three categories- were also tested: Age, one's own educational level and type of work (working with 'people', 'things' or 'data'). Gender specific analyses were performed as a tendency of interaction effects between gender and patterns of changes were found.

Pattern of changes seemed to have an independent contribution and showed the highest odds ratios in the analyses of increased work load for women, increased development possibilities, decreased job security, and salary in relation to effort for both women and men and increased control in the analyses on men (table 2). However, the confidence intervals were wide as an effect of a rather small sample. In the other aspects of working conditions no significant associations with pattern of changes were found.

Table 2. An overview of the results of analyses of the associations between variables on the organizational level and consequences for the working conditions as the dependent variables (significant odds ratios are marked with *).

Dependent variables	Independent variables							
	Pattern of changes		Employer		Proportion of women in staff		Type of work object	
	Women	Men	Women	Men	Women	Men	Women	Men
Increased work load	*				*			
Increased control		*		*	*		*	
Increased development	*	*		*				
Decreased salary	*		*					*
Decreased job security	*							

Besides pattern of changes, 'employer', 'proportion of women at the work site', and 'type of work' were associated with the consequences for one's own working conditions. The results show that lean production seem to be associated with the most negative consequences for women in three aspects as well as the most positive consequences regarding development possibilities. In the analyses on men, pattern of changes was less important. However, it seems as the centralizing pattern is associated with the most negative consequences for men as they reported the least increase of control compared to the others. The results also indicate that the risk of negative consequences is higher in the public sector than in the private for men, in female dominated work sites and when working with 'people' for women.

The individually related explaining variables did not show any significant associations with perceived consequences except age group in the analyses on men. The middle aged men reported the most positive consequences of the organizational changes.

The five patterns of changes were compared with regard to the dimensions included in the job strain model (Karasek & Theorell 1990) by means of analyses of variance (ANOVA, SPSS procedure). The results showed that the patterns of changes were significantly associated with skill discretion, decision latitude, and the demand/control ratio. The "best" conditions were found in the "stable" work sites and the most deteriorated in "lean production" work sites for women and in the "result monitoring" work sites for men. As perceived consequences of organizational changes might be affected by the level of demands, control, and skill discretion, this was tested by means of logistic regressions. When the levels of demands, control or skill discretion were included as independent continuos variables in the analyses of increased work load, control, and development possibilities respectively, the associations with patterns of changes remained significant or were strengthened. This means e.g. that those reporting a high level of job control more often than others reported increased control possibilities. Even if the direction of the associations cannot be interpreted in this cross-sectional study, it could be hypothesized that organizational changes function as a selection mechanism that reinforce both negative and positive psychosocial working conditions. It might mean that inequity in working conditions increases between groups. For example, employees in the public sector would experience more negative consequences in relation to the private, working with people in relation to working with things, middle aged in relation to the youngest men in the working force and so forth. This hypothesis should be tested in further studies.

5.   CONCLUSIONS

The main conclusions are:
- work sites in the public sector have been exposed to more extensive changes than the private
- knowledge of conditions on the organizational level regarding changes seems to have an impact on how the consequences for the working conditions are perceived by the employees

- both negative and positive consequences for the working conditions are recognized
- patterns of changes seem to be associated mainly with work load, development and control possibilities, job security and salary in relation to effort
- patterns of changes seem to be more important for women's working conditions than for men

Above all, patterns of changes independently contribute in explaining the variance in work load, development and control possibilities. Furthermore, it seems as organizational changes directed at lean production systems have a great impact on the psychosocial working conditions particularly for women.

The results of the present study cannot be generalized to the whole Swedish working population. It is a cross-sectional study and the sample is small and not randomly selected as the aim was to match women and men and cover a wide variety of organizations and types of work. However, the fact that data was collected from different sources and levels, and the combination of qualitative and quantitative analyses, facilitates the interpretations made regarding how organizational changes are perceived by a variety of employees in Swedish work life of today.

On the basis of the results so far we intend to further elaborate methods for assessment and analyses that can be used in large scale studies of working conditions and health and preferably in longitudinal studies. External assessments of working conditions that were collected in the MOA-study are now being analyzed. The dimensions used to assess organizational changes by interviewing managers of the work sites included in the MOA-study were formulated as questionnaire items which were responded by the study persons. These items will be validated by comparing the answers with the information given by the employer at the same work site. The items on consequences of changes used in the MOA-study are included in the latest version of the Stockholm Public Health Questionnaire (1998). These data are now analyzed and related to the information of the psychosocial working conditions from the same individuals four years ago and their health status today. If we gain more knowledge from longitudinal studies, we might be able to draw further conclusions on the importance of organizational changes as early indicators of health hazards and health promoting challenges in work life.

REFERENCES

Aronsson, G., Sjögren, A. 1994. *Samhällsomvandling och arbetsliv. Omvärldsanalys inför 2000-talet* [Social change and working life: A pre-millennial analysis]. Fakta från Arbetsmiljöinstitutet.

Bejerot, E., Söderfeldt, B., Aronsson, G., Härenstam, A., Söderfeldt, M. 1998. Changes in control systems assessed by publicly employed dentists in comparison with other professionals. *Acta Odontologica Scandinavica* 56:30-35.

Czarniawska, B. & Sevón, G., (eds.), 1996. *Translating Organizational Change*. Berlin, New York, de Gruyter.

Fenwick, R. and Tausig, M. 1994. The Macro Economic Context of Job Stress. *Journal of Health and Social Behavior*, 35:266-282.

Härenstam, A., Bejerot, B. 1995. *Styrsystem, effektivitet och arbetsvillkor*. [Management , efficiency and work environment]. In: Westlander et al (eds.) På väg mot det goda arbetet [On the way toward good working conditions], Solna: Arbetslivsinstitutet, pp. 123-147.

Härenstam, A., Wiklund, P., Westberg, H., Ahlberg-Hultén, G. and the MOA-Research Group. 1998. Struggling for Human Dignity and a Position in Work Life. A Qualitative Analysis of Interviews with Swedish Women and Men in a Variety of Work and Life Situations. *First International ICOH Conference on Psychosocial Factors at Work*. August 24-26, 1998. Copenhagen, Denmark. Book of abstracts. The Danish Working Environment Fund.

Johnson, J.V. & Hall, E. M. 1996. Dialectic Between Conceptual and Causal Inquiry in Psychosocial Work-Environment research. *Journal of Occupational Health Psychology* 1:362-374.

Karasek, R. & Theorell, T. 1990. *Healthy Work*, New York, Basic Books

Kohn, M. L. & Schooler, C. 1983. *Work and Personality*: An Inquiry Into the Impact of Social Stratification. Norwood, NJ: Ablex.

Kristensen, T. 1995. The Demand-Control-Support Model: Methodological Challenges for Future Research. *Stress Medicine* 11:17-26.

Le Grand, C., Szulkin, R., Thålin, M. (eds.), 1993. *Sveriges Arbetsplatser - Organisation, personalutveckling, styrning*. [Work places in Sweden – Organization, staff development and management]. Stockholm, SNS Förlag.

Røvik, K A. 1998. *Moderne organisasjoner. Trender i organisasjonstenkningen ved tusenårskiftet* [Modern organizations. Trends in organization research in the millennial shift]. Bergen, Fagbokforlaget.

Sandberg, Å. 1997. *Ledning för alla? Om perspektivbrytningar i företagsledning.* [Management, work and trade unions in change]. In Sandberg Å (ed.). Ledning för alla. SNS Förlag, Stockholm.

Söderfeldt, B., Söderfeldt, M., Jones, K., O'Campo, P., Muntaner, C., Ohlson, C. G. & Warg, L. E. 1997. Does Organization Matter? A Multilevel Analysis of the Demand-Control Model Applied to Human Services. *Social Science and Medicine* 44:527-534.

Notes
[1] There is a vast literature on this matter, see for example, Czarniawska B & Sevón G, eds, 1996; Røvik K A, 1998; Sandberg Å. ed., 1997.
[1] See for example Aronsson G & Sjögren A, 1994, Sandberg Å 1997.
[1] The full name of the study is: Modern work and living conditions for women and men. Development of methods for epidemiological studies. It is an interdisciplinary study performed at the Departments of Occupational Health in Stockholm and Örebro with financial

support from the Swedish Public Health Institute and the National Work Life Institute, grant nr 95-0331. This interdisciplinary research project is aimed at organisational, psychological, ergonomical and chemical/physical conditions and is designed to develop methods for population-based studies tailored to the work life conditions for women and men in Swedish work life of today.

ENCLOSURE IN HUMAN SERVICES: *The Panopticon of Dentistry*

[1]Eva Bejerot & [2]Björn Söderfeldt
[1]*National Institute for Working Life, S-171 84 Solna, Sweden:* [2]*National Institute for Working Life, Solna, and Center for Oral Health Sciences, Lund University, Malmö, Sweden*

Abstract: There are a number of indicators of increased work-environment problems within human services. The trend in the dental profession provides one example of this. The objectives of this study were to find indicators of differences between ideal and reality in dentists work in the Swedish Public Dental Health Service (PDHS). 160 dentists in the PDHS answered an open-ended question. Textual analysis was conducted in the form of line-by-line categorization, searching for sensitizing concepts. Enclosure and visibility emerged as two such concepts. The results were interpreted in Foucauldian terms, in particular through the metaphor of the Panopticon, the perfect prison of the 18th century. The work of Hirschman offers a path to a broader understanding of dentists' work situation. Individuals' reactions to negative circumstances may be to leave their organization (exit), to protest (voice), or to do neither (loyalty). Operationalization of enclosure within Hirschman's framework shows that in the case of dentists only the loyalty option remains available.

1. BACKGROUND

The Public Dental Health Service (PDHS) is an example of a public human service organisation in Sweden. Here, work conditions have been the subject of debate for a very long time. The focus has been on management in dentistry, in the light of the almost constant dissatisfaction among dentists with pay, pace of work and management style. Also, the possibilities of establishing oneself as a private practitioner have been very limited during the last 25 years, due to the construction of the dental insurance system introduced in 1974. Just recently, January 1999, this restriction was removed since it was contradictory to the European Union rules for a free market. Public dentistry will, however, continue, particularly in rural areas where dentists do not establish private practices. Public dentistry is also considered important in strengthening competition in the dental sector, and as a basis for setting prices. About half of the dentists in Sweden work in the PDHS, and a majority of these dentists are women working part-time, while the majority of the male dentists work in private practice.

Health Effects of the New Labour Market, edited by Isaksson *et al.*
Kluwer Academic / Plenum Publishers, New York, 2000.

A dentist in the PDHS will use more than 90 percent of the eight-hour day working directly with patients. All work is registered on the individual level and filed in a computerised control system, usually on a county council level. This control system is based on time studies, with a fee-for-service system, and reporting of work at a 5-minute level (Bejerot & Theorell 1992). The computerised control system makes each individual dentist totally visible. The system enables comparisons to be made between individual performance and choice of treatment and also comparisons between clinics and between private and public dentistry. These comparisons lead to a convergence of the methods of working. The dentists who deviate in regard to income/hour (too low) or treatment time/patient (too long) have their attention drawn to this deviation (in regular meetings with the head of the clinic). The control system may be seen as a way of standardising the dentists' work.

In a questionnaire answered by 4000 academicians, including dentists in the PDHS, changes in managerial control systems and their effects on the work environment of employees were analysed. The results showed that there is a marked difference in how different professional groups are affected by the same changes in managerial control systems. Those who work with things or data (for example engineers and economists) have a more advantageous development compared to those who work with "life" (for example physicians and teachers). Thus, the *content of work* was of significance for which effect managerial changes had on work conditions (Bejerot *et al* submitted).

Also, dentists in the PDHS were found to be a particularly vulnerable group. They reported both extensive changes in the management control system, and also marked deterioration of work conditions (ibid.). The changes in management control systems were divided into two different dimensions of Human Resource Management (HRM) technologies, which were interpreted as mirroring "hard" and "soft" HRM models, i.e. strategies based on "management by objectives" and "management by dialogue". A clear duallity was apparent in changes of managerial control systems in the PDHS.

In an analysis of the properties of "healthy work" among professionals, aspects as intellectually stimulating work, freedom and independence, initiative taking appreciated and harmony between work and personal values were studied. The result showed considerable differences between various types of occupations. In regard to dentists, the difference between ideal and reality differed considerably between dentists in the PDHS and those in private practice. Differences were particularly evident with regard to independence and encouragement in taking initiative (Aronsson *et al* in press). It seems probable that the reason for these lie in factors such as work organisation and leadership style.

To summarise, the working conditions of dentists in PDHS are characterised by a restricted labour market, detailed managerial control systems and a strong element of competition. This can be regarded in the light of the development in New Public Management (NPM), which has often been described as characterised by an increase in decentralisation, monitoring of results, internal pseudo-markets and external contractors. Some countries, such as Great Britain, Australia, New Zealand and Sweden (Hood 1995, Olson *et al* 1998), are considered to have implemented NPM to a large extent. This transformation has also brought about a change in relations between employers and employees, moving from the collective doctrines in the traditional Industrial Relations towards more informal strategies according to Human Resource Management (HRM) (Guest 1987). In HRM the emphasis is on the individual and his or her resources, and also relations and loyalty to the organisation. In the view of its advocates adopting an HRM strategy will lead to harmony, and benefit all organisational "stakeholders", the individual worker as well as the organisation and society. However, we have not found much research on what consequences these models, which were originally constructed for industry, have had on the work conditions in human service organisations.

The objective of this study was to make a further analysis of the differences between ideal and reality in dentists' work in PDHS, with focus on the effects of HRM and with a special eye on enclosure in human services.

2.   THE STUDY

A questionnaire was administered to 757 dentists in Sweden. The response rate was 68 percent. Of respondents, 312 worked in the PDHS. An open question was posed at the end of the questionnaire. *"If you recall the view you had of the dental profession when you were a student, what is different to what you had expected?"* 160 of the 312 dentists gave a reply of some length, more than just a few words. Here, textual analysis was conducted in the form of line-by-line categorisation, searching for sensitising concepts.

The open question was made to catch the discrepancy between ideal and reality. Although the question was not designed to illustrate the impact of management control systems or changes in work conditions, the responses, in the dentists' own words, provide insight into everyday difficulties and thereby facilitate understanding of management and work-related problems.

Various responses to the question were initially sorted under the main headings "Better than expected" and "Worse than expected", with most ending up under the heading "Worse" (table 1). They were then given subheadings in the process of search for sensitising concepts (categories that would "open" the material). Eventually, "effort and rewards", "meaning of work", and "enclosure" became these concepts, which guided the further process of search and interpretation.

Table 1. Categorisation of dentists answers (n=160) to the open question
"If you recall the view you had of the dental profession when you were a student, what is different to what you had expected?"

	Better than expected	*Worse than expected*
Demands		Physical effort
		Mental effort
		Contradictory demands
Material rewards		Status
		Money
Immaterial rewards	Relations with patients	Development possibilities
	Delivery of care	Freedom and discretion

To give some flavour to the results, listen to the "voices" from the PDHS. First, some comments from the area of effort and rewards.

"Much more mental and physical stress. Salaries are low; we used to have almost the same salaries as physicians, there is a big difference now. "The pace of work has increased more and more. After 14 years, I feel totally worn out."

Many comments concerned contradictory demands: professional pride and loyalty to patients on the one hand, and economic necessities on the other. They suggest that management and employees in the PDHS do not share the same view on the priorities and basic aims of their activities. These comments also apply to the area of the meaning of work.

"I had not expected to be hunting for money in the way we do today. I thought we would be able to care for patients, even if their financial situation did not permit any great outlay on dental treatment."

"It is very important to do a good odontologic job. But I feel that I am under pressure from my employers to increase quantity and takings.

One of the dimensions that become apparent from the analysis is control and confinement.

"I had no idea that there would be so much control, via time reports, takings /hour, median treatment times, and so on. It is as if you were fettered to the chair."

"You stand in your booth, work according to every ten- or fifteen-minute booking. I don't think you should work with people in this way.

The comments above concern organisational and physical enclosure, marked by restricted work content and a detailed reporting system. Another form of enclosure described by the dentists is the narrow range of competence and limited opportunities for development.

"I never thought there would be so few chances for development and that the intellectual stimulation would be so small."

"Much higher pace of work and little further education, and small chances of changing your job."

Thus, dentists displayed evidence of enclosure on three dimensions: in time-space, in competence, and on the labour market.

3. DISCUSSION

The management control system of the PDHS can be regarded as a technology that enables enclosure and extensive employee visibility. The results can be interpreted on the basis of two conceptual frameworks. The influential work of Hirschman (Hirschman 1970) offers a path to a broader understanding of dentists' work situation. Individuals' reactions to negative circumstances may be to leave their organisation ("exit"), to protest ("voice"), or to do neither ("loyalty"). Also, modern work organisation can be characterised in Foucauldian terms, in particular through the metaphor of the Panopticon, the perfect prison of the 18th century (Foucault 1977).

So let us summarise some of the causes of the vulnerability of dentists, and put the results into Hirschman's concepts of "exit, voice and loyalty". First, the electronic surveillance system makes the individual dentists' performance visible. The system promotes competition between dentists, and also undermines the voice-option of the "losers" in this competition, i.e. the dentists who work somewhat slowly or hesitate to charge high sums for treatment. They are the individuals who will feel the greatest pressure from these comparisons. But the legitimacy of their protests will be undermined by their low status in the organisation.

Secondly, the enclosure in time-space, competence and the labour market permit few exit-possibilities for dentists in the PDHS. Operationalisation of enclosure within Hirschman's framework shows that – in the case of dentists – only the loyalty option remains available. The contradictory demand between economy and loyalty towards the patient is an area of frustration in dentistry. Doing a good job constitutes the meaning of work and is the main source of job satisfaction. The price of this contradiction is paid by the well being of the dentist's (Bejerot 1998).

In trying to capture the whole picture, the Panopticon-metaphor proved to be helpful. It was Jeremy Bentham (1748-1832), one of the early philosophers of political liberalism who first outlined a model for the perfect prison. He called it a Panopticon (all-seeing), and it could be applied to schools, work places, and hospitals as well as prisons. A Panopticon has a central rotunda, with a peripheral building forming a ring around it. The rotunda has large windows overlooking the ring, which divides into cells. No cell inhabitant can see his neighbour, but anyone at the centre can look into all the cells. The prisoner has no means of avoiding the eye of the authorities, as the rotunda windows have venetian blinds; he never knows when he is the object of surveillance.

Michel Foucault, a historian and philosopher used the Panopticon as a metaphor for the modern disciplinary society. He writes of the creation of a new form of social power, which he regards as having crystallised in the eighteenth century. This, he describes as a "capillary form of power" – a power which "reaches into the very grain of individuals" – a power technology that solves the problem of surveillance.

> "All that is needed, then, is to place a supervisor in a central tower and shut up in each cell a madman, a patient, a condemned man, a worker or a schoolboy. By the effect of back lighting, one can observe from the tower, standing out precisely against the light, the small captive shadows in the cells of the periphery. They are like so many cages, so many small theatres, in which each actor is alone, perfectly individualised and constantly visible. The panoptic mechanism arranges spatial units that make it possible to see constantly and to recognise immediately. (...) Full lighting and the eye of a supervisor capture better than darkness, which ultimately protected. Visibility is a trap" (Foucault 1977 p. 200).

Indeed, the combination of modern management and information technology solves a central problem; namely the conflict between the need for detailed supervision on the one hand and the cost of building up a supervisory system on the other. In this context, a number of work-life researchers have been inspired by the work of Foucault. The way new technology is used by managers to increase control over employees has been called the "Information Panopticon" (Zuboff 1988), or the "Electronic Panopticon" (Sewell & Wilkinson 1992). Formulating the experiences of dentists in a Foucauldian conceptual framework provides clarification of the problems in this sector, as well as in other human services.

The control system in PDHS cannot be regarded as a curiosity, an extreme model that is not relevant to studies of other human services. On the contrary, there is at present a development and implementation of similar models in several areas of care in Sweden, from help for elderly to psychiatry. Modern management is often introduced within a framework of harmony; "What is good for the organisation, is also good for the employee". The key words have a positive tone; dialogue, customer orientation, quality, team-work, feed-back, training and development appraisal. Who could be against that? But in reality the soothing words might very well be "the velvet glove on an iron fist" (Willmott 1993). The study of PDHS was inspired not only by the concepts of Foucault and Hirschmans, but also by those of Critical Management Studies (Legge 1995, Alvesson 1996), particularly in the statistical part of the study (Bejerot *et al* 1999, submitted). Sisson's (1994) work on rhetoric and reality in HRM is an example of how the tension between rhetoric and reality may be described (table 2).

Table 2. Sisson's model of rhetoric and reality in HRM (Source: Sisson 1994 p.15)

Rhetoric	Reality
Customer fist	Market forces supreme
Total Quality Management	Doing more with less
Flexibility	Management can do what is wants
Core and periphery	Reducing the organisation's commitments
New working patterns	Part-time instead of full-time jobs
Empowerment	Making someone else take the risk and responsibility
Training and development	Manipulation
Employability	No employment security
Recognising contribution of the individual	Undermine the trade union and collective bargaining
Team work	Reduces the individuals' discretion

The results of the present study confirm Sisson's analysis.

In human service the employees need to obtain better work conditions, and for this it would be an advantage to strengthen their voice options. More knowledge about the rhetorical element in modern management should have an emancipatory and democratising effect. The current trend in Sweden towards heterogeneity in the public sector provides increased exit possibilities for groups, which were previously limited to a single employer. However, this increasing exit opportunity is not necessarily connected to an improved voice capability.

A long-term strategy for increasing exit could be to broaden the basic training in human service professions, and try to obtain a "double competence". The basic training for dentists, for instance, could be combined with a short training in some alternative field such as business economics, preventive public health, social work or pedagogics. The advantages of a double competence within human service professions would be:

- That individuals could increase their possibilities of development and choice of careers, and be less vulnerable in their professional life.

- A broader content of work and more contacts with the outside world would be positive factors in the development of professions and would also improve the possibilities for voice.
- Education for human service professions would be a more interesting choice for young people.

ACKNOWLEDGEMENT

This study was supported by a grant from the Swedish Work Environment Fund.

REFERENCES

Alvesson, M., and Willmott, H. 1996, Making sense of management. A critical introduction. Sage, London.

Aronsson ,G., Bejerot, E., and Härenstam, A. 1999, Healthy work - ideal and reality among public and private employed academicians in Sweden. Public Personnel Management (in press, June).

Bejerot, E., and Theorell T. 1992, Employer control and the work environment: A study of the Swedish Public Dental Service. International Journal of Health Services 22: 669-88.

Bejerot, E. 1998, Dentistry in Sweden: Healthy work or ruthless efficiency? Arbete och Hälsa 1998:14, Solna: Arbetslivsinstitutet.

Bejerot, E., and Söderfeldt, B., Härenstam, A., Aronsson, G., and Söderfeldt, M. 1999, Perceived control systems, work conditions, and efficiency among Swedish dentists: interaction between two sides of Human Resource Management. Acta Odontologica Scandinavica 57: 46-54.

Bejerot, E., and Söderfeldt, B., Härenstam, A., Aronsson, G., and Söderfeldt, M. (Submitted). Towards healthy work or ruthless efficiency? The effect of managerial changes on professional work with life or things.

Foucault, M. 1977, Discipline and Punish: The Birth of the Prison. Allen Lane, London.

Guest, D. 1987, Human Resource Management and Industrial Relations. Journal of Management Studies 24(5):503-21.

Hirschman, A. 1970, Exit, Voice, and Loyalty. Responses to Decline in Firms, Organizations, and States. Harvard University Press, London.

Hood, C. 1995, The "New Public Management" in the 1980s: Variations on a theme. Accounting, Organizations and Society 20: 93-109.

Legge, K. 1995, Human Resource Management. Rhetorics and Realities. Macmillian Press, London.

Olson, O., Guthrie, J., and Humphrey, C. 1998, Global Warning! Debating International Developments in New Public Financial Management. Cappelen, Oslo.

Sewell, G., and Wilkinson, B. 1992, Someone to watch over me: Surveillance, discipline and the just-in-time labour process. Sociology 26(2): 271-289.

Sisson, K. 1994, Personnel management: paradigms, practice and prospects. In K. Sisson (ed.) Personnel Management (2nd edn). Blackwell, Oxford, pp. 3-50.

Willmott, H. 1993, Strength is ignorance; slavery is freedom: managing culture in modern organizations. Journal of Management Studies 30: 515-52.

Zuboff, S. 1988, In the age of the smart machine. The future of work and power. Basic Books, New York.

THE IMPACT OF ORGANIZATIONAL CHANGES ON THE PSYCHOLOGICAL CONTRACT AND ATTITUDES TOWARDS WORK IN FOUR HEALTH CARE ORGANIZATIONS

René Schalk and Charissa Freese
WORC at Tilburg University, The Netherlands

Abstract: This chapter presents the results of a longitudinal study in four health care organizations in the Netherlands, examining changes in psychological contracts and the consequences of these changes during a process of organizational transformation. The general hypothesis tested in this study is that changes in the organization affect psychological contracts of employees, and that changes in the psychological contract affect workplace attitudes at three points in time (with six-month intervals) during a process of organizational change, employees of the four organizations were asked to fill in a questionnaire, measuring the mutual obligations of employer and employee (the psychological contract), attitudes (affective commitment, intention to turnover), and the employees' perceptions of the organizational changes and the change process. Data for all three measurement points were available for 155 employees. The results show that in these organizations the organizational changes were not of the 'turn key' type, but that there was a continuous process of change affecting employees at different points in time. Furthermore, some employees perceived the changes as positive, while others were not satisfied with the changes and the process of implementing them. The evaluation of change at a certain point in time affects the psychological contract of employees, and consequently influences their attitudes towards work. By means of in-depth interviews with 29 employees the existence of typical patterns of change in the psychological contract (balancing, revision, and abandonment) has been examined. Balancing and revision were the most prominent patterns found, next to some cases of abandonment.

Key words: organizational transformation, psychological contract, workplace attitudes

1.   INTRODUCTION

Organizations today are confronted with many changes in their environment, due to growing competition, globalization of markets, the introduction of new technologies, changing governmental regulations, etcetera. Many organizations try to cope with these developments by changing the

Health Effects of the New Labour Market, edited by Isaksson *et al.*
Kluwer Academic / Plenum Publishers, New York, 2000.

internal organization (which means restructuring, changes in jobs) and/or refiguring the organizational boundaries (by downsizing, merging, acquisitions).

Organizational change as referred to here is the deliberate introduction of novel ways of thinking, acting and operating within an organization as a way of surviving or accomplishing certain organizational goals (Cummings & Worley, 1993).

These organizational changes often have impact on the employment relationship between the employer and the employees, because the changes are likely to affect what the organization will offer to the employees involved and/or what the organization expects from the employees.

Many authors in Work and Organizational Psychology, and more generally across the management sciences, have portrayed the various and deeply rooted changes to working relationships between employers and employees over recent years (Anderson & Schalk, 1998). What has been most important for many people at work has been the simultaneous loss of job security coupled with increasing demands from employers for them to be more flexible, innovative, and willing to contribute to the organization 'above and beyond the letter' of their formal job descriptions or contracts of employment (Anderson & Schalk, 1998). Anderson and Schalk (1998, see Table 1 presents the following overview of past and emergent forms of the 'typical' working relationship.

Table 1. Past and emergent forms of employment relationships

Characteristic	Past form	Emergent form
Focus	Security, continuity, loyalty	Exchange, future employability
Format	Structured, predictable, stable	Unstructured, flexible, open to (re)negotiation
Underlying basis	Tradition, fairness, social justice, socio-economic class	Market forces, saleable abilities and skills, added value
Employer's responsibilities	Continuity, job security, training, career prospects	Equitable (as perceived), reward for added value
Employee's responsibilities	Loyalty, attendance, satisfactory performance, compliance with authority	Entrepreneurship, innovation, enacting changes to improve performance, excellent performance
Contractual relations	Formalized, mostly via trade union or collective representation	Individual's responsibility to barter for their services (internally or externally)
Career management	Organizational responsibility, inspiraling careers planned and facilitated through personnel department input	Individual's responsibility, outspiraling careers by personal reskilling and retraining

There is a general trend in organizations to move from the 'past' form of the employment relationship towards the 'emergent' form. This process, which in fact means creating 'new deals' between employers and employees, is not an easy one.

In the implementation phase of organizational changes, when change can be observed by everyone in the organization, discrepancies are most likely to occur: the match or mismatch between organizational goals and individual goals becomes prominent at this stage (Schalk, Campbell & Freese, 1998). Any mismatch may result in resistance to change, and may have negative effects on employee attitudes and behavior.

Because of the change and the processes during change, the nature of the relationship between the individual employee and the organization will change. Examples are changes in working conditions or working environments, employment contracts, relationships, the primary processes, etc. These changes directly influence individual employees and their perceptions and expectations about the relationship with the organization. Often the mutual obligations between employer and employee are explicitly or implicitly redefined in this process. This means that the psychological contract (e.g. Rousseau, 1995, 1996) will be affected.

The concept of the psychological contract was first introduced by Levinson, Price, Munden, Mandl, and Solley (1962) and Argyris (1960). They used the concept of the psychological contract to exemplify the importance of the mainly implicit and unspoken mutual expectations between an employee and the organization. In their view, some expectations in the contract (e.g. regarding salary) are conscious, but others are not, and are revealed only indirectly. Yet, all expectations are supposed to determine the relationship between organization and employee.

Rousseau (1990) has defined the psychological contract as the employee's perception of the reciprocal obligations existing with their employer. The main focus here is on the employee's perspective, limiting the psychological contract to an intra-individual level. Psychological contracts are operationalized with two sets of terms, i.e. employee-focused and employer-focused obligations, both of which are seen from the employee's perspective (Rousseau, 1990). Obligations are beliefs, held by an employee or employer, that each is bound by promise or debt to action or course of action in relation to the other party (Rousseau, 1990). Employment obligations constitute the psychological contract (Robinson, Kraatz & Rousseau, 1994).

In our view, this concept of the psychological contract is a useful starting point to examine processes occurring within employees during organizational change, and the consequences for employee attitudes and behavior.

From an organizational or managerial point of view, a key issue in planning for action in implementing organizational change is how to motivate commitment to organizational change. This includes at least three major processes: communication, support, and participation (Cummings & Worley, 1993). Effective communication can take away at least part of the feeling of uncertainty and lack of information about the change, reducing speculation and unfounded fears (Covin & Kilmann, 1990; Bronson, 1991; Covin, 1993; Young & Post, 1993). When interest is shown in their feelings and perceptions (support), employees are more likely to be less defensive and more willing to share their concerns and affairs (Covin & Kilmann, 1990; Shaw, Fields, Thacker & Fisher, 1993). By involving organizational members directly in the planning and implementation process of change, one cannot only overcome resistance, but also make high quality changes and take the needs of individual members into account in the changes (Bronson, 1991; Darcy & Kleiner, 1991; Cummings & Worley, 1993).

Organizational changes may influence the psychological contract of employees in a number of ways. First, the bare fact that something will change in the organization may already generate an experienced violation of (employer) obligations. Employees may become insecure about the future and expect that more violations are likely to occur. Secondly, the change itself may have consequences for the work situation of employees when their role and task is affected, and they have to adapt to new circumstances and changed demands. In the third place, the way changes are implemented (communication, participation, and support in the change process) will have consequences for the psychological contract (Schalk, Campbell & Freese, 1998).

Here we will discuss some results of a longitudinal study in four health care organizations in the Netherlands, examining changes in psychological contracts and their consequences during a process of organizational transformation. The general hypothesis tested in this study is that changes in the organization affect the psychological contract, and that changes in the psychological contract affect attitudes towards the organization (commitment and intention to turnover).

We will examine causal models to test these relationships and, more specifically, examine changes in psychological contracts and attitudes over time using the results of in-depth interviews with 29 employees.

The in-depth interviews were focused on assessing typical patterns of changes in the psychological contract as described by Roe and Schalk (see Schalk & Freese, 1997). To explain the dynamic processes of changes in the psychological contract, and particularly the features of sudden change, Roe & Schalk have proposed a model that assumes that the employee observes the actual behavior of the organization and of himself/herself and compares this with the behavior to be expected on the basis of the psychological contract.

Roe & Schalk's model states that the employee compares the actual behavior of the organization and his or her own behavior with what would be expected on the basis of the psychological contract. This means that the employee monitors and evaluates whether deviations from agreed mutual obligations occur within the framework of the existing psychological contract.

In case of minor deviations, the person may take corrective actions without changing the psychological contract. In case of major deviations, the person will take corrective actions as well, but these actions result in a change of the psychological contract. The psychological contract serves as a cognitive model of monitoring behavior, and remains in use as a basis for action, until it becomes clear to the employee (for example, from unexpected events or by a gradual drift which leads to critical boundaries being overstepped) that it has lost its validity, which means that the contract no longer holds in the individual's thinking due to change or revision.

According to Roe & Schalk, there are three typical patterns of variations in organizational and individual behavior. Variations in the perceived behavior of the organization and/or the individual that remain within 'acceptance limits' are without consequences for the psychological contract, and thus for commitment, and subsequent behavior. Positive deviations of the organization's behavior are likely to be followed by positive deviations on the individual side, while negative deviations would have the opposite effect. This pattern is called *balancing*.

If the perceived behavior of the organization and/or the individual reaches or exceeds the 'acceptability levels', changes in consequences are expected. In this case one would expect the person to reconsider the contract as well as to show a decline or improvement in commitment, and subsequent behaviors (Kotter, 1973). Furthermore, clarification about and re-negotiation of the contract is to be expected. This pattern is called *revision*, as it may lead to a revised contract.

If the deviation exceeds the limits of the existing contract, the contract is likely to break down. Accordingly, one may expect commitment to drop strongly, and behavioral responses to be extreme. Open conflicts, emotional expressions, and signs of aggression and depression may occur as well (Rousseau, 1990). Often the employee will quit or be fired by the organization. This condition is called *abandonment*.

2.   METHOD

2.1   Sample

Employees of four health care organizations participated in this study. Three provide home care for persons with (mental or physical) health problems and their families, and one of them also provides counseling and advice related to health issues. One organization hosts elderly people who are not able to care for themselves because of mental or physical problems.

In the Netherlands, because of the need of reducing the costs of health care and changing demands of clients, health care organizations are going through a lot of changes. Two of the organizations were involved in a merging process and a radical restructuring process according to the 'business process redesign' (BPR) approach, one was in a process of restructuring tasks and cutting a middle management layer, and the home for elderly people was in a process of restructuring tasks.

At three points in time (with six-month intervals) employees were asked to fill in a questionnaire. At point one, 869 employees were approached of whom 448 responded (response rate 52%). At point two, the respondents at time one who were still employed with the organization (N = 411) were asked to fill in the same questionnaire. The response rate was 60% (245 employees). Complete questionnaire data for all three measurement points which are used here were available of 155 employees, of whom 99 (64%) were employed with the two merging organizations, 38 (24%) in the other home care organization and 18 (12%) in the elderly care organization.

Mean age of the sample was 39.1 years (S.D. 7.8), mean tenure with the organization 7.8 years (S.D. 5.6), and mean tenure in the current job 6.2 years (S.D. 5.2). Most employees in the sample were female (97%), with 90% having a partner. More than half of the employees (57%) had children, and for 79%, their income was the second income in the family. There were 21 (14%) employees with supervisory tasks, and most of the employees had part-time jobs (mean number of working hours 22.1, S.D. 9.5), in a tenured position (96%). Most employees (83%) were satisfied with their current contract.

Our analyses are based on data of respondents who completed questionnaires on all three measurement points. This group might not be representative for the total sample. We examined whether there were differences between the respondents who filled in all three questionnaires (N = 155) and respondents who filled in one or two questionnaires (N = 293) with respect to age, gender, education, children, main earnership, supervisory job, organization, department, job, type of employment (temporary/permanent and number of working hours), tenure in job and organization.

The sample we use here consists of employees with relatively more supervisory jobs, with a higher education, and more working hours. With respect to the other characteristics, no significant differences were found. Thus, the data used are from a sample which can be considered as representative with respect to such factors as gender, age, tenure, organization, department, and job, but includes more higher educated employees with more supervisory jobs and more working hours.

2.2   Instruments

The questionnaire sent to the employees three times consisted of six parts:

Part 1:   general questions about demographic characteristics (such as age, gender, education) (only at time 1), and (changes in) job, contract, home situation;

Part 2:   global assessment of the relationship with the organization and features of this relationship;

Part 3:   assessment of employer obligations and experienced violations of employer obligations;

Part 4:   assessment of employee obligations;

Part 5:   affective and continuance commitment, intention to turnover;

Part 6:   questions about the changes and experiences in the change process.

In this chapter, results are reported for the following scales and variables:

1.   Assessment of employer obligations (43 items; 7 point scale, 1 = less than expected, 7 = more than expected; for example: "To have work that is varied", "Achieve progress in my field of work", "Possibilities to work together in a pleasant way", "That people receive information needed", "(Financial) additional rewards for performance or special occasions, bonuses and advantages");

2.   Assessment of employee obligations (21 items, 5 point scale, 1 = I feel absolutely not obligated to do this, 5 = I feel very strongly obligated to do this; for example: "Protect the organization's image", "Follow the organizations norms and policies", "Only being absent when you are really ill"); (Items mainly based on Rousseau & Tijoriwala (unpublished) and Manning (1993).

3.   Affective commitment (8 items; 7 point scale, 1 = absolutely do not agree, 7 = I fully agree, for example: "I really care about the fate of this organization"); (items mainly derived from the "Organizational Commitment Scale" (Mowday, Steers & Porter, 1982)).

4.   Intention to turnover (8 items; 7 point scale, 1 = absolutely do not agree, 7 = I fully agree, for example: "I often think about quitting");

5.   Change and change perception (4 questions: "Did something change in the past six months in your work or the organization policy?" (1 = yes, 2 = no), "What kind of changes were there?" (eight categories: job, tasks, (formal) contract, team composition, supervisor, organization (personnel) policy, organizational structure; 1 = yes, 2 = no), "Are you satisfied with the change implementation?" (1 = no, 2 = no change, 3 = yes), "Are you (mentally) preoccupied with the change?" (1 = no, 2 = yes, somewhat, 3 = yes, very much).

2.3   Design

The design of the study was to present the questionnaire before the implementation of changes (time 1: pre-test), approximately one month after change implementation (time 2, first post-test) and seven months after the change implementation at time 3 (second post-test). The questionnaires were sent to employees in the period 1996-1998 with intervals as described, on different points in time related to the situation in the four participating organizations.

To get more information on the process of changes in psychological contracts over time, 29 employees were interviewed. They had volunteered for an interview by indicating their willingness to do so on the questionnaire. All interviews were held after the period in which the questionnaires were distributed. Main aim of the interviews was to assess typical patterns of change in psychological contracts.

3.   RESULTS

Table 2 gives the means, standard deviations and reliabilities of psychological contract and attitudes scales, and Tables 3 and 4 represent the results for 'change and change perception' variables. Table 2 shows that the reliabilities of scales vary between .79 and .95. The mean scores on scales point out that, on the average, employees in our sample have positive feelings about their work situation, characterized by high affective commitment (mean above 5 on a 7-point scale) and low intention to turnover (mean about 2.75 on a 7-point scale).

Table 2. Means, standard deviations and reliabilities of psychological contract and attitudes scales

Scale	T1 Mean	T1 s.d.	T1 alpha	T2 mean	T2 s.d.	T2 alpha	T3 Mean	T3 s.d.	T3 alpha
Employer obligations	4.06	.92	.94	4.07	.84	.94	3.95	.88	.95
Employee obligations	3.87	.35	.80	3.83	.39	.85	3.83	.39	.85
Affective commitment	5.24	.78	.79	5.12	.79	.83	5.00	.81	.84
Intention to turnover	2.69	1.00	.86	2.77	.92	.86	2.81	1.04	.88

The table also shows that the fulfillment of employer obligations is experienced as slightly better than expected (mean about 4 on a 7-point scale). The employees have high scores on employee obligations (mean slightly below 4 on a 5-point scale). It has to be noted that these positive outcomes might be related to the fact that the data are obtained from employees with 'stronger' contracts (more working hours, more supervisory jobs, and higher education). There is a trend in the scores over time on the three measurement points on all scales in the negative direction.

Table 3. Changes during the organizational transformation

Question	Response category	T1	T2	T3
Did something change in the past six months in your work or the organization policy?	yes	78.7%	66.5%	58.1%
What kind of changes were there?	job	7%	5%	7%
	tasks	20%	20%	21%
	contract	29%	18%	20%
	team	44%	16%	9%
	supervisor	46%	31%	17%
	org. policy	9%	4%	7%
	org. structure	47%	31%	25%
	other	8%	12%	10%

Table 3 presents the results on the changes. At each measurement point a majority of the employees indicates that something has changed in their work or organization policy in the last six months. The score is highest at time 1. With respect to the type of changes, most prominent changes at time 1 were related to organizational policy or structure, team composition, and the person of the supervisor. At times 2 and 3, changes in organizational structure and policy were mentioned most often.

Table 4. Change perception

Variable	T1		T2		T3	
	Mean	s.d	Mean	s.d	Mean	s.d
(mental) preoccupation with change	1.75	.76	1.57	.73	1.52	.69
Satisfaction with change implementation	2.12	.81	2.04	.71	1.91	.67

The satisfaction with change implementation decreases over time, as well as the (mental) preoccupation with the change process (see Table 4).

To test the hypothesis that changes in the organization affect psychological contracts, and that changes in the psychological contract affect attitudes towards the organization, three causal models were tested, using a computer program for testing linear structural equation models (AMOS).

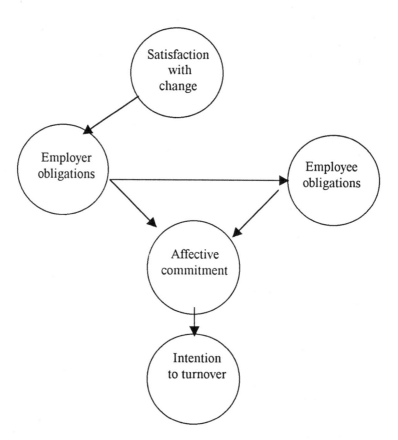

Figure 1. The causal model tested by AMOS at time 1, 2 and 3

The Analysis of MOment Structures (AMOS) program is comparable to programs like LISREL or EQS and provides parameter estimates for causal relationships and 'fit' measures of causal models as a whole with data from non-experimental studies.

Table 5. Estimates of linear structural relationships and model fit measures

Relationship	T1 Est	T1 SE	T1 CR	T2 est	T2 SE	T2 CR	T3 Est	T3 SE	T3 CR
Satisfaction with change → employer obligations	.27	.09	3.02	.34	.09	3.72	.20	.11	1.92
Employer obligations → employee obligations	.11	.03	3.52	.13	.04	3.41	.11	.04	3.23
Employer obligations → affective commitment	.28	.06	4.27	.30	.07	4.41	.39	.06	6.10
Employee obligations → affective commitment	.56	.17	3.36	.61	.14	4.20	.56	.14	3.86
Affective commitment → intention to turnover	-.88	.08	-11.66	-.78	.07	-11.25	-.97	.07	-14.44
Chi square	10.96			11.86			7.06		
Df	5			5			5		
P	.05			.04			.22		
GFI	.97			.97			.98		
AGFI	.92			.91			.95		
RMR	.04			.03			.03		

The models tested implied that change satisfaction at a certain point in time influences the perception of employer obligations, which influences the perception of employee obligations. Both employer and employee obligations (the psychological contract), in turn, were supposed to influence affective commitment to the organization, which was supposed to influence the intention to turnover. Figure 1 represents this model.

Table 5 provides the parameter estimates, standard errors, and the 'critical ratios' of the linear structural relationships in the model. The critical ratios are comparable to t-ratios and should exceed 2 to be considered as significant. Table 5 also lists the 'fit' measures of the tested causal models. A causal model can be considered as having a good fit if the Chi Square is not significant, the Goodness of Fit-Index (GFI) is greater than .95, and the Root Mean Square Residual (RMS) is lower than .05.

Table 5 shows that almost all assumed relationships turn out to be significant. Overall, the models have a good fit with the data, which indicates that the assumed relationships are found in the data.

The interviews provide additional information about the change processes, which occurred over time. Of the 29 employees interviewed, 13 indicated significant changes in how they perceived the obligations of the organization towards them and/or their obligations towards the organization. Sixteen employees reported no fundamental changes in the psychological contract. Three employees showed a typical abandonment pattern, one of them had already quit at the time of the interview, one was actively looking for another job, and one looked for another job and had diminished her number of working hours. In other employees, revision and balancing patterns were found, although the boundary between revision and balancing was not always clear.

4.   DISCUSSION

The design of the study did not work out as it was meant to be. The change process in the participating organizations proved to be a continuous process, which, as the results show, had in fact already started before the first measurement point (see Table 3). Therefore, assessing the effect of 'the' (turnkey) change was not possible.

Table 3 shows that 'the change' implemented in the organizations had very different consequences as experienced by the employees. Some of the employees experienced no change at all, others negative or positive changes. For example, a change of supervisor or team composition may be perceived as positive, whereas changes in organizational structure may be perceived as negative. Also, different patterns of alternating positive, negative, or no change over time appeared.

It is important when looking at change processes in organizations to realize that changes may have either a positive or a negative influence on employees.

The results of tests of the causal models show the effects at a certain point in time of satisfaction with change of the psychological contract, and of the psychological contract on affective commitment, and, after that, intention to turnover. Thus, employees seem to react to changes when they become salient for them, and strongest reactions appear at that time.

The results of the interviews suggest that, in the course of time, at least with employees who stay with the organization (as the employees in our sample), revision or balancing processes in the psychological contract in most cases lead to a (new) balanced psychological contract with the organization, that is, if what the organization does in the change process does not cross the 'tolerance limits' of the contract. When asked in the interviews what would be 'crossing the limit' of their psychological contract with the organization, employees indicated that for them this would be the case if, for example:

- Work would have a negative effect on their health;
- working would no longer be satisfying or stimulating;
- if their feelings were hurt by the organization;
- if the quality of care for clients would be affected too much.

This would lead to abandonment of the contract.

In short, the results of this study lead to the following conclusions:

1. Employees react to changes when they become salient for them;
2. Change may have different effects for employees, and there are differences in the perception of the change as more positive or more negative;
3. Satisfaction with change is most closely related to the psychological contract, which, in turn, is most closely related to affective commitment, and, after that, intention to turnover.
4. Balancing, revision, and abandonment as typical patterns of change in the psychological contract occur.

The results of this study show that using the psychological contract may be a useful way of looking at processes during organizational changes. Therefore it is important, when managing change processes, to include information on the psychological contract before the change process into the strategy to manage the change, and to communicate, support, and provide opportunities for participation to employees to enable them to balance or revise their psychological contract, and to prevent the occurrence of abandonment processes.

These are only the first results of this study. Further analysis will be necessary to further address the effects of different kinds of changes, and the interrelations between the constructs measured, and the link between quantitative and qualitative data.

ACKNOWLEDGEMENTS

We would like to extend our thanks to Charlotte Vermond, the interviewer of the in-depth interviews, and to Dr. Marcel Croon for his statistical advice.

REFERENCES

Anderson, N. & Schalk, R. (1998). The psychological contract in retrospect and prospect. *Journal of Organizational Behavior*, 19 (SI), 637-647.

Argyris, C. (1960). *Understanding organizational behavior*. London: Tavistock Publications.

Bronson, L. (1991). Strategic change management. *Organization Development Journal*, 9, 61-67.

Covin, T.J. (1993). Managing workforce reduction: A survey of employee reactions & implications for management consultants. *Organization Development Journal*, 11, 67-76.

Covin, T.J. & Kilmann, R.H. (1990). Participant perceptions of positive and negative influences on large-scale change. *Group and Organization Studies*, 15, 233-248.

Cummings, T.G. & Worley, C.G. (1993). *Organization development and change*. Minneapolis: West Publishing Company.

Darcy, T. & Kleiner, B.H. (1991). Leadership for change in a turbulent environment. *Leadership and Organization Development Journal*, 12, 12-16.

Levinson, H., Price, C.R., Munden, K.L., Mandl, H.J. & Solley C.M. (1962). *Men, management and mental Health*. Cambridge: Harvard University Press.

Manning, W.E.G. (1993). *The content of the psychological contract between employees and organizations in Great Britain in the early 1990s*. PhD thesis, University of London.

Mowday, R.T., Porter, L.W. & Steers, R.M. (1982). *Employee-Organization linkages: the psychology of commitment, absenteeism, and turnover*. New York: Academic Press.

Robinson, S.L., Kraatz, M.S. & Rousseau, D.M. (1994). Changing obligations and the psychological contract: a longitudinal study. *Academy of Management Journal*, 37, 137-152.

Rousseau, D.M. (1990). New hire perspectives of their own and their employer's obligations: a study of psychological contracts. *Journal of Organizational Behavior*, 11, 389-400.

Rousseau, D.M. (1995). *Psychological contracts in organizations. Understanding written and unwritten agreements*. Thousand Oaks: Sage.

Rousseau, D.M. (1996). Changing the deal while keeping the people. *Academy of Management Executive*, 10, 50-58.

Schalk, R., Campbell, J.W. & Freese, C. (1998). Change and employee behaviour. *Leadership and Organization Development Journal*, 19, 3, 157-163.

Schalk, R. & Freese, C. (1997). New facets of commitment in response to organizational change: research trends and the Dutch experience. In: Cooper, C.L. & Rousseau, D.M. (Eds.). *Trends in Organizational Behavior, Vol. 4*. Chichester: John Wiley, pp. 107-123.

Shaw, J.B., Fields, M.W., Thacker, J.W. & Fisher, C.D. (1993). The availability of personal and external coping resources: Their impact on job stress and employee attitudes during organizational restructuring. *Work and Stress,* 7, 229-246.

Young, M.B. & Post, J.E. (1993). Managing to communicate, communicating to manage: How leading companies communicate with employees. *Organizational Dynamics*, 22, 31-43.

ALTERNATIVE WORK ARRANGEMENTS
Job Stress, Well-being, and Work Attitudes among Employees with Different Employment Contracts

[1]Magnus Sverke, [2]Daniel G. Gallagher, and [1]Johnny Hellgren
[1]*Department of Psychology, Stockholm University, 106 91 Stockholm, SWEDEN*
[2]*Department of Management, James Madison University, Harrisonburg, VA 22807, USA*

Abstract   In recent years there has been increased employer use of alternative forms of employment contracts to supplement more traditional employment arrangements. Using data from Swedish health-care workers (N=711; 86% women), this study compares full-time and part-time permanent employees with contingent workers and sets out to answer the following questions: Do workers on non-traditional work schedules experience more or less (1) job related role stress, (2) involvement in the organization, and (3) well-being? Contingent workers were found to experience more job insecurity and role ambiguity but also lower levels of somatic complaints as compared to core employees. On a general level, contingent workers expressed levels of job involvement and organizational commitment almost comparable to full-time employees while part-time workers held less favorable work attitudes. The results also revealed gender differences among contingent workers –women on temporary contracts expressed substantially more job insecurity and somatic complaints but also felt more involved in their jobs and more committed to the organization than men. Given that there exists a variety of contingent employment arrangements and that the occupational status of these differ, additional research is needed to increase our understanding of the consequences of different forms of alternative work arrangements.

1.   INTRODUCTION

The concept of flexibility has become a key issue in organizational strategies and the use of alternative work arrangements is on the rise. Employers in virtually every industrialized country of the world are moving, in varying degrees, toward increased flexibility in how they staff their organizations (Purcell & Purcell, 1998; Sparrow & Marchington, 1998). Most importantly, there has been an increased interest in employing workers on the basis of short or fixed term contracts rather than on the basis of implicit long-term contracts in order to "gain the fluid capabilities of flexibility and outside knowledge produced by the ready movement of labor in and out of organizations" (Sherer, 1996, p. 115). The most visible example is the growth of the temporary worker industry through which

Health Effects of the New Labour Market, edited by Isaksson *et al.*
Kluwer Academic / Plenum Publishers, New York, 2000.

employers hire workers through an intermediary organization (temporary firm) for a specified period of time. In the aftermath of downsizing, many laid-off workers are replaced by temporary workers to carry out work when needed (Howard, 1995; Purcell & Purcell, 1998), and one estimate suggests that 80 to 90 percent of all organizations make use of non-permanent workers (Brewster & Tregaskis, 1997). In Sweden, the use of non-permanent workers increased from 10 percent in 1989 to 14 percent in 1995 (Statistics Sweden, 1997), largely as a function of the legalization of temporary firms in 1992 (SOU 1997:58). A majority of these temporary employees are women (Isaksson & Bellagh, 1999).

However, despite the growth in alternative work arrangements and despite the tremendous amount of literature on the topic of temporary work, research has typically focused on the extent of temporary work, reasons for the growth, human resource management practices concerning temporary workers, and the effects for the organization (Beard & Edwards, 1995; Pfeffer & Baron, 1988). So far, only limited research attention has been directed at investigating the attitudes and work experiences of temporary workers or in contrast to more "regular", non-temporary workers. We frequently have to rely on anecdotes and unasserted evidence when it comes to how individuals are affected by fixed term employment contracts. One area which might be particularly ripe for empirical inquiry deals with the potential implications of alternative work arrangements for the safety and well-being of individuals and the organizations that employ them (Rousseau & Libuser, 1997).

In this chapter, we will compare temporary and core health care workers with respect to a number of role stress factors, work attitudes, and health indicators. We begin with a discussion of the definition of alternative work arrangements followed by a brief review of its potential implications for the individual before we present the study and our findings.

2.   ALTERNATIVE WORK ARRANGEMENTS DEFINED

There exists a plethora of denominations of alternative work arrangements. The trend toward increased use of workers on temporary, fixed term contracts has been referred to by such terms as externalization (Pfeffer & Baron, 1988), peripheralization (Dale & Bamford, 1988), or flexibilization (Sparrow & Marchington, 1998) of the workforce. Clearly, such terms have implicit connotations concerning the consequences of temporary work. For instance, the term "flexibility" is unclear and "comes with the sort of intellectual and moral 'baggage' that might, in another forum, provide a fertile ground for textual analysis" (Tregaskis, Brewster, Mayne, & Hegewisch, 1998, p. 62). Following McLean Parks, Kidder, and Gallagher (1998), we take the position that the term "contingent work" might be more encompassing and less implicative of a value judgement.

Regardless of the term used to describe this trend, it is clear that the growth of temporary employment contracts is a function of multiple employer objectives, such as lower labor costs, increased temporal flexibility, and reduced responsibilities for management and supervision of employees (Pfeffer & Baron, 1988; Reilly, 1998). The intensified market competition has spurred employers to reduce pay roll costs by employing workers only in periods of high demand (Atkinson, 1984). In an environment characterized by rapid technological change, organizations may lack employees with needed skills, yet are reluctant to make a long term commitment to hiring and training workers in areas where particular skills are needed (Kochan, Smith, Wells, & Rebitzer, 1994). Hence, many companies contract for needed services (e.g., installation or revamping of an office information management system), provided by skilled professionals on a short term or project basis, without expectation of either party of the traditional long term employment arrangement (Matusik & Hill, 1998).

Although still a majority of contingent workers are women and many temporary jobs are in what may be called traditional female occupations (Aronsson & Göransson, 1998), this emerging trend suggests that the face of contingent workers has changed – from the traditional view of temporary workers as secretaries, office workers, and manual day laborers to now include a growing range of professional skill, such as computer information specialists, engineers, legal staff, and nurses (Davis-Blake & Uzzi, 1993). This emerging category of temporary workers has been referred to by some writers as the "elite temporaries" (Diesenhouse, 1993).

The above reasoning calls for the realization of two important points. First of all, despite the increased attention on the growth of alternative or contingent work arrangements, the "traditional", implicit long term worker-employer relationship still remains the prevailing form of employment contract. But contingent employment contracts are growing at a faster rate than traditional contracts in many nations. Second, contingent work is not a unitary concept. Rather, there exists a variety of contractual employment arrangements which could be categorized as contingent (see McLean Parks et al., 1998).

One such contingent employment arrangement concerns temporary-help workers hired through temporary firms (e.g., Adecco, Manpower, Olsten, Randstad). The client organization contracts with the temporary firm to provide workers for a specified period of time, and while work is conducted in the client's facilities the temporary worker is assigned and paid by the temporary firm. A second and often more extensive form of contingent work is the use of in-house and direct-hire workers. Simply stated, the employer may operate its own internal or in-house, employer-based registry or temporary pool, where qualified workers are listed with the organization and called into work when they are needed for short-term work assignments or to fill vacancies. Often they do not have the full range of benefits, but they may get higher hourly pay rates. In-house contingent workers may often view registry work with the employer as a means of getting access to more permanent jobs when they become available. For employers, the use of their own temporary pool cuts costs, but can also be used as a means to screen potential hires.

Other forms of contingent work involve consultants, independent contractors, and subcontracted workers. Consultants provide professional services to organizations on a short-term or project basis. Similar to temporary-help employees, consultants are employed by the supplier organization (i.e., consulting firm) but provide services for the client organization. Unlike temporary firm workers in many countries, the consultant has an ongoing employment relationship with the consulting firm. Independent contractors represent one of the largest and fastest growing sectors of contingent employment arrangements. They provide needed services to an employer on the basis of an individual service contract, normally on a project basis (e.g., free-lance writers, computer programmers, software writers, translators, etc.). Unlike consulting firm employees, independent contractors are predominately self-employed and hence have their own worker-client relationships. The notion of subcontracted workers involves that work is outsourced or transferred to another organization whose employees perform the tasks on or off the premises of the client company (e.g., cafeteria/food services, security work).

Clearly, there exist more types of contingent employment arrangements and, in addition, a large variation within each form. However, the basic point is that contingent work comes in multiple forms and that the nature of employment relationship differs (i.e., worker-employer, worker-employer-client, worker-client). Although all work is to some extent contingent, we maintain that a minimum requirement for work to be classified as contingent is that it is fixed term or limited in duration. Thus, "the contingent workforce consists of any worker that does not have either an implicit or explicit understanding that employment will be continuous or ongoing" (McLean Parks et al., 1998, p. 701).

It is not unusual to see part-time workers counted within the ranks of contingent workers. Even if this contractual arrangement, from a managerial perspective, may be seen as a valuable form of flexibility (Tregaskis et al.,

1998), "Part-time working is not necessarily confined to the contingent workforce" (Purcell & Purcell, 1998, p. 44). Rather, many organizations view part-time employees as part of the core, and part-time jobs are used for operational rather than cost-reducing reasons.

In accordance with a recent review of the literature by Barling and Gallagher (1996), we take the position that part-time work is less a form of contingent employment but an alternative to full-time employment. Similar to contingent work, part-time employment allows employers increased flexibility in meeting uneven work scheduling (especially in service and retail sectors). More similar to full-time work, though, many part-time work arrangements are based on an implicit ongoing employment relationship and a traditional and identifiable employer-employee relationship. Furthermore, as noted by Barling and Gallagher (1996), research over the past twenty years has demonstrated limited attitudinal and behavioral differences between workers employed on full and part-time schedules. Whether contingent workers are more like full-time or part-time core workers is an empirical question, which we will address.

3.   IMPLICATIONS OF CONTINGENT WORK

According to a widely held assumption, contingent workers are not generally considered "part of the corporate family" (Belous, 1989, p. 6). The limited and short-term nature of contingent contracts reduces employer incentives to provide temporary workers with the on-the-job training and socialization necessary for skill development (Kochan et al., 1994). Contingent workers, therefore, are less integrated in the organization and less familiar with work practices than permanent employees.

A typical consequence of this externalized relationship with the organization is that contingent workers may represent a threat to workplace safety. Two recent studies (Kochan et al., 1994; Rousseau & Libuser, 1997) summarize safety-related concerns which have surfaced in the U.S. petrochemical and mining industries. Both Kochan et al. (1994) and Rousseau and Libuser (1997) show that the use of subcontracting firms and casual workers to perform jobs traditionally performed by "regular" company employees can produce a segment of an on-site workforce that is not as stringently trained and supervised in workplace safety practices as are traditional full-time employees. Furthermore, the transitory nature of contingent employment can result in a lack of familiarity with standard operating and safety procedures. A second potential consequence of contingent work is job insecurity and work stress. Contingent workers may be a "threat" also to themselves as a result of a less predictable work situation. Fixed term employment arrangements involve unpredictability not only with respect to the number of work hours and income but also concerning the nature of task assignments and – at least for some forms of contingent work – the employer for whom work will be conducted. Job insecurity refers to a perceived uncertainty concerning the continuation of employment itself or features of the job (Greenhalgh & Rosenblatt, 1984; Hellgren, Sverke, & Isaksson, in press), and such insecurity is almost by definition associated with contingent work (Beard & Edwards, 1995). Some writers even go so far as to define job insecurity as an objective phenomenon inherent in contingent work "without reference to a worker's perceptions, [but] rather considered as an independently determined probability that workers will have the same job in the foreseeable future" (Pearce, 1998, p. 34).

In a similar vein, even if variable working-hours can provide better opportunities to balance home and work responsibilities (e.g., Reilly, 1998), it is plausible that the temporary and short term nature of contingent work may result in increased role stress and impaired well-being. Although this issue has received scant research attention (for exceptions, see Krausz, Brandwein, & Fox, 1995; Martens, Nijhuis, van Boxtel, & Knottnerus, 1999), it could be expected that role related stress and ambiguity (and resulting personal and organizational dysfunctions) may be more pronounced for contingent workers. In general, newcomers to an organization go through a period of role ambiguity and stress, which is often reduced with organizational experience, training, and mentoring. However, temporary workers frequently find themselves in "new" positions and, hence, undergo a continuous process of organizational and job introduction and learning.

Due to the temporary nature of the employment contract, both the organization and co-workers may be less willing to invest time and effort in assisting contingent employees in the understanding of their role responsibilities (Kochan et al., 1994). Further, within many organizations, contingent workers may be assigned the jobs which other organizational members are either unwilling or unable to perform (Rousseau & Libuser, 1997). In one respect, a temporary worker may be assigned stressful or even mundane tasks that more permanent employees within the organization may avoid. In the case of more demanding assignments that permanent workers are unable to perform, contingent workers may find themselves without sufficient co-worker or managerial support for the resolution of role related stresses and ambiguities.

Finally, because temporary workers have "less stake in the contingent job, their co-workers or the organization" (Pearce, 1998, p. 36), they are generally expected to express less favorable job attitudes and less commitment to the organization. However, in contrast to this, research has generally found that there is no attitudinal difference between contingent workers and their fellow-workers employed on permanent contracts (Krausz et al., 1995; Pearce, 1993).

It is also possible that the implications of contingent work may differ between men and women. In general, gender differences appear to be consequential for undertanding organizations (Pfeffer, 1983). Not only are there large gender differences in employment contracts, but women seem to express more negative reactions to contingent work as compared to men (Aronsson & Göransson, 1997, 1998).

4. RESEARCH OBJECTIVES

The purpose of this study was to conduct an exploratory investigation to address the types of issues related to individual differences which might exist between core employees and contingent workers with regard to how they perceive their role characteristics (job insecurity, role ambiguity, role conflict, and role overload), work attitudes (job involvement and organizational commitment), and self reported measures of individual health (mental distress and somatic complaints).

The study also differentiates between regular employees on the basis of full-time and part-time employment status. Such a distinction provides the opportunity to determine the extent to which employment and health related attitudes and experiences differ by both the permanency of employment relationship (temporary/non-temporary) and the degree of hourly attachment to a particular job (full-time/part-time). Through this approach we will also have the opportunity to determine the extent to which the employment related experiences of contingent workers are more similar to full-time or part-time employees.

In addition, the study also tests for gender differences. Through this, we hope to shed some light on how the consequences of contingent work may differ between men and women.

5.   RESEARCH DESIGN

5.1   Setting and Sample

The sample for this study was made up of the total workforce of an urban Swedish emergency hospital undergoing organizational change (e.g., restructuring, outsourcing, and minor layoffs). Since the late 1980s, the Swedish health care sector has been characterized by radical change in order to cut costs and improve competitiveness. Various reforms regarding political government of the health care industry and internal management of hospitals have been implemented (SOU 1993:38). These changes have been motivated by political considerations as well as by economic decline and budgetary restrictions in the public sector (Öhrming & Sverke, 1996). Creation of quasi-markets, furtherance of competition between producers of health care, and introduction of an increased freedom of choice for patients and their relatives have served as important ingredients in the changed conditions for the health care industry (Jonsson, 1993). In this respect, a distinction has been made between purchasers (politicians) and providers (e.g., hospitals) of care. For the large hospitals these changes have, despite the declining financial situation, involved increased flexibility regarding the organization of the health care provided (Spri, 1994).

We used mail questionnaires to assess the study variables. Questionnaires were distributed to all 1,185 core employees and contingent workers at the hospital. Altogether, 762 participants returned their questionnaires in the self-addressed envelopes that were provided, for a response rate of 64 percent. The study is based on 711 individuals who reported their employment status. Of these, 358 were employed on permanent full-time contracts, 230 were permanent part-time employees, and 123 were contingent workers (of which 35 were in-house temporaries contracted on an hourly basis, 77 were direct-hire workers with a limited contract, and 11 had other forms of contingent employment arrangements).

Table 1 presents the characteristics of these three employment categories. As can be seen from the table, contingent workers were younger and had shorter experience of their occupation and organization as compared to full-time and part-time employees. Females were over-represented among the part-time employees. In contrast to those employed on full-time contracts, on average part-time employees worked to an extent corresponding to 71 percent of full-time and contingent workers 89 percent of full-time. In terms of occupational dispersion, the contingent worker category contained a comparatively large proportion of physicians. Nurses were over-represented among part-timers while administrative and support personnel had an above average representation among workers employed on a full-time contract.

Table 1. Sample description

| Variable | Employment contract | | | | df | χ_2/F |
	Full-time	Part-time	Contingent	Total		
Age	46.19	44.43	36.35	43.92	2,708	46.36***
Gender (female), %	84.08	93.48	81.30	86.64	2	15.83***
Occupational tenure	18.14	17.57	9.12	16.46	2,688	44.77***
Organizational tenure	15.45	14.95	6.39	13.91	2,671	45.33***
Work hours, % of full-time	100.00	70.52	88.87	88.52	2,683	503.58***
Occupational group					4	32.25***
Physician, %	12.72	1.35	16.53	9.68		
Nurse, %	63.91	79.37	66.94	69.50		
Administration/support, %	23.37	19.28	16.53	20.82		

*** $p < .001$

5.2   Measures

We compared the three employment categories with respect to a number of role stressors, health indicators, and work attitudes. Unless stated otherwise, responses on the study variables were obtained on a 5-point Likert scale ranging from 1 (strongly disagree) to 5 (strongly agree). Variable indices were constructed using mean values of the items comprised by the respective measures.

5.2.1   Role stressors

Job insecurity was measured using a scale designed to reflect an overall concern about the future existence of one's present job (Ashford, Lee, & Bobko, 1989). Rather than asking respondents how unlikely or likely they believe it is that they will lose their jobs, we redrafted the ten items into statements (e.g., "It is likely that I may be laid off permanently"). The scale demonstrated satisfactory internal consistency (α = .80). *Role ambiguity* was assessed using a combination of items from Caplan (1971) and Rizzo, House, and Lirtzman (1970). The index contained four items (e.g., "I know exactly what is expected of me") with a reliability estimate of .75. *Role conflict* was measured using a slightly modified version of the Rizzo et al. (1970) scale. The five items (e.g., "I do things that are apt to be accepted by one person and not accepted by others") evidenced satisfactory reliability (α = .75). *Role overload* was assessed with three items (e.g., "It fairly often happens that I have to work under a heavy time pressure") developed by

Beehr, Walsh, and Taber (1976). The scale demonstrated adequate reliability ($\alpha = .80$).

5.2.2   Work attitudes

Job involvement was assessed with a six-item short-form version of the Kanungo (1982) scale (e.g., "The most important things that happen to me involve my present job"). The coefficient alpha reliability was .82. *Organizational commitment* was measured using a short-form four-item version of Allen and Meyer's (1990) affective commitment scale (e.g., "This organization has a great deal of personal meaning to me") with a reliability estimate of .65.

5.2.3   Health indicators

Mental distress was assessed with the General Health Questionnaire (GHQ; Goldberg, 1979), which is a screening test designed for detecting non-psychiatric disorders. We used the 12-indicator version (GHQ-12) which has been shown to evidence adequate psychometric consistency and uni-dimensionality in studies of employment-related and occupational problems (Banks, Clegg, Jackson, Kemp, Stafford, & Wall, 1980). Responses to the questions (e.g., "Have you recently lost much sleep over worry?") are given on a four-point scale ranging from 0 (never) to 3 (always). The coefficient alpha reliability was .83. We measured *somatic complaints* using a ten-item index in which the respondents indicated how frequently (1=never; 5=always) they had suffered from various symptoms (e.g., muscular tension, headache, stomach problems) in the past 12 months. This symptom checklist, which was developed by Andersson (1986) and slightly modified by Isaksson and Johansson (1997), evidenced satisfactory internal consistency ($\alpha = .79$).

6.   FINDINGS

Let us begin by examining the univariate and bivariate statistics. These results are presented in Table 2.

The overall mean values for job insecurity, role ambiguity, and role conflict were relatively low (around 2 on the 1-5 scale) while the average level of role overload was 3.56. Mean levels of job involvement and organizational commitment were below the scale midpoint (2.44 and 2.67, respectively). The average levels of well-being were on the low to medium side with 1.74 on the 0-3 GHQ scale and 2.14 on the five-point somatic complaints measure.

Our model is based on the assumption of correlated dependent variables. As can be seen from Table 2, all role stressors were significantly and positively interrelated. There was also a strong positive association between the two work related attitudes as well as between the two health indicators. In addition, the general trend of these bivariate relationships suggests that high levels of role stress are associated with lower levels of work attitudes and, in turn, with impaired well-being. There were a few exceptions to this trend – job involvement was unrelated to most role stressors and both health indicators, and organizational commitment was unrelated to job insecurity and role overload. Table 2 also shows that employees employed on a part-time contract evidenced lower levels of job insecurity and job involvement as compared to other workers; contingent work, on the other hand, was associated with higher levels of job insecurity and role ambiguity as well as lower levels of somatic complaints.

Our next step involved comparing the three forms of employment contract with respect to mean levels in role stressors, work attitudes, and health indicators. We also tested for gender differences even if the number of men was relatively small and these results therefore must be interpreted with caution. Given the demographic differences between worker categories, we employed multivariate analysis of covariance (MANCOVA) procedures with age and occupational tenure as covariates. (The results reported below refer to a strict 3 x 2 model without interaction effects because adding the employment contract by gender interaction did not generate a significant multivariate effect, $F[16,1298] = 0.12$, $p > .05$). Mean values for men and women with different employment contracts are reported in Table 3.

Table 3. Mean values in role stressors, work attitudes, and health indicators for female and male workers with full-time, part-time, and contingent employment contracts

| | Employment contract | | | | | | Gender effect | | Contract effect | |
| | Full-time | | Part-time | | Contingent | | Univariate | Stepdown | Univariate | Stepdown |
	Female	Male	Female	Male	Female	Male	F	F	F	F
Role stressors										
Job insecurity	2.07	1.98	2.01	1.92	2.44	2.09	2.99	2.99	7.60***	7.60***
Role ambiguity	1.81	2.09	1.82	1.83	2.01	2.01	6.09*	6.11*	3.76*	3.60*
Role conflict	2.37	2.45	2.32	2.19	2.24	2.75	1.32	1.74	0.72	2.93
Role overload	3.66	3.39	3.50	3.36	3.50	3.50	0.02	0.04	1.47	0.60
Work attitudes										
Job involvement	2.55	2.61	2.26	2.35	2.54	2.21	0.07	0.26	8.41***	8.52***
Organizational commitment	2.70	2.71	2.60	2.61	2.73	2.39	0.01	0.00	3.34*	3.94*
Health indicators										
Mental distress	1.75	1.73	1.73	1.63	1.78	1.58	1.19	1.01	0.95	0.51
Somatic complaints	2.16	2.00	2.22	1.97	2.10	1.59	11.80***	14.79***	3.03*	4.89**

* $p < .05$ ** $p < .01$ *** $p < .001$

Degrees of freedom for univariate F-tests: Gender (1,658); Employment contract (2,658)

6.1 Employment contract differences

There was a significant multivariate effect of employment status ($F[16,1302] = 4.11$, $p < .001$), thus indicating that there were overall differences in study variables between full-time, part-time, and contingent workers.

To examine this multivariate difference in more detail, we used univariate follow-up tests. In terms of role stressors, the follow-up univariate tests showed that workers on full-time, part-time, and coningent employment contracts differed only with respect to job insecurity ($F[2,658] = 7.60$, $p < .001$) and role ambiguity ($F[2,658] = 3.76$, $p < .05$). Hardly surprising, the contrast tests revealed that contingent workers experienced higher job insecurity than both full-time ($t = 3.23$, $p < .001$) and part-time employees ($t = 3.86$, $p < .001$). Contingent workers also reported more role-related ambiguity than full-time ($t = 2.12$, $p < .05$) and part-time employees ($t = 2.74$, $p < .01$).

There were significant univariate differences between employment contracts also in job involvement ($F[2,658] = 8.41$, $p < .001$) and organizational commitment ($F[2,658] = 3.34$, $p < .05$). The contrast tests indicated that contingent workers, on a general level, expressed significantly higher levels of job involvement as compared to part-time employees ($t = 3.15$, $p < .001$). They also expressed less commitment to the organization as compared to both full-time ($t = 2.15$, $p < .05$) and part-time employees ($t = 2.56$, $p < .05$). With respect to the health indicators, there was a significant univariate difference between groups only for somatic complaints ($F[2,658] = 3.03$, $p < .05$). This difference could be attributed to contingent workers reporting fewer somatic complaints as compared to both full-time ($t = 2.14$, $p < .05$) and part-time employees ($t = 2.44$, $p < .05$).

Given that our model is based on the assumption of a role stress – work attitudes – well-being relationship, and given the observed bivariate relationships between variables, we also employed the Roy-Bargman stepdown procedure which accounts for related dependent variables. In this procedure, once a variable has been tested for group differences it is transferred over to the covariates, thereby allowing it to be related to the next variable to be tested. Variables were entered in the order they are listed in Table 3. The significant effects remained for job insecurity ($F[2,658] = 7.60$, $p < .001$), role ambiguity ($F[2,657] = 3.60$, $p < .05$), job involvement ($F[2,654] = 8.52$, $p < .001$), organizational commitment ($F[2,653] = 3.94$, $p < .05$), and somatic complaints ($F[2,650] = 4.89$, $p < .01$). None of the previously non-significant variables reached significance.

Table 2. Variable intercorrelations, means, standard deviations, and reliabilities

Variable	1	2	3	4	5	6	7	8	9	10	11	12	13	M	SD	alpha
1 Age	1.00													44.06	10.42	–
2 Gender (female)	.11	1.00												–	–	–
3 Occupational tenure	.69	.13	1.00											16.5	9.69	–
4 Job insecurity	-.09	.05	-.05	1.00										2.09	.77	.80
5 Role ambiguity	.11	-.07	-.09	.13	1.00									1.87	.76	.75
6 Role conflict	-.07	-.06	-.06	.28	.38	1.00								2.35	.87	.75
7 Role overload	-.05	.06	-.02	.09	.13	.41	1.00							3.56	1.02	.80
8 Job involvement	.19	-.01	.09	.03	-.11	-.00	.02	1.00						2.44	.83	.82
9 Organizational commitment	.27	.02	.14	-.03	-.24	-.14	-.05	.69	1.00					2.67	.88	.79
10 Mental distress	.00	.06	.04	.25	.32	.35	.31	.01	-.09	1.00				1.74	.38	.83
11 Somatic complaints	-.02	.14	.00	.20	.19	.34	.31	-.00	-.11	.56	1.00			2.14	.68	.79
12 Part-time work	.03	.14	.08	-.08	-.05	-.03	-.05	-.15	-.05	-.02	-.07	1.00		–	–	.47
13 Contingent work	-.32	-.07	-.33	.16	.08	-.00	-.03	.01	.01	.00	-.09	-.30	1.00	–	–	.36

For correlations $> .08$, $p < 0.05$. – not applicable. Scale range: variables 4-9 and 11 (1-5); variable 10 (0-3).

6.2 Gender differences

There was a significant multivariate effect also for gender ($F[8,651] = 3.40$, $p < .001$). However, significant univariate effects were obtained only with respect to role ambiguity ($F[2,658] = 6.09$, $p < .05$) and somatic complaints ($F[1,658] = 11.80$, $p < .001$). When the stepdown procedure was employed to account for correlations between the dependent variables, the effects remained significant for both role ambiguity ($F[1,657] = 6.11$, $p < .05$) and somatic complaints ($F[1,650] = 14.79$, $p < .001$), and no other variable reached significance.

The contrast test indicated that men (on full-time contracts) reported significantly higher role ambiguity than women ($t = 2.47$, $p < .05$) while women, in general, reported more somatic complaints than men. This latter gender difference was especially prevalent among contingent workers. Visual inspection of Table 3 also indicates that, among those employed on contingent work schedules, women also tend to experience more job insecurity, less role conflict, more job involvement, and more organizational commitment than their male counterparts, but these results should be interpreted with caution given the small number of men with temporary jobs in the sample.

7. DISCUSSION

We opened this chapter by noting that contingent work is becoming increasingly frequent in most industrialized countries and emphasized the importance of learning more about if and how contingent workers differ from "core" employees. From the perspective of the health care organization examined in this study, the general absence of significant differences is good news. The three forms of employment contract differed only in the levels of job insecurity, role ambiguity, job involvement, organizational commitment, and somatic complaints.

Most interestingly, the primary difference was not so much between contingent and core workers but rather between part-time employees, on one hand, and full-time employees and contingent workers, on the other.

7.1 Are Contingent Workers Similar to Anyone Else?

One of the few differences we found concerned job insecurity, and this difference could be attributed to contingent workers reporting higher levels of insecurity as compared to the permanent full-time and part-time employees. This difference is hardly surprising given that contingent work, almost by definition, involves such insecurity (Beard & Edwards, 1995). In contrast to research suggesting job insecurity to result in inflated stress and impaired work attitudes and well-being (Ashford et al., 1989; Hartley, Jacobson, Klandermans, & van Vuuren, 1991), however, an intriguing finding of the present study is that the comparatively high level of job insecurity among contingent workers did not also manifest itself in other factors.

Although research has typically considered contingent workers – as a function of low opportunities for on-the-job training and socialization – to experience their work situation as stressful and conflicting (e.g., Kochan et al., 1994; Rousseau & Libuser, 1997), contingent workers reported only slightly more role ambiguity than core workers, and we did not find differences in role conflict or role overload between workers with different employment contracts. However, our results are in accordance with the study of Krausz et al. (1995) which found that temporary-help employees did not differ from permanent employees with respect to inter-role and intra-role conflict.

There are at least two potential explanations for this partial lack of differences. From the individual's perspective, it could well be that the possibility to balance work with other factors, such as family responsibilities, outweighs pressures and demands at work (Howard, 1995; Reilly, 1998). From an organizational perspective, it is possible that the demands on core employees increase with the presence of temporary workers (McLean Parks & Kidder, 1994; Rousseau & Libuser, 1997). For instance, Pearce (1993) found that organizations using contingent workers may actually shift greater responsibility for critical tasks to permanent workers. It is therefore possible that the role responsibilities of full-time and part-time permanent employees may be shifting and, hence, more ambiguous when they work together with contingent employees, and that such shifts counterbalance potentially high levels of role stress in the contingent workforce.

We did find significant differences between the three forms of employment contract in terms of work related attitudes, but here the primary distinction was between part-time employees, who reported lower levels of job involvement and organizational commitment, and full-time employees and contingent workers, who expressed more favorable attitudes to the job and the organization. While it could be argued that contingent workers in general will not hold as favorable work attitudes as core employees because they are less integrated in the organization (e.g., Beard & Edwards, 1995), also other studies have found that they do not differ from permanent employees. For instance, Krausz et al. (1995) reported similar levels of work involvement among permanent and temporary-help employees, and Kidder (1996) found no differences in normative commitment between full-time and temporary nurses.

It is possible that our finding of more positive work attitudes among full-time and contingent workers may in part reflect hours on the job. On average, contingent employees worked to an extent corresponding to 88.87 percent of full-time as compared to 70.52 percent for part-time employees. Another potential explanation concern the occupation status of the groups. Full-timers and contingent workers tended to contain above average proportions of physicians and administrative and support staff while part-timers primarily worked in nursing occupations.

There was also an overall difference between the three forms of employment contract with respect to somatic health complaints. In contrast to previous research which has found that employees with a fixed contract express more somatic complaints and more mental distress as compared to employees with non-flexible working conditions (Martens et al., 1999), however, we did not find contingent workers to differ from full-time employees with respect to physical and mental health problems. Rather, part-time employees reported more somatic complaints than their fellow-workers.

While it is possible that this result stems from part-time work generating health problems, it is equally plausible that this result is a function of attributes of part-time work such that, for instance, some people prefer part-time work because of health problems (Barling & Gallagher, 1996). Research also suggests the importance of a match between preferred and actual work hours (Armstrong-Stassen, Horsburgh, & Cameron, 1994). A recent study, also conducted on hospital employees (Krausz, Sagie, & Bidermann, in press), found that part-time nurses who were satisfied with, and felt in control over, their work hours were better off and reported less burnout as compared to those who wanted shorter hours than they currently were working. In analogy, it could be that the contingent workers in the present study took temporary work because it gives them more control over their schedules – when and how much they work – but obviously such an assertion requires empirical examination.

7.2   The Role of Gender

Our results also revealed some interesting gender differences. In general, regardless of employment contract, men reported slightly more role ambiguity and women expressed more somatic complaints. This latter difference was especially prevalent among contingent workers. In addition, our results indicate that women on temporary employment contracts tend to experience more job insecurity and role conflict than their male counterparts, but also higher levels of job involvement and organizational commitment.

Clearly, these results must be interpreted with caution given the small number of men in the sample. It is also possible that the gender differences in part reflect differences in age and occupational status between workers with differing employment contracts. Still, however, the results are in congruence with previous research. For instance, research suggests that depression is more widespread among women (Eaton & Kessler, 1981) and a meta-analysis by Haring, Stock, and Okun (1984) found men to be slightly happier. It appears that "women experience, on average, both positive and negative emotions more strongly and frequently than men" (Diener, Suh, Lucas, & Smith, 1999, p. 292).

Our data suggest that gender differences in alternative work arrangements require more research. Indeed, both our findings and the cautions we listed suggest the need for further investigation. For instance, do men and women on part-time and temporary jobs differ systematically with respect to factors such as age, education, and occupational status? Do they differ in their reasons for working part-time and on contingent contracts? Are there systematic differences between men and women for different forms of contingent work? If so, what are the consequences for job stress, work related attitudes, and subjective well-being?

8.   CONCLUSIONS

In summary, the results of the present study imply that contingent workers are similar to anyone else, suggesting that they are as well integrated into their jobs and the organization as core, full-time employees. There are a number of plausible explanations for this general finding. First of all, the contingent workers we studied typically work on long-term fixed contracts. Their average tenure with the organization was six years which suggests that they may, in fact, hold their temporary job status longer than permanent workers in other industries. Related to this, the contingent workers in the sample are made up primarily by what we would call in-house temporaries and direct-hire temporaries. This would explain why they have a long working history with a single employer, a fact which makes them much different from other types of contingent workers such as independent contractors and temporary firm workers. Hence, the organization also has a greater incentive to integrate and support these workers within the organization (cf. McLean Parks et al, 1998). As noted by Sparrow (1998), flexibility of contract has to be accompanied by various other types of flexibility in order to reach managerial goals, and such a strategy could be a partial explanation to the findings.

Second, it is entirely possible that our results may be affected by the "professional" nature of the sample. For instance, Leinberger and Tucker (1991) argued that skilled workers in knowledge-based organizations are advantaged and not easily substituted. As health care professionals, both the regular (full-time and part-time) and temporary employees may be more directed and accustomed to role characteristics associated with the profession rather than a particular organization (Pozner & Randolph, 1980). Along similar lines, the nature of the health care professional work may be more easily transferred from one organization to another. Hence, the stress associated with changing employers may be less problematic for contingent workers in highly professional jobs. Clearly, however, this argument calls for an extension of the research to occupations which may be less professionally oriented to examine if there is likely to be a greater difference between core employees and contingent workers in terms of role stressors, work attitudes, and health indicators.

We also see a need to extend the present research to determine if the nature of the temporary contract makes a difference. Although implicit or explicit assumptions concerning differences based on the degree of integration into the organization have characterized the literature (e.g., Beard & Edwards, 1995; McLean Parks & Kidder, 1994), such comparisons are facilitated by the conceptualization and categorization of contingent work arrangements recently provided by McLean Parks et al. (1998). Of particular interest to health-care work might be the contrast of workers from employer-operated in-house pools (as in the present study) as compared with contingent workers hired via third-party temporary-help firms.

Along lines similar to research done by Krausz et al. (1995) and Pearce (1998), it would also be helpful to confirm the extent to which the work attitudes and well-being of contingent workers vary by the voluntary vs. involuntary choice of temporary work. Alternatively stated, similar to comparisons between part-time and full time-work (Armstrong-Stassen et al., 1994; Barling & Gallagher, 1996), are workers who voluntary choose temporary employment arrangements more positively receptive of their roles compared to workers who are employed as temporaries due to the lake of a suitable permanent alternative? The growing body of research which suggests that the voluntary choice of alternative employment arrangements might be more important than employment status *per se* clearly warrants further examination.

Finally, workers' tolerance for role stress as well as the levels of organizational attachment and job involvement may be a function of their motivations for undertaking temporary work. In particular, a worker who sees temporary employment as a means of permanent entry to an organization may have a higher level of job involvement and organizational commitment than a worker who is satisfied with the prospect of moving from one temporary assignment to another (Beard & Edwards, 1995; McLean Parks et al., 1998). Along similar lines, job related ambiguity and conflict may produce a more problematic employment situation for the worker who is seeking a "temp to perm" career compared with the contingent worker who may be indifferent to a long term assignment with a particular employer, and such differences would be manifested also in their work attitudes and well-being.

In conclusion, the results of the present study suggest that contingent work, although characterized by insecurity concerning future employment, may not have consequences that differ dramatically from traditional full-time work. Along with the enduring trend of organizational restructuring, downsizing, and flexibilization, alternative work arrangements are likely to continue to grow and affect the daily lives of rapidly increasing numbers of workers. While our study contributes to the understanding of the consequences of contingent work for the individual, we acknowledge the need for additional research investigating different forms of contingent work in more detail.

ACKNOWLEDGEMENTS

The research reported here was supported by a grant from the Swedish Council for Work Life Research.

REFERENCES

Allen, N. J., and Meyer, J. P., 1990, The measurement and antecedents of affective, continuance and normative commitment to the organization. *Journal of Occupational Psychology, 63*, 1-18.

Andersson, K., 1986, Utveckling och prövning av ett frågeformulärsystem rörande arbetsmiljö och hälsotillstånd. Rapport 2: 1986, Yrkesmedicnska kliniken, Örebro.

Armstrong-Stassen, M., Horsburgh, M.E., and Cameron, S.J., 1994, The reactions of full-time and part-time nurses to restructuring in the Canadian health care system. In *Academy of Management Best Paper Proceedings 1994* (D.P. Moore, ed.), Dallas, Texas, 14-17 August.

Aronsson, G., and Göransson, S., 1997, Fast anställning men inte det önskade jobbet [Permanent employment but not the preferred job]. *Arbetsmarknad & Arbetsliv, 3*, 193-205.

Aronsson, G., and Göransson, S., 1998, Tillfälligt anställda och arbetsmiljödialogen: En empirisk studie [Contingent workers and the work-environment dialogue: An empirical study]. *Arbete och Hälsa*, 1998:3.

Ashford, S., Lee, C., and Bobko, P., 1989, Content, causes and consequences of job insecurity: A theory-based measure and substantive test. *Academy of Management Journal, 32*, 803-829.

Atkinson, J., 1984, Manpower strategies for flexible organizations. *Personnel Management*, August, 28-31.

Banks, H.M., Clegg, W.C., Jackson, R.P., Kemp, N.J., Stafford, M.E., and Wall, D.T., 1980, The use of the general health questionnaire as an indicator of mental health in occupational studies. *Journal of Occupational Psychology*, 53, 187-194.

Barling, J., and Gallagher, D.G., 1996, Part-time employment. In *International review of industrial and organizational psychology*, vol. 11 (C. L. Cooper and I. T. Robertson, eds.), Wiley, Chichester, UK.

Beard, K.M., and Edwards, J.R., 1995, Employees at risk: Contingent work and the experience of contingent workers. In *Trends in organizational behavior*, vol. 2 (C.L. Cooper and D.M. Rousseau, eds.), Wiley, Chichester, UK.

Beehr, T.A., Walsh, J.T., and Taber, T.D., 1976, Relationship of stress to individually and organizationally valued states: Higher order needs as a moderator. *Journal of Applied Psychology, 61*, 41-47.

Belous, R.S., 1989, *The contingent economy: The growth of the temporary, part-time, and sub-contracted workforce*, National Planning Associates, Washington, DC.

Brewster, C., and Tregaskis, O., 1997, The non-permanent workforce. *Flexible Working*, 2, 6-8.

Caplan, R.D., 1971, Organizational stress and individual strain: A social-psychological study of risk factors in coronary heart diseases among administrators, engineers, and scientists. Institute for Social Research, University of Michigan, University Microfilms No. 72/14822, Ann Arbor, Michigan.

Dale, A., and Bamford, C., 1988, Temporary workers: Cause for concern or complacency? *Work, Employment and Society*, 2, 191-209.

Davis-Blake, A., and Uzzi, B., 1993, Determinants of employment externalization: A study of temporary workers and independent contractors. *Administrative Science Quarterly*, 38, 195-223.

Diener, E., Suh, E.M., Lucas, R.E., and Smith, H.L., 1999, Subjective well-being: Three decades of progress. *Psychological Bulletin, 125*, 276-302.

Diesenhouse, S., 1993, In a shaky economy, even professionals are "temps". *New York Times*, May 16, F5.

Eaton, W.W., and Kessler, L.G., 1981, Rates of symptoms of depression in a national sample. *American Journal of Epidemiology, 114*, 528-538.

Goldberg, D., 1979, *Manual of the General Health Questionnaire*, National Foundation for Educational Research, Windsor.

Greenhalgh, L., and Rosenblatt, Z., 1984, Job insecurity: Toward conceptual clarity. *Academy of Management Review*, 3, 438-448.

Haring, M.J., Stock, W.A., and Okun, M.A., 1984, A research synthesis of gender and social class as correlates of subjective well being. *Human Relations, 37*, 645-657.

Hartley, J., Jacobson, D., Klandermans, B., and van Vuuren, T., 1991, *Job insecurity: Coping with jobs at risk*, Sage, London.

Hellgren, J., Sverke, M., and Isaksson, K., in press, A two-dimensional approach to job insecurity: Consequences for employee attitudes and well-being. *European Journal of Work and Organization Psychology.*

Howard, A., 1995, *The changing nature of work*, Jossey-Bass, San Francisco, CA.

Isaksson, K., and Bellagh, K., 1999, Anställda i uthyrningsföretag: Vilka trivs och vilka vill sluta? [Temporary firm employees: Who are satisfied and who want to quit?], *Arbete och hälsa*, 1999:7.

Isaksson, K., and Johansson, G., 1997, *Avtalspension med vinst och förlust*, Folksam, Stockholm.

Jonsson, E., 1993, *Konkurrens inom sjukvården: Vad säger forskningen?* (Competition in the health care industry: What can research tell us?), IKE, Stockholm.

Kanungo, R.N., 1982, Measurement of job and work involvement. *Journal of Applied Psychology*, 67, 341-349.

Kidder, D.L., 1996, PhD Thesis *On call or answering a calling? Temporary nurses and extra-role behaviors*. University of Minnesota.

Kochan, T.A., Smith, M., Wells, J.C., and Rebitzer, J.B., 1994, Human resource strategies and contingent workers: The case of safety and health in the petrochemical industry. *Human Resource Management*, 33, 55-77.

Krausz, M., Brandwein, T., and Fox, S., 1995, Work attitudes and emotional responses of permanent, voluntary, and involuntary temporary-help employees: An exploratory study. *Applied Psychology: An International Review*, 44, 217-232.

Krausz, M., Sagie, A., and Bidermann, Y., in press, Actual and preferred work schedules and scheduling control as determinants of job related attitudes. *Journal of Vocational Behavior.*

Leinberger, P., and Tucker, B., 1991, *The new individualists*. Harper Collins, New York.

Martens, M.F.J., Nijhuis, F.J.N., van Boxtel, M.P.J., and Knottnerus, J.A., 1999, Flexible work schedules and mental and physical health: A study of a working population with non-traditional working hours. *Journal of Organizational Behavior*, 20, 35-46.

Matusik, S.F., and Hill, C.W.L., 1998, The utilization of contingent work, knowledge creation, and competitive advantage. *Academy of Management Review*, 23, 680-687.

McLean Parks, J., and Kidder, D.L., 1994, "Till death us do part...": Changing work relationships in the 1990s. In *Trends in organizational behavior*, vol. 1 (C.L. Cooper and D.M. Rousseau, eds.), Wiley, Chichester, UK.

McLean Parks, J., Kidder, D.L., and Gallagher, D.G., 1998, Fitting square pegs into round holes: Mapping the domain of contingent work arrangements onto the psychological contract. *Journal of Organizational Behavior*, 19, 697-730.

Öhrming, J., and Sverke, M., 1996, Etablerade sjukhus och nya driftsformer: Delrapport från en tvärvetenskaplig studie av S:t Görans Sjukhus AB och Södertälje sjukhus (Established hospitals and new modes of management: Part report from an interdisciplinary study of two Swedish emergency hospitals). Stockholm: *School of Business Research Reports 1996: 10.*

Pearce, J.L., 1993, Toward an organizational behavior of contract laborers: Their psychological involvement and effects on employee coworkers. *Academy of Management Journal*, 36, 1082-1096.

Pearce, J. L., 1998, Job insecurity is important, but not for the reasons you might think: The example of contingent workers. In *Trends in organizational behavior*, vol. 5 (C.L. Cooper and D.M. Rousseau, eds.), Wiley, Chichester, UK.

Pfeffer, J. (1983). Organizational demography. In *Research in organizational behavior*, vol. 5 (L.L. Cummings and B.M. Staw, eds.), JAI Press, Greenwich, CT.

Pfeffer, J., and Baron, N., 1988, Taking the work back out: Recent trends in the structures of employment. *Research in Organizational Behavior*, 10, 257-303.

Pozner, B.Z., Randolph, W.A., 1980, Moderators of role stress among hospital personnel. *The Journal of Psychology*, 105, 215-224.

Purcell, K., and Purcell, J., 1998, In-sourcing, out-sourcing, and the growth of contingent labour as evidence of flexible employment strategies. *European Journal of Work and Organizational Psychology*, 7, 39-59.

Reilly, P.A., 1998, Balancing flexibility: Meeting the interests of employer and employee. *European Journal of Work and Organizational Psychology*, 7, 7-22.

Rizzo, J.R., House, R.J., and Lirtzman, S.I., 1970, Role conflict and ambiguity in complex organizations. *Administrative Sciences Quarterly*, 15, 150-163.

Rousseau, D.M., and Libuser, C., 1997, Contingent workers in high risk environments. *California Management Review*, 39, 103-123.

Sherer, P.D., 1996, Toward an understanding of the variety in work arrangements: The organization and labor relationships framework. In *Trends in organizational behavior*, vol. 3 (C. L. Cooper and D. M. Rousseau, eds.),. Wiley, Chichester, UK.

SOU 1993:38. Reformerad landstingsmodell: En kartläggning och analys av pågående förnyelse, ur *Hälso- och sjukvården i framtiden: Tre modeller* (Health care service in the future: Three models). Fritzes, Stockholm.

SOU 1997:58. *Personaluthyrning*. Fritzes, Stockholm.

Sparrow, P., 1998, The pursuit of multiple and parallel organizational flexibilities: Reconstituting jobs. *European Journal of Work and Organizational Psychology*, 7, 79-95.

Sparrow, P.R., and Marchington, M., 1998, Is HRM in crisis? In *Human resource management: The new agenda* (P.R. Sparrow and M. Marchington, eds.), Pitman, London.

Spri, 1994, *Stockholmsmodellen: Beslutsbefogenheter och ekonomiskt ansvar* (The Stockholm Model: Decision-making authorities and financial responsibilities). Spri, Stockholm, Report 381.

Statistics Sweden, 1997, *Arbetskraftsundersökningen 1996* [The Swedish Labour Force Survey 1996], Statistics Sweden, Stockholm.

Tregaskis, O., Brewster, C., Mayne, L., and Hegewisch, A., 1998, Flexible Working in Europe: The evidence and the implications. *European Journal of Work and Organizational Psychology*, 7, 61-78.

TELEWORK IN PERSPECTIVE – NEW CHALLENGES TO OCCUPATIONAL HEALTH AND SAFETY

Michael Ertel, Eberhard Pech and Peter Ullsperger
Federal Institute for Occupational Safety and Health, - Subdivision „Health effects of stress and psychosocial factors", P.O. Box 5, D-10266 Berlin, Germany

Abstract: The emerging information society gives rise to new, flexible work styles of which telework can be regarded as a typical example. In order to explore the impact of „flexible" working conditions on well-being and health, a questionnaire was designed and administered to 1.400, highly skilled freelancing teleworkers in the media sector. The following results are based upon the data of the first part of a longitudinal study. The response rate amounted to 15 %, which not only poses methodological problems but also highlights the challenge researchers and practitioners face when trying to access a dispersed workforce. The results point to some ambivalence in the work situation of the freelancers under study. High work motivation, high skill utilization and task variety are coupled with a high level of time pressure, recurrent fluctuations in the amount of work and conflicting work demands (i.e., demands for high performance and tight deadlines) and long working hours. When disconnected from supportive networks, teleworkers with challenging demands will have difficulties in setting limits to their workload and in recovery. So importance should be attached to detect early signs of potential health risks, particularly in young workers. Moreover, theoretical concepts for studying work organization in relation to health risks have to be revised to account for the health aspects of flexible work styles.

1.   INTRODUCTION AND OBJECTIVE

The emerging information society is characterized by an increasing pace of technological and organizational change (e.g., new methods of production, new information technologies, teleworking). With regard to teleworking, it has been emphasized that more flexibility about timing and structure of work is beneficial particularly in terms of less commuting, increased productivity and closer integration of work and home. However, conceptual clarification is needed as what the term "flexibility" really means. Theorell (1996) pointed out that it is necessary to differentiate between organizational flexibility and the individual's flexibility. Rissler (1994) demonstrated negative long-term health consequences resulting from

Health Effects of the New Labour Market, edited by Isaksson *et al.*
Kluwer Academic / Plenum Publishers, New York, 2000.

excessive workload in high-tech jobs. The objective of this paper is to shed some light on the impact of "flexible" working conditions on well-being and health. It is a pilot study and as such the first part of an ongoing research project with a longitudinal design. We regard telework as a typical example of the new, flexible work styles that is of specific relevance, because information technology is increasingly being used at home as well as in the office or at other places. So it becomes less important that employees work in the same environment.

Teleworking is a flexible way of working which covers a wide range of work activities, all of which entail working remotely from an employer, or from a traditional place of work, for a significant proportion of working time (...).

The work often involves electronic processing of information, and always involves using telecommunications to keep the remote employer and employee in contact with each other (Gray et al 1995).

However, telework is not primarily a technical phenomenon; it must rather be seen in a broader context of organizational restructuring (e.g., heightened competition, mergers, take-overs, privatizations, downsizing, transformation of permanent employment into short-term contracts, portfolio careers, etc.). It can often be regarded as "an intermediary stage on the road to entrepreneurship" (Haddon 1994). Particularly in the case of self-employment, telework will be associated with a shift of responsibilities from the (former) employer to the worker, primarily with regard to
- the ergonomic design of the workplace,
- time management,
- health and safety at work, social security,
- and the balance between work and private life.

That is why this type of "flexible" working makes specific demands on the workers (Sonnenberg 1997). As a growing proportion of the workforce will be self-employed, we focused in the first study of this kind in Germany on working conditions of freelancing/self-employed teleworkers.

2.   MATERIAL AND METHODS

The data were gathered on the basis of a questionnaire which was designed in cooperation between our research group and representatives of the union of media workers in Germany. It represents an adapted version of the questionnaire "Health at the VDU workplace" (Gesundheit am Bildschirmarbeitsplatz - GESBI) (Ertel, Junghanns, and Ullsperger 1994).

The questionnaires were administered to freelancing teleworkers, who are members of that union, in Munich (Bavaria).   Two weeks before the questionnaires were sent to the freelancers, preliminary information on the project was given in a separate letter so that the participants would be well informed in advance. Up to November 1998, the response rate amounted to 15 %. Of the 210 questionnaires returned, 52 % were from women and 48 % from men (Figure 1).

The data represent the self-reported assessment of the work situation and related issues by the respondents. Quantitative data were analyzed using SPSS.

Additionally, some qualitative data were integrated. Bivariate and multivariate analyses were carried out.

Sample structure

210 freelancers (journalists for newspapers, TV and radio,
                    multimedia designers, photographers etc.)

Education: 90% completed high school or university

Gender: 52% female; 48% male

Age: <35 years: 28%; 35 – 44 years: 41%;
             >45 years: 31%

Figure 1. Sample Structure resulting from the returned questionnaires

3.   RESULTS

With people spending a significant proportion of their working time at home, the question arises whether they have got a suitable workplace and if they work under ergonomically acceptable conditions. So we asked, *"From whom were you assisted in designing your workplace at home?"* There was neither any assistance by members of work councils or unions and clients/employers, nor by occupational health and safety specialists. A quarter of teleworkers (24 %) got support from friends and colleagues and 83 % answered that they informed themselves (on these matters). Even more striking, almost all (97%) of respondents answered that there was neither a control nor a "check-up" of their workplace by an expert. More than two thirds (68 %) have a separate working room, but only 30 % prepared for working at home by acquiring specific skills as regards the ergonomic design of a workplace.

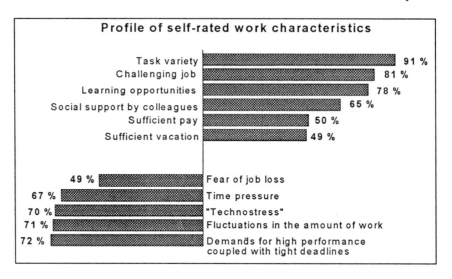

Figure 2. Profile of self-rated work characteristics

The profile of some important work characteristics (Figure 2) offers interesting insights into the work situation of the freelancing teleworkers. On the one hand, the data show that they have a high degree of self-control over the work process. On the other hand, "Technostress" (the term refers to the experience that technology demands immediate response) (Weil and Rosen 1997) and fluctuations in the amount of work (e.g., combinations of high work intensity with unemployment or enforced leisure) constrain the flexibility experienced by teleworkers. A related question refers to working time. C. Cooper recently demanded that there should be "more systematic research on the impact of working hours on health and well being, a well as on how these hours affect productivity" (Cooper 1996). In comparison with many company-based workers, freelancing teleworkers have a less structured work-and-home-environment, they are able to set their own work patterns. While being free to organize their breaks at a pace that suits them; they may often tend to work long hours (without making regular breaks), particularly when there are deadlines to meet. Moreover, there are no legal restrictions on working hours for freelance workers, who are paid for work accomplished and not for time spent. So we hypothesized that freelance teleworkers would work comparatively longer hours than the average of 40 hours. 56 % of freelancers report working more than 8 hours per day and 63 % report working over 40 hours per week (Figure 3).

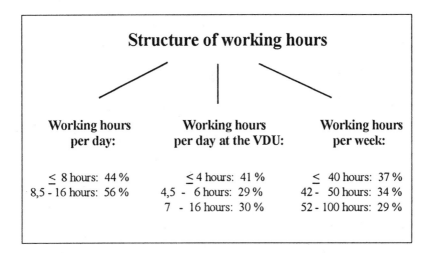

Figure 3. Structure of working hours

75 % of freelancers report that they do not register and document their working time. On closer inspection, it appears that self-rated workload is sensitive to the duration of working hours. Moreover, there is evidence of an intrusion of work on private life as a result of long working hours (Figure 4).

Impact of working hours on workload and leisure

	Self-rated workload "too high":	Work spills over into leisure
≤ 40 hours (37 %)	16 %	41 %
42 - 50 hours (34 %)	39 %	65 %
52 - 100 hours (29 %)	57 %	80 %

Figure 4. Impact of working hours on workload and leisure

As potential health effects of job demands may be moderated by (individual) coping styles, we included in our analysis the concept of *disturbed relaxation ability*. Scheuch (1997) hypothesizes that the erosion of traditional career patterns and of occupational structures and social networks may foster the development of this "personality trait". It can be regarded as a specific behaviour pattern (of coping with job demands), that mediates between external stressors and (individual) symptoms of stress. The category "disturbed relaxationability" was constructed from the following items (translated from the original German version) (Rothweiler et al 1993).

1. My work sometimes gets me going to such an extent that I can't bring myself to stop.
2. I often have trouble falling asleep because problems in my job keep going through my mind.
3. Time and time again I find it difficult to find the time for my personal needs (e.g. haircut, etc.)
4. Even on holiday I find myself spending time thinking about problems in my job.
5. I often put so much effort in my work that I feel I will never be able to carry on like that for the rest of my life.
6. I find it difficult to switch off after work.

Research on cardiological rehabilitation demonstrated that disturbed relaxation ability is an important work-related risk factor for coronary heart disease. According to Richter (1994), disturbed relaxation ability is correlated with elevated blood pressure and with delayed recovery of stress-related physiological parameters. It predicts long-term stress outcomes. Disturbed relaxation ability was found to have significant and consistent correlations with length of working hours per week (Figure 5), adding to the evidence that long working hours (e.g. over 50 hours per week) adversely affect health (Sokejima and Kagamimori 1998).

Working hours (per week) and disturbed relaxation ability

	Disturbed relaxation ability:
≤ 40 hours (37 %)	19 %
42 - 50 hours (34 %)	37 %
52 - 100 hours (29 %)	49 %

Figure 5. Working hours per week and disturbed relaxation ability

A more detailed exploratory analysis by CHAID (Chi-squared Automatic Interaction Detector) identifies the highest risk for disturbed relaxation ability among freelancers, whose work situation is characterized by constant pressure for high performance coupled with regular information overload. Conversely, the group of freelancers, who occasionally or seldom experience pressure for high performance and at the same time often have learning opportunities in their job, do not at all suffer from disturbed relaxation ability; that is, 100% of that subgroup are able to relax (Figure 6).

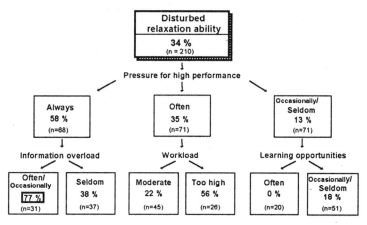

Figure 6. Predictors of disturbed relaxation ability (as computed by CHAID)[1]

---

[1] Explained in technical terms, CHAID performs an exploratory analysis. It divides the sample into distinct groups based on categories of the "best" predictor of a dependent variable. It then splits each of these groups into smaller subgroups based on other predictor variables. This splitting process continues until no more statistically significant predictors can be found. The subgroups that CHAID derives are mutually exclusive and exhaustive, that is, subgroups do not overlap, and each case is contained only in one subgroup (Magidson 1993).

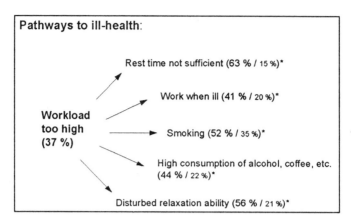

Figure 7. Pathways to ill health (* p< .05)

Referring to the mechanisms that connect working conditions and health, there is a variety of pathways that can lead to ill health. All these measures are strongly correlated with the magnitude of self-rated workload. The category "**Rest time**" deserves particular attention, as it reflects duration of working hours, work rhythm and work intensity. 63 % of freelancers, whose workload is "too high", report that their rest time is not sufficient - in contrast to 15 % of those, whose workload is moderate (Figure 7). Figure 8 shows that insufficient rest time is an important factor in the incidence of health complaints.

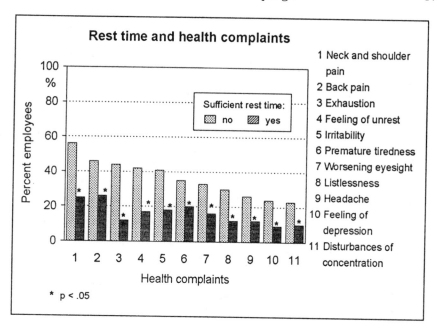

Figure 8: Rest time and health complaints

In order to create a more stable measure that reflects work-related proneness/ susceptibility to ill-health on the basis of a self-report instrument, we used cluster analysis (K-means) of a number of altogether 23 health complaints to divide the respondents into two distinct groups. The one group, representing 70 % of all cases, was categorized as being relatively healthy ("low level of health complaints"), whereas the other group, representing 30 % of all cases, were categorized as being susceptible to ill-health ("high level of health complaints"). In a following step, the new category "high level of health complaints" was taken as a dependent variable in the exploratory tree analysis conducted with CHAID.

The exploratory analysis (Figure 9) identifies the most important predictors of the dependent variable "high level of health complaints". It shows that freelancing teleworkers who do not have a balance between work and private life and at the same time are under constant pressure for high performance, are most likely to develop ill-health (68%). Conversely, only 3% of respondents who experience a balance between work and private life and at the same time never or seldom work when ill, are likely to develop ill-health.

The latter predictor highlights the issue of **undetected/hidden sickness**, which is sometimes labeled "presenteeism". That leads in a consecutive step to the last part of the analysis, where "Work when ill" is taken as a dependent variable.

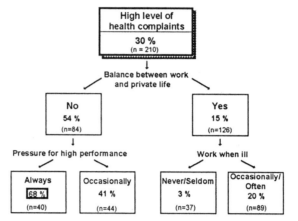

Significant distinctions produced by SPSS-Modul CHAID (Chi-squared Automatic Interaction Detector) p < .05

Figure 9: Predictors of a high level of health complaints (as computed by CHAID)

The tree diagram in Figure 10 shows that particularly female respondents whose (self-assessed) workload is too high, tend to work in case of illness.

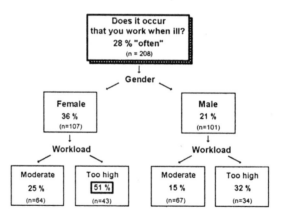

Significant distinctions produced by SPSS-Modul CHAID (Chi-squared Automatic Interaction Detector) p < .05

Figure 10: Predictors of "presenteeism" (as computed by CHAID)

4.   DISCUSSION AND OUTLOOK:

The objective of this paper was to highlight some important work-related health risks among a category of young, highly skilled and self-employed teleworkers in the media sector. Opportunities and risks are differentially distributed among different groups of workers in the "new working life". With work gradually leaving "traditional" (on-site or centralized) workplaces, workers will face health risks that may be overlooked when there is no control of workplace regulations and a lack of shared work experience that once formed the basis of social support at work. Under the conditions of the "new working life", people can no longer rely on organizational structures that provided stability and a protective environment. The problem is that working conditions (particularly the ergonomic design of workplaces, work rhythm and working hours spent) and work-related behaviour patterns (e.g. work when ill) tend to become "invisible" or inaccessible from the perspective of occupational health and safety . A new, rather ambivalent work ethic and a new work culture emerge, where people are "willing to sacrifice sleep for fast cycle time, but they demand fun and flexibility in exchange" (Cox 1997). There are reports of software companies in the USA, where being married is regarded as a "disadvantage" and where employees are "expected to be single or live a single's lifestyle" (Cringely 1996).

We believe that it is necessary to sensitize employees and free-lancers alike to the risk of this "boundaryless" workstyle to their family life, their social networks, and their health. In this context, the issue of the "affective meaning of job demands" (Payne, Jabri, and Pearson 1988) must be addressed, in order to make health and safety an issue under the new conditions of working life.

The specific characteristics and problems of a new work culture are reflected in the disproportionately low return rate of 15% of our sample. From a methodological point of view, this certainly limits the generalizibility of our results to settings beyond this single case study. One possible explanation for this low participation rate lies, as already mentioned, with the specific work culture in which the freelancers are embedded. They have a high sense of professional autonomy, internalized the idea of individual achievement and are constantly exposed to market fluctuations. It is therefore reasonable to assume that the majority of these "new workers" relies on solutions at the individual level and is not eager or inclined to take part in a kind of collective action. A second set of explanations for the low turnout possibly lies in resignation on the part of those freelancers who hardly manage to make ends meet. This interpretation was offered by our partners of the union of media workers. People who have difficulty in earning their living can't be expected to engage in activities which do not appear to be of immediate use to them. A third explanation lies with the overall motivation of the freelancers. Given their high workload, they just might be too exhausted - and less motivated - to continue working by reflecting their work situation in a questionnaire. This underscores the magnitude of the challenge we face in trying to gain access to a dispersed workforce. Although our partners themselves thought a return rate over 10 % to be a success - given that it took the respondents approximately 1 hour to fill in the questionnaire - our expectations were not met. Discussing with our partners of the union of media workers, we came to the conclusion that the self-selection bias in our sample results in a considerable underestimation of the problems we encountered (in particular as regards length of working hours, workload in general, health complaints and social security). So we may encounter also in this context the growing problem of polarization in work life and in society as a whole (Starrin, Rantakeisu and Hagquiwt 1997). Those who can't derive self-esteem from their work, because working conditions are unsatisfactory or humiliating, tend to retire from social life. This is in keeping with the observation that "with increasing demands on effectiveness and increasing threats of becoming unemployed, employees will be more and more reluctant to report problems at work" (Theorell 1997). On the other hand, those who enjoy comparatively favourable working conditions will be prone to actively engage in social activities which may result in future improvements.

However, these obstacles do not generally render questionnaire-based studies invalid. Rather it is imperative to thoroughly prepare the research process; in particular, more emphasis must be put on assuring the respondents of the anonymity and the confidentiality of their answers. To gather self-assessed reports on workload, coping behaviour and health complaints will remain a necessary precondition of health-oriented job redesign. However, the ever-increasing trend towards individualization will inevitably lead to a greater variability of working conditions and thus pose problems for epidemiological research. Keeping the limitations of the present pilot study in mind, we think that it is necessary to continue with that type of research. Modified approaches will be needed to access freelance workers, e.g., with questionnaires presented on the Internet, which will be part of the research design of the follow-up of our study.

REFERENCES

Cooper, C.L. (1996). Working hours and health, *Work & Stress*, Vol. 10(1), pp.1-4.

Cox, A.M. (1997). Wide awake on the New Night Shift, in: *Fast Company* 4/1997

Cringely, R.X.(1996). *Accidental Empires*. How the boys of Silicon Valley make their millions, battle foreign competition, and still can't get a date. Harmondsworth: Penguin.

Ertel, M.; Junghanns, G.; Ullsperger, P. (1994). *Gesundheit am Bildschirmarbeitsplatz* (GESBI). Bremerhaven: Wirtschaftsverl. NW, (Schriftenreihe der Bundesanstalt für Arbeitsmedizin: Forschung; 12.003)

Gray, M. et. al. (1995). *Teleworking Explained*. Chichester: Wiley, p. 2

Haddon, L.; Lewis, A (1994). The experience of teleworking: an annotated review, in: The *International Journal of Human Resource Management* 5:1 Feb, pp. 193-223

Magidson, J. (1993). *SPSS for Windows*. CHAID. Release 6.0. Chicago (SPSS Inc.)

Payne, RL; Jabri, MM; Pearson, AW. (1988). On the importance of knowing the affective meaning of job demands, in: *Journal of Organizational Behaviour*, 9, pp. 149-158

Richter, P.: Job content and myocardial health risks - consequences for occupational prevention, in: Vartiainen, M.; Teikari, V. (eds.) (1994). *Change, learning and mental work in organizations*. Helsinki: University of Technology, Report No. 157, pp. 19-33

Rissler, A. (1994). Extended Periods of Challenging Demands in High Tech Work - Consequences for Efficiency, Quality of Life, and Health, in: Bradley, G.E.; Hendrick, H.W. (Eds.): Human Factors in Organizational Design and Management - IV. Amsterdam: North-Holland, pp. 727-732

Rothweiler, E. et.al. (1994). Self-report coronary-prone behaviour: a replicated comparison between east german (GDR) and scottish student, in: Person. individ. Diff., Vol. 15, No. 2 pp. 155-161

Scheuch, K. (1997). Psychomentale Belastung und Beanspruchung im Wandel von Arbeitswelt und Umwelt, in: Borsch-Galetke, E.; Struwe, F. (Eds.): 37. Jahrestagung der Deutschen Gesellschaft für Arbeitsmedizin und Umweltmedizin e.V. Hüthig: Fulda, pp. 65-80

Sokejima, S.; Kagamimori, S. (1998). Working hours as a risk factor for acute myocardial infarction in Japan: a case-control study, in: *BMJ*, 317, pp. 775-789.

Sonnenberg, D. (1997). The „new career" changes: understanding and managing anxiety, in: *British Journal of Guidance & Counselling*, Vol. 25, No. 4, pp. 462-472

Starrin, B.; Rantakeisu, U.; Hagquist, C. (1997). In the wake of recession - economic hardship, shame and social disintegration, in: *Scand J Work Environ Health*; 23 suppl 4, pp. 47-54

Theorell, T. (1996). Flexibility at Work in Relation to Employee Health in: Schabracq, M.J.; Winnubst, J.A.M.; Cooper, C.L. (Eds.): *Handbook of Work and Health Psychology*. Chichester: Wiley, pp. 147-160

Theorell, T. (1997). How will future worklife influence health ? in: *Scand J Work Environ Health;* 23 suppl 4, pp. 16-22

Weil, M.W.; Rosen, L.D. (1997). TechnoStress: coping with technology. New York : Wiley.

THE RELATIONSHIP BETWEEN PRECARIOUS EMPLOYMENT AND PATTERNS OF OCCUPATIONAL VIOLENCE
Survey Evidence from Thirteen Occupations

[1]Claire Mayhew and [2]Michael Quinlan
[1] National Occupational Health and Safety Commission, Sydney, Australia; [2] School of Industrial Relations and Organisational Behaviour, University of New South Wales, Sydney, Australia.

Note: The views expressed in this paper are those of the authors and do not necessarily reflect those of the National Occupational Health and Safety Commission (NOHSC).

Abstract: There is increasing recognition that the growth of precarious employment in industrialised countries affects the incidence of occupational injuries. As yet there has been little research into connections between precarious employment and occupational violence. This study provides Australian evidence on patterns of workplace violence in occupations dominated by contingent workers. The study examined surveys of workers in thirteen occupations. The surveys included male and female dominated occupations, enabling exploration of the relationship between gender, work characteristics and occupational violence. Qualitative data allowed exploration of the origins and situational characteristics. In several surveys a control group of non-precarious workers enabled comparisons to be made between contingent and traditional workers. The studies revealed marked differences in levels of violence across occupations although low level violence in the form of abuse was common in most and there was a significant level of actual physical assault amongst four occupational groups. In two of the three occupations where direct comparisons were possible precarious workers were at greater risk of occupational violence. There is also reason to believe that managing occupational violence is more difficult where precarious employment is involved. Overall, our study provides some evidence that precarious employment can exacerbate occupational violence problems.

1.   INTRODUCTION

The last 20 years have witnessed significant changes to labour market structures in most industrialised countries. It is increasingly being recognised that the growth of contingent or precarious forms of employment, including

Health Effects of the New Labour Market, edited by Isaksson *et al.*
Kluwer Academic / Plenum Publishers, New York, 2000.

183

temporary/casual, part-time, self-employed and micro small business, leased and subcontract workers, as well as organisational restructuring processes (like privatization, downsizing and outsourcing) can have significant implications for work organisation. These changes may, in turn, have effects on occupational health and safety (OHS). A growing body of international research (using a range of methodologies) has found that contingent workers experience higher rates of work-related injury and disease than non-contingent workers undertaking similar tasks (Aronsson 1998, Foley 1998, Mayhew *et al* 1997, Mayhew and Quinlan 1997, 1999). Similarly, there is growing evidence that downsizing and outsourcing by organisations can lead to an overall deterioration in injury, disease and sickness-related absenteeism (Salminen *et al* 1993, Blank *et al* 1995, Rebitzer 1995, Rousseau and Libuser 1995, Saksvik 1996, Vahtera *et al* 1998, Netterstrom and Hansen 1998). Several researchers have drawn a connection between organisational restructuring and bullying or aggressive behaviour in the workplace (see McCarthy *et al* 1995). It has also been suggested that workers with casual or insecure jobs (including those in employment programs) were especially vulnerable to bullying or intimidation (Working Women's Centre of South Australia, 1998). However, we are unaware of attempts to systematically explore possible connections between precarious employment and occupational violence.

Our paper tries to remedy this gap. It is possible to hypothesise links between precarious employment and occupational violence. Indeed, a number of the factors in precarious employment that are seen to contribute to injury and disease may be equally conducive to occupational violence. First, in relation to outsourcing the combination of reward pressures and disorganisation can lead to situations where competition work or delays to task completion due to other workers can lead to friction and violence (for evidence of this in the building industry see Mayhew and Quinlan, 1997). The growth of precarious employment has also partly involved the expansion of informal, isolated, smaller and less regulated workplaces (like small business and home-based work) where aggressive forms of behaviour are more liable to flourish undetected. Second, women still make up the majority of contingent workers and young workers (especially adolescents) constitute a significant source of the expansion in temporary and part-time workers. Both may be especially vulnerable to subjugation in the workplace or find it difficult to cope with violent situations (such as robberies). Third, contingent workers are frequently found in jobs and industries where the risk of occupational violence may well be high including taxi drivers, clubs and pubs, fast food and late night retail outlets.

2.   THE NATURE OF OCCUPATIONAL VIOLENCE

2.1   What is Occupational Violence?

Irrespective of how narrowly or broadly it is defined, workplace violence is not a new phenomenon. Long ignored, occupational violence has recently received prominent attention from the media and OHS agencies in a number of countries (especially the USA see OSHA 1998, Oregon OSHA 1998) as well as the ILO (Chappell and Di Martino 1998). At this stage there is limited research into the incidence of occupational violence (see Jenkins 1996, Nelson and Kaufman 1996, Einarsen *et al* 1998) and no clear agreement as to what is meant by the term. In the USA attention has focused on homicide at work Occupational violence can also include verbal abuse, threats, physical violence, sexual harassment, 'activities that create an environment of fear', stalking, bullying amongst workers or between managers and workers, and behaviours that lead to stress or avoidance behaviour in the victim. In this paper we have defined occupational violence as the attempted or actual exercise by a person of any physical force or threatening statements or behaviour which gives a worker reasonable cause to believe he or she is at risk.

A number of factors may be identified as contributing to occupational violence (see Chappell and Di Martino 1998:51-78). These include broad social factors/government policies such as rising levels of unemployment and inequality; widespread substance abuse; laws and social norms about gun ownership and the carrying of weapons (like knives); de-institutionalisation of the mentally ill; and the breakdown of extended family and community support groups. Other factors include changes to working/trading hours (leading to more people working at night or in isolation) and the changing gender composition of the workforce (placing more women in occupations likely to involve violence like police/security forces). Industries or activities may attract certain types of violence due to the nature of their activity (like prisons and law enforcement) or location (such as shops, chemists or clinics located near the haunts of drug addicts or disaffected minorities). For some types of retail establishment, a combination of trading hours, cash flows, location and security may make them a prime target for armed robbery. Other workplace factors include working in isolation or in a moving workplace (as with taxi drivers), exchange of money, guarding valuable property, working in community-based settings or with unstable and volatile persons. More specific workplace factors include management style and work arrangements, and the insecurity or pressures associated with organisational restructuring. Crowded or poorly designed workplaces and disorganised work-processes, as well as production and payment system pressures, can be sources of friction and hostility.

A useful typology is to separate occupational violence into three categories:

a) employee/employee or manager/employee occupational violence;

b) randomised member of the public/employee occupational violence e.g. during armed hold-ups (which attracts much media attention); and

c) client initiated occupational violence, which may be systemic in some human services, law and justice, and health occupations. (M. Parker, pers.comm.)

a)   Internal organizational occupational violence

This includes mobbing or bullying (Leymann 1990 and Zapf and Leymann 1996) as well as assaults that originate between or amongst managers and workers. Authoritarian management styles, downsizing and increasing job insecurity can be associated with bullying or confrontational styles of management as well as greater friction amongst employees (Babiak 1995, and McCarthy *et al* 1995). It can also lead to disgruntled workers who feel cheated of their entitlements and self-esteem, and may exacerbate stress on those who are bereaved or suffer a mental illness (Mullen 1997:23-24). Over-crowded or poorly designed workplaces, where insufficient account has been taken of peaks in activity (as in restaurants), or sites where overlapping activities have not been carefully scheduled (as with multiple subcontractors on a building site) can initiate friction and hostility. This is especially the case where a performance-based payment system means any interruption to work results in a loss of earnings.

b) Randomized member of the public/employee occupational violence

Retail outlets e.g. all night chemists may be prime targets because of their trading hours, location and comparatively low levels of security. Occupational violence associated with jobs where close contact between workers and the public is required may be increased with alcohol-affected customers occurs e.g. in the taxi or hospitality industries. Staff cuts resulting in service delays may also be a source of customer- initiated hostility. These patterns may change over time as increased security measures by some traditional targets for robbery such as banks and betting agencies cause criminals to focus on other commercial activities involving cash transactions (such as fast food outlets). The incidence of violent activity may be concentrated in particular localities (some city suburbs), and amongst distinct groups in society.

(c) Client-initiated occupational violence

Specific industries are at risk due to the very nature of their activities e.g. prisons, juvenile detention, remand centres and other law enforcement activities; drug-treatment establishments, hospitals and social security advice/application centres. The changing gender composition of the workforce may affect perceived vulnerability and the potential for violence, e.g. female public servants in juvenile protection programs may be targeted. Further, some detained individuals may deliberately or inadvertently adopt behaviour that is violent or conducive to arousing fear amongst others in the workplace. Changes to working arrangements including increased late night shifts or working in isolation can increase the risk of assault hospital workers may also be the targets of violent mentally ill, emotionally unstable, or drug/alcohol addicted patients (Mullen 1997).

2.2   Evidence on the extent of occupational violence

Attempts to establish the extent of occupational violence are fraught with difficulties, and is significantly influenced by definitions adopted. For phenomenon such as bullying, verbal abuse and threats of violence there is only a limited amount of recent survey evidence (see for example Eirnarsen and Skogstad 1996 and Eirnarsen et al 1998).

One area of violence where fairly compelling data is starting to emerge is workplace homicide. In the USA homicide has become a leading source of death at work. Between 1980 and 1990 it was the third most significant cause of workplace death, accounting for 7,600 fatalities or 12% of all job-related deaths (NIOSH 1995). Examining US data for the years 1980 to 1992, Jenkins (1996, cited in Chappell and Di Martino 1998:38) found the incidence of occupational homicide was highest in the retailing, public administration and transport industries. In terms of occupations, taxi drivers were the most at-risk group followed by sheriffs, police, garage workers and security guards. By 1994 homicide was the second leading cause of death to American workers, and had risen to 16% of the 6,588 fatal work injuries in the United States (BLS 1995). Of these fatalities, 179 were supervisors or proprietors in retail sales, 105 were cashiers and 49 were managers in restaurants. In recent years homicide has become the single most important cause of death at work amongst females in the USA.

Many of these deaths arose as a result of robberies in retail establishments. Unfortunately, the US data makes no direct link to precarious employment although these arrangements are pervasive in a number of 'at risk' occupations (notably taxi driver) and industries (such as retailing).

Australia has experienced a far lower rate of workplace homicide. The second work-related fatality census (Driscoll et al 1998:53) covering the period 1989 to 1992 found occupational homicides accounted for around 2% of all traumatic work-related deaths in Australia. The most at risk industries were 'community services' – including police and medical services (24%), 'wholesale and retail trade' (22%), and 'recreation, personal and other services' including brothels (20%). The most at risk occupations were 'managers and administrators' (24%), 'sales and personal service workers' including prostitutes (20%), and 'para-professionals' including police officers (13%). Guns were in involved in 49% of occupational homicides, knives in 22% and another weapon in 18%. The assailant was most commonly a customer, client or patient (31%), a stranger (29%), a co-worker or former co-worker (7%), and in 33% of cases there was an unknown or 'other' assailant. The most common motive was robbery (27%), pre-meditated murder (13%), in the course of another assault (13%), and in 27% of cases the motive was unknown. Assailants were usually male (71%), While most victims were employees (62%), the self-employed and micro small business owners were over-represented compared with their proportion in the labour force (36%). (Pers. comm. T Driscoll 1 June 1998).

Evidence on less serious forms of occupational violence is fragmentary. In the USA NIOSH collected information on occupational violence as part of the BLS Annual Survey of Occupational Injuries and Illnesses. In 1992 this survey identified 22,400 assaults resulting in days off work. Unlike homicides, non-fatal assaults were distributed more equally amongst men (44%) and women (56%), with the majority occurring in the service (64%) and retail (21%) industries. Other surveys, such as the US National Crime Victimisation Survey indicate a far higher level of workplace assault.

Comparative international data are rare. A survey of 15,800 workers in the EU (EFLILWC 1998) found 9% had been subjected to intimidation at work: 3 million EU workers had been subjected to sexual harassment, 6 million to physical violence and 12 million to psychological violence. Interestingly from our perspective. Chappell and Di Martino were able to break the survey data down according to gender and employment status. This revealed that workers in precarious employment reported sexual harassment 50% above the all-worker average, and those in precarious employment expired more bullying).

Overall, existing indicate the phenomenon is widespread and may be increasing in some occupations and industries where precarious employment is prevalent. Scientific studies of occupational violence have found increased risks for:

– taxi drivers, particularly abuse and threats from passengers (HSE 1991 cited in Chappell and Di Martino 1998:46, Dalziel and Soames 1997, Mayhew 1999);

- a survey of hospitality and bar workers found verbal abuse was experienced by more than 50% and assaults by 11%, with bouncers especially at risk (Mayhew *et al* 1996);
- nursing and other hospital staff working with mentally ill clients have reported threats, abuse and actual attacks for many years (Grainger 1997:544, Nordin 1995 cited in Chappell and Di Martino 1998:47);
- teachers, particularly those working in secondary schools, have reported a significant increase in abuse and threats from students (ILO *Press Release* 20 July 1998);
- electricity workers who are disconnecting power have been subjected to violence from clients;
- Bullying management styles have been associated with changing work arrangements, downsizing, re-structuring, and increasing job insecurity (McCarthy *et al* 1995). Babiak (1995) concluded that restructuring provided career advancement opportunities for 'industrial psychopaths'.

The injury data indicate that forms of occupational violence are common for workers in constant contact with the public, particularly when cash is on hand, in the evening and where alcohol is available. In half the cases just mentioned the at-risk groups were precariously employed. For example, Kinney (1993:292) states *'Homicides among adolescent workers are rising as a result of late-night employment in the service sector ... As service establishments stay open longer at night, fatalities are certain to increase'*.

3. SURVEY EVIDENCE ON PRECARIOUS EMPLOYMENT AND OCCUPATIONAL VIOLENCE

We have conducted a number of surveys of precariously employed and workers. Here we present findings from six surveys of workers in thirteen occupations (taxi, childcare, building contractors, cabinetmakers, demolishers, transport, hospitality, newsagents, garage mechanics, printers, clothing manufacture, café and restaurant, and fast food workers) undertaken in Australia between 1993 and 1998. In each survey randomly-selected workers were asked a series of questions about their experiences of violence on-the-job, using three indicators of violence: abuse, threats, and physical assaults. Interviews for all six studies were conducted on a face-to-face basis, using a questionnaire with closed and open-ended questions, together with a semi-structured interview schedule. (Individual names and site locations were not recorded on the questionnaire or interview transcripts.) In each of the studies interviewees were asked: "Have you ever been verbally abused, threatened or assaulted on the job or on the way to or from work since [date 12 months earlier]". Interviewees were then required to check one of the response boxes: [ ] no, [ ] verbally abused, [ ] threatened, [ ] assaulted; and to "describe" the incident in narrative data. The most recent study of young casual workers marginally differed from earlier studies in that on-site occupational violence incidents were in a separate question to those which occurred on the journey to or from work. Further, "hold-ups/snatch and grabs" were provided with a separate possible response box on the questionnaire.

The surveys included male and female dominated occupations, enabling some exploration of the relationship between gender, work characteristics and occupational violence patterns. Qualitative analysis explored the origins, nature and situational characteristics of violent incidents. The majority of the workers interviewed occupied precarious jobs (e.g. self-employed contractors, home-based workers and casual fast food workers). In few occupations a control group of non-outsourced/less precarious workers was also surveyed, providing a basis for comparing the incidence of occupational violence between contingent and traditional employee workers.

Table 1 summarises the survey findings. Occupational violence was found to be a significant issue in almost all surveyed groups, although there were marked differences between the occupational groups in terms of the percentage of interviewees who had been the victim of verbal abuse, threats, and physical assault incidents.

The surveys also revealed variations in the origins and natures of violence amongst the various occupational groups. The occupational violence pattern variations are discussed separately below.

First, the 1998 survey of 304 young casual workers employed in company-owned and franchised stores of a multinational fast food chain (covering three states) found that verbal abuse at work was very common (48%) particularly from disgruntled or short-tempered customers, but the incidence of threats and physical assaults was minimal. Only three incidents involved occupational violence *between* store employees; all the rest were customers or robbers. Occupational violence incidents on the way to or from work were minimal. Reported 'hold-ups' and 'snatch and grab' incidents were more common in one state (NSW) but no other variations in occupational violence were found between the states or between company-owned and franchised outlets. A very similar pattern of occupational violence incidents was found in the 1996/97 survey of 70 owner/managers of small-scale café and restaurant businesses in the wider Brisbane region (see 'Barriers' discussion below). That is, low level occupational violence (particularly verbal abuse) may be an endemic risk for workers in food outlets.

Table 1. Occupational violence incidents experienced by 1,438 workers in 13 occupational groups (% of each sample)

Study title	Year done	Employment status	Total no inter-viewed	Abuse	Threats	Physical attack	Held up or snatch & grab
Young casual[1]	1998	Precarious	304	48.4	7.6	1.0	2.3
Interventions[2]	1997		331				
Contractors		Precarious		12.7	5.3	2.7	
Cabinet-makers		Precarious		14.7	4.7	2.0	
Demolishers		Precarious		29.0	6.4	3.2	
Barriers[3]	96/97		248				
Garage		Precarious		9.7	4.2		
Café		Precarious		45.7	15.7	1.4	
Newsagent		Precarious		62.9	11.4	1.4	
Printing		Precarious		37.1	2.9	2.9	
Taxi drivers[4]	1993	Precarious	100	81.0	17.0	10.0	
Clothing mfg[5]	97/98		200				
Factory-based		Secure		4.0	1.0	1.0	
Outworkers		Precarious		49.0	23.0	7.0	
Outsourcing[6]	1995		255				
Childcare		Secure & precarious		50.0 (15.0)	13.0 (2.5)	11.0 (-)	
Hospitality		Precarious		57.0 (53.0)	46.0 (30.0)	11.0 (7.0)	
Transport		Secure & precarious		47.0 (13.0)	6.0 (13.0)	- (13.0)	
Building		Precarious		15.0 (56.0)	- (17.0)	- (-)	

1) Mayhew & Johnstone in press, p.131.
2) Mayhew *et al* 1997.
3) Mayhew 1997. p.76.
4) Mayhew 1999.
5) Mayhew & Quinlan 1998 p.108.
6) Mayhew *et al* section 4.6. The first figure shown is the percentage of employees; the number in brackets is the comparable % for outsourced workers in the same industry sub-group.

Second, the 1997 'interventions' study of 331 workers (150 building contractors, 150 cabinetmakers, and 31 demolishers) in small businesses found that contractors did not experience significant levels of occupational violence. The cabinetmakers also reported violent incidents infrequently, and then only in relation to payment for services discussions, disputes with ex-employees or, if they were working on a building site, the foreman. However demolishers experienced higher levels of verbal abuse (29%) although only 6% had been threatened, and very few assaulted in the immediate past year. That is, only amongst demolishers was a significant level of occupational violence identified.

Third, the 1996/97 'barriers' study involved 248 owner/managers of businesses with less than five employees, including owner-managers of garages (n=73), café/restaurants (n=70), newsagencies (n=70), and small scale printing workshops (n=35). Occupational violence patterns were distinctly different in each of the four groups studied. Violence on-the-job was a rare event for *garage* owner/managers with around 10% verbally abused in the immediate past twelve months. In contrast, lower-level occupational violence was common for small-scale *cafe and restaurant* owner/managers with nearly half having been verbally abused and a significant proportion threatened in the past year (some had been both verbally abused and threatened). However, just over half had never experienced any occupational violence incidents. Most physical threats to cafe and restaurant owner/managers came from customers – who were sometimes alcohol-affected. Some threats accompanied a robbery. Occupational violence was also an endemic problem for newsagent owner/managers, with 63% having been verbally abused (nearly always by customers). The level of physically threats was also high with around 13% of newsagent owner/managers experiencing hold-ups on their premises involving themselves, a spouse or a child. Of all four groups studied during this research project, newsagents had the highest level of robbery-related occupational violence. Amongst the *printer* owner/managers interviewed, verbal abuse was relatively common with 37% citing incidents, one was threatened, and one had been physically assaulted. Again, customers, and payment and quality disputes, were associated with occupational violence incidents.

Fourth, in the 1993 taxi study, 100 drivers were interviewed about their occupational violence experiences in the immediate past twelve-month period. Overall, this occupational group had the highest level of occupational violence of any of the studies with 81% verbally abused, 17% threatened with an assault, and 10% assaulted by a passenger(s). The types of injury suffered varied considerably from upper body lacerations and fractures (e.g. broken jaw, broken nose) to 'torn shirt'. In some cases there was no actual physical injury but the mental effects were considerable, for example: *'threatened to kill me Sunday'*. The majority of drivers (91%) were precariously employed and were paid according to a percentage of takings, 6% of the interviewed population were owner/drivers, and 3% held taxi leases. The qualitative data clearly indicated that the ability to exercise choice over shifts worked was a core determinant of exposure to risk.

Owner/drivers had the greatest choice and hence drove on the most rewarding and safest shifts (during daylight hours and often on the 'airport' and other business 'runs'). In contrast, the subcontract drivers had less choice and worked at times that 'fitted in' with taxi owners, other jobs or study commitments. As a result the subcontract drivers frequently worked twelve-hour shifts, often drove during the evening/night on the 4pm to 4am shift, and more frequently carried young male alcohol-affected customers. Hence it is hardly surprising that the casual taxi drivers experienced more verbal abuse, threats, and assaults than did the owner/drivers.

A number of risk factors were identified: the majority of assailants were male (83%) and young (75% under age 30). The majority of assaults (72%) occurred between 6pm and 5 am, with alcohol a factor in 59% of incidents. Most followed a 'hail' from the street (46%) or from a taxi rank (36.5%), particularly in the inner and near city suburbs (33%). While customers from disadvantaged subgroups who were desperate for money were perceived to be higher risk, attacks were infrequently associated with fare evasion (15%) – except when fare evaders (or 'runners') were chased by drivers. Four underlying factors enhanced the level of risk. First, the supply and demand equation for taxi work was found to be unbalanced because of an over supply of service providers and a shortage of customers. Second, taxi vehicles were primarily purchased on the basis of cost, not safety (i.e. standard sedans remain much cheaper than the London style cabs), although the supply of safety shields, emergency lights, and improved radio systems were becoming common. Third, widespread acquiescence to aggressive customer behaviour was identified, with muted state responses. Fourth, inadequate police resources were available to investigate assaults that resulted in only minor injuries, and brief court-imposed sentences were believed to encourage further occupational violence incidents.

The fifth study undertaken in 1997/98 involved interviewing 100 randomly selected factory-based clothing workers and 100 outworkers (incapable of being randomly selected), both groups being predominantly female. Factory-based clothing worker employees experienced relatively low levels of occupational violence compared to the other groups studied. In marked contrast, clothing outworkers commonly experienced occupational violence with 49% being verbally abused in the immediate past year, 23% threatened, and 7% assaulted. The qualitative data indicated that the occupational violence experiences of outworkers occurred in a wide range of situations, and were sometimes racially based from the general public during pick-up/delivery of clothing products. The majority of outworkers were recently arrived immigrants from East Asia with a limited command of English while factory-based workers had mostly arrived in earlier waves of migration from southern or eastern Europe. Most occupational violence incidents experienced by outworkers came from 'middlemen' and were usually economically based. There was an over-supply of home-based workers seeking work from middlemen who were, in turn, pressured by retailers to minimise production costs. Harassment, abuse and outright assaults were endemic to the subcontracting system, and ethnic factors can be best viewed as a compounding influence. For example when one outworker tried to get payment for work completed, the middlemen: '... *yelled and abused me like I was animal; then didn't pay me'* . Outworkers are in a very powerless and difficult position and while occupational violence appears to be an increasingly serious problem for outworkers, it remains largely hidden.

Sixth, the 1995 'outsourcing' study included child-care (n=95), hospitality (n=76), transport (n=43), and building (n=41) workers. Because both employee and outsourced workers were interviewed for each group, comparisons could be made on the basis of employment status. The data indicated that, overall, occupational violence was a major OHS issue. Across all 255 workers in the four groups studied, 48% of employees had been verbally abused, compared with 33% of self-employed/outsourced workers. Around 10% of employees and 7% of outsourced workers reported being threatened. About 4% of employees reported being assaulted in the immediate past year, compared with 2% of outsourced workers. An important consideration is that in those industry sectors where outsourcing was common and increasing, the working conditions and levels of security had also diminished for more permanent workers, for example, in the hospitality industry.

Overall, it was found that the patterns were markedly different in the different industry sectors. In the child-care industry, the qualitative data indicated that most verbal abuse came from parents, as did most threats (sometimes following demands from non-custodial parents who wanted to remove their children). On the other hand, children initiated most physical assaults, often during tantrums. For hospitality workers, verbal abuse from customers was virtually the norm for both self-employed and employee workers. One possible explanation for the high level of occupational violence in a tourist destination like the Gold Coast (where many interviews were conducted) was the high itinerant population of holidaymakers. This environment is more conducive to 'binge drinking' in the absence of peer group pressure which helps control behaviour in hotels and clubs with a more established and regular clientele. Hotel and casino bouncers often face unenviable situations given the volatility of some drunk or abusive clients, and the use of casual workers without proper training to undertake these tasks exacerbates the risk. Transport workers interviewed generally experienced lower levels of occupational violence, although serious incidents were more pronounced amongst self-employed drivers and frequently involved altercations with other drivers. Some of the building workers interviewed experienced frequent lower-level occupational violence incidents and the problem appeared to be more pronounced amongst outsourced workers (see Table 1).

In summary, the patterns of occupational violence identified through these studies of precarious workers are that occupational violence is common. It appears to be most pronounced in working situations where close contact with the public is required, where alcohol/drug affected clients/customers may be served, where there is strong competition for work, and if the potential for robbery exists. In the occupations we examined it appears that:

– employee/employee and manager/employee occupational violence was comparatively infrequent. Major exceptions to this were clothing outworkers and truck drivers;

– robbery-related occupational violence is an important problem in specific sectors of the retail industry, many of which are small businesses; and

– client/customer-initiated occupational violence is a significant problem in the childcare and hospitality industry.

4.   VARIATIONS BETWEEN PRECARIOUS WORKERS AND SECURE EMPLOYEES

Indicating that occupational violence is a widespread phenomenon amongst a number of precarious occupations is useful but only the first step in establishing a better understanding of the relationship between precarious employment and occupational violence. Obviously, there is a need to extend these studies and benchmark them against findings in relation to other industries. Further, in seeking to explore the impact of precarious employment there is a need to make direct comparisons between secure and precarious workers undertaking the same tasks. In terms of our initial hypotheses we are able to make several observations. In the taxi study it was noted that there was some evidence that a competition for work and the allocation of less safe schedules to casual drivers exacerbated the risks they faced. However, the comparison sample was too small to make more definitive observations. Only in two of the studies could occupational violence data be reliably compared on the basis of employment status: the clothing manufacture study completed in 1998, and the 1995 'subcontracting/outsourcing' study.

The 1997 Clothing manufacture study presented quite distinct pictures of occupational violence for different employment sectors in the industry. In this study it is fairly clear that precariously employed workers – the outworkers – experienced far more occupational violence and this could, to a very large degree, be attributed to changes in work organisation associated with outsourcing. While racial prejudice was undoubtedly associated with some of this occupational violence, 'middlemen' from their own language community perpetrated the vast majority of incidents. The poor bargaining position of these women in the labour market, their subjugated position in families and communities, and the dominance of middlemen within language groups, enhanced the potential for occupational violence to endure with little reprimand.

Evidence from the 1995 'outsourcing' study is less compelling, partly due to the smaller sample size for some groups and less pronounced distinctions in employment status as well as the critical influence of industry-specific factors in shaping the pattern of occupational violence. For child-care workers the incidence of all forms of occupational violence was far higher for those who were employees. Employees were frequently abused (50%), threatened (13%), and assaulted (11%) in the immediate past year. In contrast, outsourced child-care workers were abused (15%), threatened (2.5%), and assaulted (0%) far less frequently. The greater vulnerability of centre-based employees to violence in comparison to home-based carers may in part be explained by the more rigid rules of centres concerning access and operating hours – a major source of client anger. Hospitality workers had a very high incidence of verbal abuse, threats, and assaults amongst both employees and outsourced workers. For employee hospitality workers, 57% had experienced verbal abuse in the immediate past year, 46% had been threatened, and 11% were physically assaulted. Similarly the outsourced/self-employed hospitality workers had frequently been verbally abused (53%), threatened (30%), and assaulted (7%). This similarity suggests that the risk factors are common across the industry. Transport workers also showed some differences between the employment status groups. Amongst employee transport workers, verbal abuse was common (47%), but threats (6%) and assaults (0%) were rare. In contrast outsourced transport workers were abused less frequently (13%), but threatened (13%) and assaulted (13%) more often in the immediate past year. (The lower numbers of transport workers interviewed means that these differences are less reliable.) For building workers there were also some marked differences between the employment status groups, with outsourced workers clearly under greater threat of an occupational violence incident. The employee builders cited low levels of occupational violence: verbal abuse (15%), threats (0%), and assaults (0%). In contrast outsourced building workers were abused far more often (56%), threatened more frequently (17%), but none had been assaulted in the immediate past year. The qualitative data indicated that competition between outsourced workers was so high that competing deadlines increased levels of verbal abuse; probably associated with task completion and payment-by-results pressures. (Again with this industry group, the lower number of workers interviewed means that these differences are less reliable.)

Drawing these findings together we can tentatively conclude that the presence of precarious workers tends to be correlated with increased occupational violence, although industry-specific risks are the prime determinant. Given that a significant proportion of the female workforce is found in precarious jobs, it is worth exploring whether there are gender differences in the pattern of occupational violence.

5.   GENDER DIFFERENCES IN PATTERNS OF OCCUPATIONAL VIOLENCE

The questionnaire and interview transcripts from most of the contingent worker studies could be separated by gender. As is widely known, Australia has one of the most strongly sex-typed workforces of any OECD country, and this was reinforced in the empirical data. Some of our studies of contingent workers were conducted in overwhelmingly male-dominated sectors (e.g. 98% of the taxi drivers interviewed were male). Hence a gender analysis of the distribution of occupational violence could not produce meaningful results. Other industry sectors predominantly employed female workers (e.g. clothing manufacture), so gender comparisons of occupational violence incidents were again of limited utility. It is in the studies where more equal proportions of male and female workers spent their working time that differences in the propensity to suffer different forms of occupational violence could be more clearly identified. In Table 2, the data from the appropriate studies are shown separated by gender.

The findings shown in Table 2 suggest that the gender division of labour is a crucial precursor to the distribution of occupational violence.

Table 2. Gender variations in occupational violence experiences of 1,338 workers in 13 different occupational groups (% of all male or female interviewees where gender was recorded)

Study title	Employment status	Abuse		Threats		assault		held up o: snatch & grab	
		m	f	M	f	m	f	m	f
Young casual[1]	Precarious	35.2%	59.9%	12.3%	5.8%	3.3%	-	3.3 %	1. %
Clothing mfg[2]									
Factory-based	Secure	6.2%	3.6%	6.2%	-	-	2.4 %		
Outworkers	Precarious	60.0%	43.0%	40.0%	25.8%	20.0%	5.4 %		
Barriers[3]									
Garage	Precarious	9.9%	-	4.2%	-	-	-		
Café	Precarious	51.1%	40.9%	23.4%	-	2.1%	-		
Newsagent	Precarious	67.6%	57.6%	16.2%	6.1%	2.7%	-		
Printing	Precarious	34.6%	44.4%	3.8%	-	3.8%	-		
Outsourced[4]									
Childcare	Secure/ Precarious	50.0%	32.0%	-	8.0%	-	6.7 %		
Hospitality	Precarious	64.7%	50.0%	52.9%	16.7%	17.6%	3.3 %		
Transport	Secure/ Precarious	31.2%	-	9.4%	-	6.2%	-		
Building	Precarious	38.7%	-	9.7%	-	-	-		

5.1   Gender variations **within** occupations

In the 1998 'Young casual worker' study a very high level of verbal abuse was cited by the fast food workers interviewed, particularly by females. Conversely, males were more liable to experience violent threats and actual physical attacks. One important comparison is the relatively similar gender breakdown of occupational violence categories amongst the 'Barriers' café/restaurant workers (although here males suffered more abuse). This similarity suggests that occupational violence from customers (particularly verbal abuse) is an endemic OHS problem for all workers in food outlets.

In the 1997/98 'Clothing manufacture' study there were few male workers. The overall level of occupational violence was very low for both males and females working in factories, but marginally higher for males in each of the categories of abuse, threats, and assaults. Of the three factory-based female workers who reported verbal abuse, two had been abused by co-workers on Just in Time (JIT) lines and one by her boss. Further, of the two female employees who had been assaulted, one attack came from her 'boss'. In contrast, as discussed earlier, occupational violence is a significant and endemic problem for most clothing outworkers (see Table 1). While the number of male outworkers is far too low to allow for meaningful comparisons with females, occupational violence is again apparently higher for males in all three categories of occupational violence assessed. For outworkers, the 'middleman' was the most frequent perpetrator of abuse, threats and assaults against both males and females. That is, for both factory-based and garment outworkers occupational violence is usually initiated *within* production chains.

The 1996/97 'Barriers' study of owner/managers of micro small businesses found marked differences between the different industry sectors in terms of both the gender division of labour and in the distribution of verbal abuse, threats, and assaults on-the-job. Amongst the 73 garage small business owner/managers interviewed, 71 were male (97%), 1 was female, and in one case gender was not recorded. Occupational violence was experienced at comparatively low levels, and no incidents were cited by the female interviewee. Occupational violence does not appear to be a major OHS issue for this occupational group, who has only intermittent contact with the public. Amongst the 70-café/restaurant owner/managers interviewed, 47 were male (67%), 22 were female (31%), and in one case gender were not recorded. The incidence of 'verbal abuse' incidents cited was relatively similar for males (51%) and females (41%). However 23% of males endured threats, and 2% had been assaulted in the immediate past twelve-month period. In contrast, no female owner/managers interviewed had been threatened or assaulted over the same period of time. That is, males suffered more serious forms of occupational violence in this industry sector, although the levels of verbal abuse directed at all workers are of concern. All incidents involved customers - who were frequently alcohol-affected.

Amongst the 70 newsagent owner/managers interviewed, 37 were male (53%), and 33 were female (47%). The incidence of 'verbal abuse' incidents cited was again relatively similar for males (68%) and females (58%). Around 16% of the male owner/managers endured threats with 3% assaulted in the immediate past twelve-month period. In contrast, only around 7% of female owner/managers interviewed had been threatened and none assaulted over the same period of time. That is, a very high incidence of verbal abuse was found for both male and female owner/managers of newsagencies. But, more severe forms of occupational violence occurred more frequently to males. Customers were nearly always the source of the incidents. Many of the more severe incidents related to robberies, especially in the early mornings (when more males than females were on-the-job). Amongst the 35 printing micro small business owner/managers interviewed, 26 were male (74%) and 9 were female (26%). Again the incidence of 'verbal abuse' incidents cited was relatively similar for males (35%) and females (44%). However 4% of males had endured threats, and another 4% had been assaulted in the immediate past twelve-month period. In contrast, no female printing owner/managers interviewed had been threatened or assaulted over the same period of time. That is, in the printing industry sector, while female owner/managers endured more verbal abuse, the more severe forms of occupational violence occurred more frequently to males. Nearly all incidents involved customers.

In the 1995 'Subcontracting/outsourcing' study there were, again, marked differences in the proportions of male and female workers in the different industry sectors. Amongst the 95 child-care workers interviewed, 3% were male and 97% female. Hence analysis on the basis of gender is probably misleading. Verbal abuse had occurred to 50% of males and 32% of females in the immediate past twelve-month period. Fully 8% of females had been threatened and 7% assaulted. No males had been threatened or assaulted. That is, in stark contrast to the café/restaurant and newsagent owner/managers in the 'Barriers' study, females cited *more severe* forms of occupational violence than did males. Amongst the 76 hospitality workers interviewed, 53% were male and 47% female. This distribution means that comparisons between male and female workers are particularly useful. Verbal abuse had occurred to around 65% of male owner/managers interviewed and 50% of females in the immediate past twelve-month period. Threats had also been received by 53% of male and 17% of female workers, and, of great concern, assaults had occurred to 18% of males and 3% of the females interviewed. That is, occupational violence appears to be a major OHS problem for all hospitality workers. All transport and building workers interviewed were male.

5.2   Gender variations <u>across</u> occupations

The male-dominated jobs identified through the 'Interventions' study (building contractors, cabinetmakers, demolishers), in the 'Barriers' research (garage mechanics), and in the 'Subcontracting/outsourcing' survey (transport and building) indicated that between 10-38% of workers had experienced verbal abuse, 4-10% had been threatened, and between 2-6% had been assaulted. That is, while verbal abuse had become almost a normal experience in these male-dominated jobs, more severe forms of occupational violence were quite irregular. Notably, none of these jobs required on-going face-to-face contact with members of the public. Self-employed workers and tradesmen dominated many of these jobs. When it occurred, the occupational violence came from customers or other tradesmen.

The female-dominated jobs assessed were in the 'Clothing manufacture' (factory-based and outworkers) and the 'Subcontracting/outsourcing' (child-care) research studies. Here the factory-based clothing workers, on the one hand, presented a stark contrast to both the clothing outworkers and the child-care workers on the other. Only around 4% of female factory-based clothing workers were exposed to verbal abuse, compared with 43% for outworkers and 32% of child-care female workers. Similarly no female factory-based clothing workers were exposed to threats, compared with 26% of outworkers and 8% of child-care female workers. Around 2% of female factory-based clothing workers were exposed to physical assaults, compared with 5% of outworkers and 7% of female child-care workers. Similar variations occurred for males in these female-dominated sectors, although males more frequently suffered more severe forms of occupational violence. In these female-dominated jobs, the occupational violence predominantly came from internal organisational supervisor/employer sources (clothing manufacture) and from parents/clients (child-care).

Jobs with significant numbers of both male and female workers included the 'young casual' worker study which was conducted in the fast-food industry, the 'Barriers' research project (café/restaurant, newsagent, and printing industry sectors), and the 'Subcontracting/outsourcing' (hospitality) industry sectors. The results of these studies together present a clear picture of the distribution of occupational violence patterns by gender for a range of contingent workers. Overall, the patterns for occupational violence are:

- Males were generally more frequently threatened and assaulted (e.g. hospitality, newsagents), but were usually less frequently verbally abused.
- Females doing the same job tasks as males were more frequently verbally abused (e.g. young casual), but less frequently threatened or assaulted.

Once the high-risk situations have been identified, the search for appropriate and reliable methods to control the situations can begin. It appears that while there are generic principles applicable to many situations (like increased security measures), industry sub-group specific strategies may need to be tailored to reduce the risks on each worksite. The strategies are likely to be most difficult to devise and implement where close client/worker contact is required.

6.   CONCLUSION

This paper reviewed the extent and severity of occupational violence amongst precarious workers. The findings were derived from surveys of a range of industry/occupational groups in Australia. However, we do not claim extensive coverage, and further work needs to be done, particularly in sectors where both men and women workers are employed. It was suggested that occupational violence could be usefully separated into three categories: (a) employee/employee or manager/employee occupational violence; (b) member of the public/employee occupational violence; and (c) client-initiated occupational violence. Our findings can be broadly summarised as follows.

Occupational violence is a significant OHS problem for precarious workers. The extent and severity of occupational violence varied markedly by industry and occupation. Primarily because of the sexual division of labour in Australia, the incidence of verbal abuse, threats, and assaults also varied markedly by gender. In the few empirical studies completed where males and females performed similar job tasks, there was a tendency for females to suffer proportionately more verbal abuse, and for males to endure a greater proportion of the more severe occupational violence categories of threats and assaults.

It is difficult to make broad generalisations about differences in levels of risk for precariously employed workers and secure employees doing the same jobs. The empirical data was limited, but there is evidence that occupational violence is higher amongst those with limited control over the risks associated with their job tasks. Competition for work, limited bargaining power and reward factors that have been seen contribute to a higher incidence of injury amongst some groups of precarious workers also appear to be conducive to occupational violence. Overall, our comparative studies between employees and precarious workers in the 'clothing manufacture', 'fast food' and 'outsourcing' studies best illuminate the complex relationship between precarious work, gender and occupational violence.

However, the situation is by no means simple and industry specific factors cannot be ignored e.g. in childcare employees suffered higher levels of violence. The primary determinant is industry sector: some jobs have intrinsically higher levels of risk because they involve close contact between workers and the public. Other confounding factors include the gender division of labour, which is quite marked in Australia. Our findings confirm the influence of factors identified in other studies, most obviously that that cash-on-hand is a precursor to many robbery-related occupational violence incidents in retail establishments, but the extent and severity is likely to be far worse in situations which require on-going face-to-face contact with the public. The risks are exacerbated when alcohol is involved. Nevertheless, the most 'at-risk' occupational groups appear to be those involving close customer/worker contact (e.g. personal services or hospitality activities.

Two final points should be made. First, the presence of precarious workers increase risks because they are less likely to possess the skills, experience, bargaining power and support from management to handle threats. Second, as the precariously employed proportion of the total workforce in an industry sector increases the labour market bargaining power of all workers may diminish and hence worker's ability to causal risks.

REFERENCES

Aronsson, G., 1998, Contingent Workers OH. paper presented to ISEOH '98 Post Congress Workshop D, Helsinki 26 September 1998.

Babiak, P., 1995, When psychopaths go to work: a case study of an industrial psychopath. *Applied Psych.: An Intl Rev.* 44: 171-188.

Blank, V., Andersson, R., Linden, A., and Nilsson, B., 1995, Hidden accident rates and patterns in the Swedish mining industry due to the involvement of contract workers. *Safety Sci* 21: 23-35.

Chappell, D., and Di Martino, V., 1998, *Violence at Work*, International Labour Organisation, Geneva.

Dalziel, J., and Soames J. R., 1997, *Taxi Drivers and Road Safety*, report to the Federal Office of Road Safety, Department of Transport and Regional Development, Canberra.

Davis, H., Honchar, P., and Suarez, L., 1987, Fatal occupational injuries of women, Texas 1975-84. *Am. J. Public Health* 77: 1524-1527.

Driscoll, T., Mitchell, R., Mandryk, J., Healey, S., and Hendrie, L., 1998, Work-related traumatic fatalities in Australia, 1989-1992, National Occupational Health and Safety Commission, Commonwealth of Australia, Canberra.

Driscoll, T., pers. comm. 1 June 1998 unpublished paper based on preliminary data from the Second Work-Related Fatalities Study, NOHSC, Sydney.

Einarsen, S., and Skogstad, A., 1996, Bullying at work: epidemiological findings in public anf private organisations. European J. Work and Orgl Psych. 5: 185-202.

Einarsen, S., Matthiesen, S., and Skogstad, A., 1998, Bullying, burnout and well-being among assistant nurses', *J. Occ. Health Safety – Aust .& NZ*, 14: 563-568.

Foley, M., 1998, Flexible Work, Hazardous Work: The Impact of Hazardous Work Arrangements on Occupational Health and Safety in Washington State, 1991-1996. In *Research in Human Capital and Development*, JAI Press.

Giuffre, P., and Williams, C., 1994, Boundary Lines: Labeling Sexual Harassment in Restaurants. *Gender and Society,* 8: 378-401.

Grainger, C., 1997, Risk management and occupational violence. *J. Occ. Health Safety – Aust .& NZ*, 13: 541-547.

ILO, 1998, Violence On the Job – a Global Problem. *International Labour Organization Press Release* (ILO/98/30), 20 July 1998.

Jenkins, E., 1996, Workplace homicide: industries and occupations at high risk. *Occ. Med*, 11: 219-225.

Kinney, J., 1993, Health hazards to children in the service industries. *Am. J. of Ind. Med.* 24: 291-300.

Leymann, H., 1990, Mobbing and psychological terror at workplaces, *Violence and Victims*, 5: 119-126

Mayhew, C., 1997, *Barriers to Implementation of Known Occupational Health and Safety Solutions in Small Business*. National Occupational Health and Safety Commission and Queensland Division of Workplace Health and Safety, AGPS, Canberra.

Mayhew, C., 1999, Occupational Violence: a Case Study of the Taxi Industry. In *Occupational Health and Safety in Australia: Industry, Public Sector and Small Business*, (C. Mayhew and C. Peterson, eds.), Allen and Unwin, Sydney, pp.127-139.

Mayhew, C., and Johnstone, R., in press, *OHS Issues for Young Casual Workers in the Fast Food Industry*, AGPS, Canberra, p.131.

Mayhew, C., and Quinlan, M., 1997, Subcontracting and OHS in the residential building sector. *Ind Rels J.* 28: 192-205.

Mayhew, C., and Quinlan, M., 1998, *Outsourcing and Occupational Health and Safety: A Comparative Study of Factory-Based and Outworkers in the Australian TCF Industry*, Industrial Relations Research Centre, University of New South Wales, Sydney.

Mayhew, C., and Quinlan, M., 1999, The effects of outsourcing on occupational health and safety: a comparative study of factory-based and outworkers in the Australian clothing industry. *Intl J. Health Services* 29. 83-107.

Mayhew, C., Quinlan, M., and Bennett, L., 1996, *The Effects of Outsourcing Upon Occupational Health and Safety*, Industrial Relations Research Centre, The University of New South Wales.

Mayhew, C., Quinlan, M., and Ferris, R., 1997, The effects of subcontracting/outsourcing on occupational health and safety: survey evidence from four Australian industries. *Safety Sci.* 25: 163-178.

Mayhew, C., Young, C., Ferris, R., and Harnett, C., 1997, *An Evaluation of the Impact of Targeted Interventions on the OHS Behaviours of Small Business Building Industry Owners/Managers/Contractors*, National Occupational Health and Safety Commission and Queensland Division of Workplace Health and Safety, AGPS, Canberra.

McCarthy, P., Sheehan, M., and Kearns, D., 1995, *Managerial Styles and Their Effects on Employees' Health and Well-Being in Organisations Undergoing Restructuring*, report to NOHSC.

Mullen, E., 1997, Workplace violence: cause for concern or the construction of a new category of fear?. *J. Ind Rels* 39: 21-32.

Nelson, N., and Kaufman, J., 1996, Fatal and nonfatal injuries related to violence in Washington workplaces, 1992. *Am. J. Ind Med* 30: 438-446.

Netterstrom, B., and Hansen, A., 1998, Outsourcing and Stress: Physiological effects on bus drivers. paper presented to ISEOH '98 Congress, September, Helsinki.

NIOSH, 1995, *Violence in the Workplace: Risk Factors and Prevention Strategies defined*, National Institute of Occupational Safety and Health, Cincinnati.

Office of Women's Affairs (OWA), 1998, *Survey of Queensland Women 1997-1998*, Queensland Government, Brisbane.

Oregon OSHA, 1998, *Guidelines for Preventing Violence in the Workplace*, Department of Consumer and Business Services, Oregon.

OSHA, 1998, *Recommendations for Workplace Violence Prevention Programs in Late-Night Retail Establishments*, OSHA 3153 US Department of Labor, Washington DC.

OSHA *News Release* 28 April 1998.

Parker, M., 22/10/98, personal communication, WorkCover Authority of NSW, Sydney.

Rebitzer, J., 1995, Job safety and contract workers in the petrochemical industry. *Ind. Rels* 34: 40-57.

Rousseau, D., and Libuser, C., 1997, Contingent workers in high risk environments. *California Management Rev.* 39: 103-121.

Saksvik, P., 1996, Attendance pressure during organisational change. *Intl J. Stress Management* 3: 47-59.

Salminen, S., Saari, J., Saarela, K., and Rasanen, T., 1993, Organisational factors influences in serious occupational accidents. *Scand. J. Work Env. Health* 19: 352-357.

Vahtera, J., Kivimaki, M., and Pentti, J., 1998, Effects of organisational downsizing on health of employees. *The Lancet* 350: 1124-1128.

Working Women's Centre of SA, 1998, *Workplace Bullying Project*, a study funded by WorkCover and the SA Health Commission Health Promotion Unit, Adelaide.

Zapf, D., and Leymann, H., (eds.), 1996, Mobbing and victimization at work, *European J. Work Orgl Psych*, 5: 161-164.

NEW WORKING TIME ARRANGEMENTS, HEALTH AND WELL-BEING

[1,2]Torbjörn Åkerstedt, [1]Göran Kecklund, [3]Birgitta Olsson and [1]Arne Lowden
[1]*National Institute for Psychosocial Factors and Health,*[2]*Department of Public Health Sciences, Karolinska institute;* [3]*Department of Business Administration, University of Stockholm*

Abstract   *The increasing demand for more effective work procedures also affects work such that the entire 24h window is exploited for work and the work pattern ceases to be stable and predictable and instead becomes directly tailored to short term variation in production/service demand (termed "flexible"). This results in increased night work, increased duration of shifts (often demanded by employees) and work hour fragmentation. We seem to know that night work and long hours are negative factors for health. However, summarizing a number of studies we find a need for reinterpretation. Thus, permanent night work may often be more acceptable than rotating hours, particularly if the night shift ends early. Long work shifts (12h) seemed to be preferable to normal (8h) ones, at least as long as not more than 2-3 shifts are worked in a row before rest and sleep was not interfered with. Furthermore, the ability to chose one's shift schedule has strong positive effects. And, finally, reduced work hours with full pay has profound effects on social functioning, but very limited effects on health. The results suggest that influence on schedules and provisions for rest may improve most work schedules.*

1.   INTRODUCTION

The increasing demand for more effective work procedures also affects work such that the entire 24h window is exploited for work and the work pattern ceases to be stable and predictable and instead becomes directly tailored to short term variation in production/service demand (termed "flexible"). This results in increased night work, increased duration of shifts (often demanded by employees) and work hour fragmentation. We know that night work in itself is hazardous to health, as is excessive work hours. Particularly the former is associated with disturbed sleep, increased fatigue and increased accident risk (Folkard, 1997; Åkerstedt, 1998). The long work shifts have not been conclusively established as fatiguing, although accident risk appears to increase beyond 10-12h.

However, we have started to wonder if long work shifts are inherently bad, and whether individual work hour flexibility, that is, "self-selection" of work hours, may counteract the effects of, for example,

Health Effects of the New Labour Market, edited by Isaksson *et al.*
Kluwer Academic / Plenum Publishers, New York, 2000.

"flexible" work hours. These issues represent some of the innovative thinking with regard to work hours the recent years. This paper will try to bring up the two issues of duration of work hours and a high degree of influence on ones work schedule. The intention is not to produce a comprehensive review of the area but rather to illustrate some important issues as a basis for discussion. For this purpose will be used two studies of individually (computer-aided) self-selected work hours, a change from 8h three-shift work to 12h shifts, and a reduction of work hours from 8 to 6h (with full pay).

2.   METHODS

The paper will simply bring up some salient points from a series of recent studies on new types of work hours – in most cases the studies have not been published yet internationally, but only in Swedish. In all studies a questionnaire on work hours, health, sleep, stress, social effects, was used - Some key variables were: attitude to work hours (range 1-5), subjective health (1-5), mental fatigue (1-5), number of days absent, sufficient time for family/activities (1-4), work load (Karasek) (1-4).

3.   SELF-DETERMINED WORK HOURS

The first issue to bring up is self-determination of work hours. Although it is seldom discussed, it seems obvious that, for most individuals, the most restricting factor in everyday life is the obligation to be at work (or to school) for a very exactly defined time span each day. Flexibility is normally not possible and the rest of life's imperatives need to be organized around this obstacle of working time. It has never been systematically studied from a stress point of view, probably because the obstacle is so obviously there and unyielding, but one may assume that the ability to determine one's own working hours would reduce much of everyday stress. Thus the ability to influence one's work situation or other aspects of life is associated with reduced stress levels (Alfredsson et. al., 1985; Karasek and Theorell, 1990).

However, flexible work hours only pertain to the start and end of a work shift – the core remains where it has always been (Wade, 1974). An alternative is to have the ability to position also the core of one's work period anywhere in the 24h cycle or even week. Traditionally, this has been a privilege of many self-employed individuals – particularly authors, painters and similar groups, but also doctors, lawyers, etc even if these groups have to consider their availability to clients/patients. To permit also other groups, in industry, health care, retail etc the same privilege has not really been seriously considered before. However, a series of spontaneous experiments are presently under way and two of these will be presented here.

3.1   Health care

The first concerns hospitals within the Swedish health care system which have adopted different types of flexible work hours. These hospitals, or rather clinics, have introduced a "credit" system of work hours. This permits the individual to select a "tailor made" combination of work shifts according to own preferences. Each hour worked yields a credit according to its attractiveness (based on negotiations) and forms the basis of the salary. The selection is carried out with the help of a computer program (Time Care®) that stores the choices, makes sure that the optimum staff level is reached for all work hours. Gaps in schedules are handled through discussion and bids and a last resort for solving incompatibilities is a "lottery" procedure organized by the program.

To study the effects of these work hours we selected a group of 292 nurses from 6 clinics (Åkerstedt et. al., 1996). This included one with the credit system and others with flexible work hours or with traditional fixed hours – night plus day shifts.   A questionnaire was used to obtain information on background (age, gender, etc), influence on work hours and work situation, social effects, sleep, stress, social support, health, etc.

The results show that a high level of influence is associated with positive attitudes to the work hours, better social functioning and satisfaction with the work situation. The clinic with the credit system had the most positive values, while clinics with traditional work hours had the most negative values. In particular, social aspects of work improved, whereas health did not show any clear differences between systems. Stepwise multiple regression showed that the main factor associated with satisfaction with the total work situation was satisfaction with work hours ($R^2=0.32$), which, in turn, was predicted by "influence on work hours" ($R^2=0.27$).

The study did not include a long term follow-up, but the results suggest very positive effects of self-determined work hours. The system is now rapidly spreading to other parts of the health care system.

3.2   Retail

To study whether the effects would be positive in other areas we followed the introduction of the same type of system in six department stores – 109 individuals and compared these with 39 individuals from a department store which retained their original scheduling procedure (Lowden and

Åkerstedt, 1999). The employees could chose which days to work and what start and stop times they would like.

A questionnaire was filled out before and one year after the introduction of the system. The results showed that self-determined work hours have strong positive effects on social well-being – time for oneself and friends – and were very popular. On the other hand, no clear effects on health (in the short run) were observed. In particular the younger seemed to appreciate the potential of the system and especially the possibility to take several days off in sequence. A negative aspect was that staffing was reduced.

It was concluded that the self-determined work hours significantly improved the situation for the employees. Apparently, the approach is possible to implement also in retail.

4.   A SHORTER WORKING DAY

We have noted above that the positioning of work hours in the 24h cycle has a profound influence on health and well-being. We have also seen that being able to choose when to work has positive effects. Studies on the most important factor would obviously be the total number of work hours. Work hours have been gradually reduced since the traditional 12h day / 6-day week. However, systematic effects on health and well-being are scarce (Harrington, 1994; Rosa, 1995). However, studies from the British munitions industry clearly indicated very positive effects on health, well being and production from a reduction of work hours from approximately 56 to 48h (Vernon, 1920). There also seems to exist a (50h) above which work hours start to have negative effects on health dubbelarbete (Theorell, 1991). However, how would a shortened working week affect us if we start reducing from the present, relatively moderate, working week of 40h?

A shorter working day has for a long time been debated as a countermeasure against excessive fatigue at work. During the recent years, however, reduction of unemployment has been introduced as the main argument for shortened work hours. With a focus on the former we have carried out a study of a reduction of daily work hours from 8h to 6h (Olsson et. al., 1999). It was part of a larger study which also included economical aspects. The project was initiated by the city of Stockholm and carried out by the Department of Business Administration at the University of Stockholm in collaboration with the National Institute for Psychosocial Factors and Health and The Department of Public Health Sciences of the Karolinska institute.

The project involved 96 individuals employed at different care centres, 1/3 of which served as a comparison group. The reduction from 8h to 6h was compensated for by employing extra personnel. The study involved three points of measurement with one year in-between – before the reduction, and 1 and 2 years afterwards. At each point in time a questionnaire was administered and a clinical investigation (blood pressure and blood samples for analysis of cortisol, prolactin, etc) was carried out.

Analysis of variance was used to evaluate the results and showed that the positive attitude to works hours had increased dramatically for the experimental group. An equally dramatic increase was seen for the variable "sufficient time for social activities"; in particular time for friends and time for own relaxation was increased. Health (absenteeism, somatic symptoms, incidence of disease, etc) was not significantly affected, apart from some positive effects on subjective sleep. The group that seemed to benefit the most from the reduction was parents with small children.

5.   A LONGER WORKING DAY

If a shorter workday has strong positive effects on attitude and social factors, then one might assume that the opposite would hold for a longer working day. This is an important issue since the interest in compressed work schedules and long shifts (in particular 12h) has increased in working life. But there is a lack of knowledge of how extended work hours (primarily 12-hour shifts) and short rests (<16 hours) affect sleep, safety and health. Or rather, the results are contradictory and often suggest improved well-being with long shifts (Harrington, 1994; Rosa, 1995).

To gain information about the effects of long shifts we initiated a study at a chemical plant which was changing from a rapidly rotating three shift (8 hours of rest between shifts) to a 12-hour shift schedule. The aim was to study the effects on sleepiness, performance, sleep and recuperation, health and attitude towards work and work hours. A questionnaire was answered by the shift workers (n=32) a few months before, and one year after the introduction of the shift change. Fourteen of these workers also participated in an intensive study of sleep/wake rhythms in both shift schedules by use of motion loggers, sleep/wake diary, and performance testing at the beginning and end of work. Another group of day-time workers at the same plant served as a control group (n=14).

Questionnaire data showed that the shift change increased satisfaction with work hours (Lowden et. al., 1996; Lowden et. al., 1998). Also positive effects on social life and a reduction of sleep complaints were reported. Feelings of discomfort were reduced at work, as well as work stress. The control of the work process increased. The 12-hour shift did not increase perceived accident risks and this was confirmed by the performance measures not showing any decrements across extended shifts. The precision at shift change hours was rated to be better but the contact between shift teams was decreased. The ability to wind down after work was made greater, the recovery from night work was better, and tiredness was reduced. Evaluations of the change showed that shift workers were most positive towards the increased amount of free days.

Data from the motion loggers demonstrated that sleep after night shift work was shortened (5.5 hr, sleep need was 7.3 hr). The quick rotation from afternoon to morning involved a sleep loss that took three days of morning shifts to recuperate from. When the quick rotation was removed, sleep increased prior to day shift (12-hour). Ratings of sleepiness during work showed a slow adaptation to night work. Most sleepiness was observed on the first night shift and particularly during the late night. Extension of work was always on parts of the day with normally high alertness (evening and afternoon). Symptoms of sleepiness were predominant on the night shifts on the 8-hour shift but also during the first morning shift that was preceded by a afternoon shift.

The reasons for the positive effects are unclear but it appears that the stability of having only two types of work hours (day and night work) to adjust to was perceived as an improvement. A second important factor was the frequently occurring days off (every two or three days) which seem to have prevented any build-up of fatigue. A third contributing factor was probably the reduced number of commutes.

The results, once again, suggest surprising advantages of long work shifts. However, it should be emphasised that results might be different in occupation with very high load, or with difficulties of taking breaks spontaneously. Also, long sequences of 12h shifts may have negative effects.

6.   RELATION TO OTHER TYPES OF WORK HOURS

In order to put our thinking of work hours into perspective it might be worthwhile to compare different types of work hour arrangements on some central variables – even if work tasks and ages may not be exactly equal. For this purpose we used our files from a number of different studies on different work hour systems and simply tabulated the "attitude to the present work hours" (1=very negative, 2=rather negative, 3=neither positive nor negative, 4=rather positive, 5=very positive), "rated subjective health" (1=very poor, 2=rather poor, 3=neither good nor poor, 4=rather good, 5=very good), and "sufficient time for social activities" (an index ranging from 1=completely insufficient, 2=insufficient, 3=not quite sufficient, 4=sufficient).

Figure 1 shows that high satisfaction scores between "rather positive" and "very positive" were given by: roster workers on *self/selected* schedule (health care-see above), *6h* day workers (care-see above), self/selected permanent *night* workers (industry), *12h* day/night workers in chemical industry (after change from 8h 3-shift work), 8h *Day* workers in a power plant, and 8h *Day* workers in the chemical industry. A second group of positive to intermediate ratings were given by: two groups of *roster* workers (in health care) with night and day work, *roster* workers in retail with day work only, *8h 3-shift* workers (chemical industry before change to 12h work shifts), *8h 3-shift* workers in the energy industry, and finally, *2-shift* workers in the auto industry (one week of morning shifts and one week of afternoon shifts).

COMPARISON OF WORK SCHEDULES

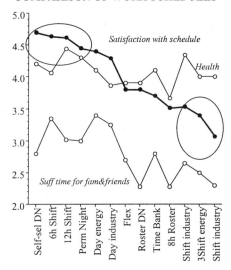

Figure 1. Mean attitude (5-1) to other work hour systems, self rated health (5-1) and sufficient time for social activities (4-1) in different groups. The most positive and negative groups are indicated by circles.

The latter group had the most negative attitude we have found this far. Apparently, the reason was the fatigue during the morning week, together with the inability to use the evening prime time optimally (due to the early rising the next day), and the negative social effects also during the afternoon week. Note that subjective health does not follow the popularity curve, but that "sufficient time for family and friends" does.

One needs to be careful when interpreting data such as the ones presented in this section, but they at least suggest that work hours can be attractive for unexpected reasons and creative work hour arrangements may have very positive effects.

7.   FINAL COMMENTS

The present paper has only sought to emphasize some new trends in with respect to the temporal aspects of working life – influence, reduced work hours and increased work shift length. The results are interesting but there is still much research to be accomplished. There are also other areas of importance where almost nothing is known and in which the present trends towards "flexibilisation" of working life leave tracks. One such area is the patterning of days off – how many days off do we need? And what is their relation to previous workload.

REFERENCES

Åkerstedt, T. Shift work and disturbed sleep/wakefulness. *Sleep Medicine Reviews* 1998,2:117-128.

Alfredsson, L. Spetz, C.-L. and Theorell, T. Type of occupation and near-future hospitalization for myocardial infarction and some other diagnoses. *Int J Epidem* 1985,14:378-388.

Folkard, S. Black times: Temporal determinants of transport safety. *Accid Anal & Prev* 1997,29:417-430.

Harrington, J. M. Shift work and health - a critical review of the literature on working hours. *Ann Acad Med Singapore* 1994,23:699-705.

Karasek, R. and Theorell, T. eds. *Healthy Work*. Basic Book, New York, 1990.

Lowden, A. Kecklund, G. Axelsson, J. and Åkerstedt, T. Övergång från 8 till 12 timmars skift. 268, Stressforskningsrapporter, 1996.

Lowden, A. Kecklund, G. Axelsson, J. and Åkerstedt, T. Change from an 8-hour shift to a 12-hour shift, attitudes, sleep, sleepiness and performance. *Scand J Work Environ Health* 1998,24 (suppl 3):69-75.

Lowden, A. and Åkerstedt, T. Självvalda arbetstider inom handeln - effekter på hälsa och välbefinnande. *Stressforskningsrapporter* 1999,in press:

Olsson, B. Åkerstedt, T. Ingre, M. Holmgren, M. and Kecklund, G. Kortare arbetsdag, hälsa och välbefinnande. *Stressforskningsrapporter* 1999,281:

Rosa, R. Extended workshifts and excessive fatigue. *J Sleep Res* 1995,4 (suppl 2):51-56.

Theorell, T. Psychosocial cardiovascular risks - on the double loads in women. *Psychother Psychosom* 1991,55:81-89.

Vernon, H. M. Industrial efficiency and fatigue. In: E.L. Collis, (Eds). *The Industrial Clinic*. John Bale and Sons, London, 1920:51-74.

Wade, M. eds. *Flexible working hours in practice*. Wiley, New York, 1974.

Åkerstedt, T. Westerlund, M. and Andersson, G. Mot bättre tider: en utvärdering av några av vårdens arbetstidsmodeller med avseende på välbefinnande och hälsa. *Stressforskningsrapporter* 1996,271:1-26.

DETERMINANTS OF THE ATTITUDE TO WORK AND SUBJECTIVE HEALTH

Göran Kecklund, Torbjörn Åkerstedt, John Axelsson and Arne Lowden
[1]National Institute for Psychosocial Factors and Health, and the Dept. for PublicHealth, Section for Psychosocial Factors, Karolinska Institutet, Box 230, Stockholm, Sweden

Abstract: Shift workers' attitude to work hours is determined by insufficient time for social activities, and ratings of poor sleep quality and sleepiness, whereas the attitude to the work situation is determined by psychosocial work factors. The aim of the present paper was to examine whether this is also seen in a group of day time workers. Secondly, we investigated whether the predicted association could be replicated when independent measures were. Finally, the relation between self-rated health and attitude questions was also examined. Sample 1 included 110 day time workers (only questionnaire data) and sample 2 included 22 three-shift workers (questionnaire and diary data). In sample 1, a negative attitude to work hours was mainly associated with insufficient time for social activities, poor sleep quality, a poor psychosocial work climate and young age. A negative attitude to the work situation was predicted by a poor psychosocial work climate, a poor self-rated health (SRH), insufficient time for social activities, and having few small children. SRH, pain, and anxiety/depressive complaints were mainly associated with the attitude to the work situation, whereas sleep quality was associated with the attitude to work hours. In the sample of three-shift workers, a negative attitude to work hours was associated with a high level of sleepiness, whereas a negative attitude to the work situation was associated with a negative attitude to work hours and low influence over work tasks. A poor sleep quality was associated with a negative attitude to work hours. The results confirmed our hypothesis that the attitude to work hours is related to insufficient time for social activities, sleep quality and sleepiness. Psychosocial work factors, in particular psychosocial support and climate as well as influence over work, and the attitude to work hours were the main predictors of the attitude to the work situation.

1. INTRODUCTION

It is well known that work hours can influence health. For example, shift work (including night work) is a risk factor for cardiovascular disease (Knutsson et al. 1986; Tenkanen et al. 1997). Overtime work and long work days are other aspects related to work hours that may increase the risk for diseases (Alfredsson and Theorell 1983; Åkerstedt 1996). However, most of the empirical support of the relation between work hours and health comes

Health Effects of the New Labour Market, edited by Isaksson *et al.*
Kluwer Academic / Plenum Publishers, New York, 2000.

from studies using self-rated health or well-being measures (Costa 1996; Åkerstedt 1996).

An interesting question is whether it is possible to develop a measure that integrates the strain that work hours cause on the subject. A simple question of the subjects' attitude to work hours could be a potential candidate for such a measure. The attitude to work hours has received little scientific attention. In a preliminary study on shift workers, we found that a negative attitude to work hours was associated with poor sleep, sleepiness and insufficient time for social activities (Åkerstedt and Kecklund 1995). The association between a low satisfaction of work hours and social problems was also found by Kundi and coworkers (1995). In their study a significant correlation between satisfaction with work hours and subjective health was also reported. Other potential determinants may be the length of the work shift, the possibility to take breaks, the timing of the shifts, and the influence (flexibility) over work hours.

In a comparison between various work hour systems, Åkerstedt found that shift workers had a more negative attitude to their work hours than daytime workers (see paper by Åkerstedt in this volume). Furthermore, it was also found that when the work schedule was improved, the attitude became more positive (Lowden et al, 1996). Those groups who had a very positive attitude to work hours also seemed to report less social problems.

The attitude to work hours co-vary strongly with the attitude to the work situation in general (Lowden et al. 1996; Åkerstedt et al. 1996). However, the attitude to the work situation is also predicted by the psychosocial situation at the work place, for example the influence over work tasks, and the social support, or the climate. Among the potential determinants that have not been examined in previous studies, gender and family situation is of great interest. The "double" work load (both paid and unpaid work at home) that represents the life situation of many women may influence their attitudes to work hours and work in general. It has been shown that a moderate amount of overtime work was associated with an increased risk of myocardial infarction in women, but not in men (Theorell, 1991). Theorell suggested that the reason for this may be related to womens traditional social role characterised of strain due to home and family responsibilities as well as due to psychosocial stress related to paid work. Another social determinant, which may influence attitudes to work is having small children, which often causes a more strenuous and stressful social situation.

Our previous studies have mainly concerned shift work groups. Thus, we don't know whether our findings are applicable on day workers as well. Furthermore, the association between the attitude to work hours and complaints about poor sleep and sleepiness may suffer from methodological problems. Since only questionnaire method have been used, the covariation between the measures may be overestimated due to similar construction of the questions and of the response alternatives (for example, the response alternatives have been based on five-point scale for all questions). The fact that the questions usually have been placed close to each other in the questionnaire may also increase the co-variation. This problem could, however, be solved by using independent measures and instruments.

The aim of the present study was to examine which factors that determine the attitude to work hours for daytime and shift workers, respectively – is the pattern of relations between variables stable for different work hour systems? Another aim was to examine the determinants of the attitude to the work situation. According to our previous findings the attitude to the work situation will be related to psychosocial work factors and, perhaps, to the attitude to work hours, whereas the attitude to work hours should be associated with insufficient time for social activities, and with complaints of sleep and sleepiness. The relation between measures of self-rated health and the attitude questions will also be examined. In the analysis of shift workers, sleep and sleepiness was measured through a diary, instead of a questionnaire (which has been used in previous studies). Can the predicted connection between sleep, sleepiness and attitude to work hours be replicated despite the change in method?

2.   METHOD

Two samples were used. The first sample (study 1) included 110 day time (83 males and 27 females) workers who worked between 07 and 16 hours in a paper mill in southern Sweden. Their work tasks were mainly maintenance and administrative work. The second sample (study 2) included 22 three-shift workers (18 males and 4 females) who worked in a power plant in the Stockholm area. Their shift schedule is presented in table 1. Age and marital status are given in the results section.

The subjects filled out a questionnaire on background (age, gender etc.), work situation, health symptoms (including sleep items), and well-being.

The following questions and indices were used in the present analysis:
- Attitudes to work hours and to the work situation (1=very negative, 2=rather negative, 3=neither negative nor positive, 4=rather positive, 5=very positive)
- Work demands (1 high – 4 low), possibility to influence work tasks (1= low, 4=high) and positive psychosocial factors related to work (the items address attitude statements of social support and the social climate at the work place, the response alternatives ranged between 1=definitely

disagree, 4=definitely agree). These scales have been developed by Theorell and coworkers (1988).

Table 1. Shift schedule [A-F=shift teams, D=day shift (07.00-16.00), A=afternoon shift (15.00-23.00), M=morning shift (07.00-15.00), **M**= morning shift (07.00-19.00), N=night shift (23.00-07.00), **N**=night shift (19.00-07.00), blank=day off, bold letters=12-hour shifts].

Team	1							2							3						
	Mo	Tu	We	Th	Fr	Sc	Su	Mo	Tu	We	Th	Fr	Sc	Su	Mo	Tu	We	Th	Fr	Sc	Su
A	D	D	D	D	D			A	A	A	A				**M**	**M**	**M**	**M**	**N**	**N**	**N**
B								D	D	D	D	D			A	A	A	A			
C	N	N	N	N											D	D	D	D	D		
D					**M**	**M**	**M**	N	N	N	N										
E	**M**	**M**	**M**	**M**	**N**	**N**	**N**					**M**	**M**	**M**	N	N	N	N			
F	A	A	A	A				**M**	**M**	**M**	**M**	**N**	**N**	**N**					**M**	**M**	**M**

Team	4							5							6						
	Mo	Tu	We	Th	Fr	Sc	Su	Mo	Tu	We	Th	Fr	Sc	Su	Mo	Tu	We	Th	Fr	Sc	Su
A					**M**	**M**	**M**	N	N	N	N										
B	**M**	**M**	**M**	**M**	**N**	**N**	**N**					**M**	**M**	**M**	N	N	N	N			
C	A	A	A	A				**M**	**M**	**M**	**M**	**N**	**N**	**N**					**M**	**M**	**M**
D	D	D	D	D	D			A	A	A	A				**M**	**M**	**M**	**M**	**N**	**N**	**N**
E								D	D	D	D	D			A	A	A	A			
F	N	N	N	N											D	D	D	D	D		

- Self-rated health (SRH; 1=very poor, 2=rather poor, 3=neither poor nor good, 4=rather good, and 5=very good).
- Indices relating to pain (back pain, stiff muscles, pain in legs or arm), gastrointestinal problems (pain in the stomach, nausea, poor apetite, hunger pangs, constipation, diarrhoea, flatulence and heartburn) and anxiety/depressive symptoms (worried, depressed, restlessness, passive, lack of initiative, listless, and feeling of meaninglessness).
- Karolinska Sleep Questionnaire (Kecklund and Åkerstedt 1992a) with the items "difficulties falling asleep"," difficulties waking-up", "not feeling well-rested", "disturbed sleep", "exhausted at wake-up time", and "sleepiness during work and free time" (the response alternatives were *never, seldom*: sometimes per year, *occasionally* : some time per month, *often*: some time per week, and *always*: several times per week). They also rated "sleep quality" (how do you sleep in general; 1=very poor, 2=rather poor, 3=neither poor nor good, 4=rather good, 5=very good), "sufficient sleep" (do you get enough sleep in general; 1=definitely too little, 2=too little, 3=somewhat too little, 4=more or less enough, 5=definitely enough), their habitual sleep need, and their diurnal type – morningness/eveningness (Torsvall and Åkerstedt 1980).

- Indices related to whether work hours interfered with social interaction (insufficient time to meet with friends, spouse and children) or with social activities (insufficient time for relaxation, household activities, organisational activities, to watch TV, hobbies, daily errands, to visit a doctor or a dentist).

In study 2, the subjects filled in a sleep/wake diary during a (42 day) shift cycle. The instrument included the Karolinska Sleep Diary (Åkerstedt et al. 1994b). A sleep quality index (SQI) was calculated for each main sleep episode using the items "sleep quality" (how was your sleep?), "ease of falling asleep", "restless sleep" and "slept throughout". The SQI (1=very poor, 5=very good) has been shown to co-vary with several physiological sleep parameters (Åkerstedt et al. 1994a). The items "sufficient sleep" (1=definitely too little sleep, 5=definitely enough sleep), "well-rested/refreshed from sleep" (1=not rested at all, 5= completely rested), and "ease of awakening" (1=very difficult to wake-up, 5=very easy to wake-up) were treated as separate components of sleep.

During every even hour (when they were awake) the subjects rated their alertness/sleepiness level on the Karolinska Sleepiness Scale (Åkerstedt and Gillberg 1990). KSS is a nine-point scale (1=very alert, 3=alert, 5=neither alert nor sleepy, 7=sleepy, but no problem to stay awake, 9=very sleepy, fighting sleep, almost impossible to stay awake) and covary with physiological sleepiness and performance. For the diary measures, a mean was computed across the entire shift cycle.

3.   RESULTS

3.1   Study 1: Day time workers

Table 2 shows the means and standard error for all variables. The variables were correlated with the attitude to work hours and the attitude to the work situation, respectively (see table 2 for results).

The attitude to work hours showed significant correlations with age, DTS, work demands, psychosocial work factors, SRH, difficulties waking-up, not being well-rested, exhausted at wake-up time, daytime sleepiness, sleep quality, sufficient sleep and both social indices. Thus, a negative attitude to the work hours was associated with low age, being an evening type, a poor psychosocial work situation, high work demands, poor health, sleep problems (except for the items difficulties initiating sleep and disturbed sleep) and insufficient time for social interaction and social activities.

Table 2. Means, standard error of the mean (±se) and correlation coefficient (r), n=110.

variables	mean±se	attitude - work hours, r	attitude - work situation, r
Age	42±1	0.43***	0.07
Gender; % males	75	0.07	0.02
Marital status, % cohabit	86	-0.16	-0.11
Children living at home, % <7 years	26	-0.02	0.16
Diurnal Type Scale (DTS, 1 evening type – 4 morning type)	2.8±0.05	0.29**	0.24*
Attitude to work hours (1 neg-5 pos.)	4.3±0.06	-	0.36***
Attitude to work situation (1 neg-5 pos)	4.0±0.07	0.36***	-
Work demands (1 high – 4 low)	2.6±0.05	0.25*	0.19*
Influence over work tasks (1 low – 4 high)	3.0±0.05	0.03	0.25**
Psychosocial work factors (1 poor – 4 good)	3.0±0.05	0.30**	0.46***
Self-rated health (SRH,1 poor – 5 good)	4.0±0.09	0.21*	0.45***
Pain index (1 always – 5 never)	4.1±0.08	0.14	0.34***
Gastrointestinal index (1 always – 5 never)	4.5±0.04	0.07	0.17
Depressive/anxiety symptoms (1 always – 5 never)	4.4±0.06	0.08	0.42***
Diff. falling asleep (1 – 5 never)	4.1±0.08	0.04	0.20*
Diff. waking-up (1 always-5 never)	3.9±0.11	0.23*	0.10
Not well-rested (1 always-5 never)	3.5±0.11	0.22*	0.30**
Disturbed sleep (1 always-5 never)	3.8±0.10	0.08	0.22
Exhausted at wake-up (1-5 never)	4.0±0.09	0.24*	0.34***
Daytime sleepiness (1 always-5 never)	3.8±0.10	0.28**	0.22*
Sleep quality (1 poor –5 good)	4.0±0.08	0.31***	0.36***
Sufficient sleep (1 never-5 definitely)	3.8±0.08	0.39***	0.23*
Habitual sleep need (hours)	7.2±0.09	-0.07	-0.03
Social interaction index (1 definitely insufficient time – 4 sufficient time)	2.8±0.01	0.38***	0.20*
Social activities index (see above)	3.1±0.06	0.42***	0.29**

*=p<0.05, **=p<0.01, ***=p<0.001

The following variables showed a significant correlation with the attitude to the work situation; DTS, work demands, influence over work tasks, psychosocial work factors, SRH, pain-index, depressive/anxiety symptoms, difficulties falling asleep, not being well-rested, exhausted at wake-up time, daytime sleepiness, sleep quality, sufficient sleep and both social indices.

A negative attitude to the work situation was associated with being an evening type, high work demands, low influence over work tasks, a poor psychosocial work climate, poor health, poor sleep (including difficulties falling asleep and not being well-rested), frequent complaints of daytime sleepiness, a feeling of not getting enough sleep, and insufficient time for social interaction and social activities. As expected, both attitude questions were highly inter correlated (r=0.36, p<0.001).

A separate analysis was made for gender and the attitudes to work. In this analysis, the variable "having children under 7 years living at home" was added as a second factor in a two-way ANOVA. The results for the ANOVA is presented in table 3. None of the effects became significant. Thus, females did not differ with respect to attitudes to work. However, females having small children did report the most negative attitude to work hours. Since this group was very small (n=7), the statistical power was weak and in larger sample the differences may be statistically significant.

Table 3. Means, standard error (±se) and p-values for a two-way ANOVA ("gender" x "small children"), n=110.

Attitudes to work hours (1 negative – 5 positive)

Having small children		2-way ANOVA
	no (means±se)	yes (means±se)	
			gender,p=0.99
males	4.3±0.1 (n=61)	4.4±0.1 (n=22)	children, p=0.42
females	4.5±0.2 (n=20)	4.1±0.1 (n=7)	interaction, p=0.18

Attitude to the work situation (1 negative – 5 positive)

Having small children		2-way ANOVA
	no (means±se)	yes (means±se)	
			gender, p=0.74
males	3.9±0.1 (n=61)	4.3±0.1 (n=22)	children, p=0.39
females	4.1±0.2 (n=20)	4.0±0.0 (n=7)	interaction, p=0.26

The attitude questions were also subjected to a stepwise multiple regression analysis (MRA). The first analysis examined the attitude to work hours as the dependent variable, and with all the other variables in table 2 as predictors (except the attitude to the work situation). Five predictors entered the regression. The first predictor to enter was the social activity index (R2=22%), followed by sleep quality (R2 increased with 9%), psychosocial work factors (+5%), age (+5%), and finally, children under 7 years (+3%). These variables explained 46% of the variance (F=15.0, p<0.001). The beta coefficients of the last step were 0.27 for social activities, 0.22 for sleep quality, 0.24 for psychosocial work factors, 0.33 for age, and 0.19 for children under 7 years.

Thus, a negative attitude to the work hours was predicted by insufficient time for social activites, poor sleep quality, a poor psychosocial work climate, young age, and few children (living at home) under 7 years. The analysis was repeated but with gender as a forced predictor. The results did not change when the effect of gender was controlled for.

The same predictors (including the attitude the work hours) were also used in a stepwise MRA with the attitude to the work situation as the dependent variable. Four predictors became significant: (1) the psychosocial work situation (R^2=16%), (2) SRH (+12%), (3) social activities (+5%), and (4) children under 7 years (+2%, R^2 total=35% explained variance, F=12.0, p<0.001). The beta coefficient for the last step were 0.26 for psychosocial work situation, 0.37 for SRH, 0.26 for social activities, and 0.16 for children under 7 years. A negative attitude to the work situation was predicted by a poor psychosocial work situation, poor health, insufficient time for social activities, and few children (living at home) under 7 years. Again, the analysis was repeated with control for gender. In this analysis, the last step (children under 7 years) was no longer significant and R^2 decreased to 33%.

In order to test whether the work related variables could predict the subjective health measures, four stepwise MRA were carried out with SRH, the pain-index, sleep quality and depressive/anxiety symptoms as dependent variables. The predictors were age, attitude to work hours as well as to the work situation, work demands, influence over work tasks, psychosocial work factors and marital status.

SRH was predicted by the attitude to the work situation (R^2=20%, beta=0.45, p<0.001). Sleep quality was predicted by the attitude to work hours (R^2=14%) and by the attitude to the work situation (+3%, p<0.001). The pain-index was predicted by the attitude to the work situation (R^2=12%) and by influence over work tasks (+5%, p<0.001). Finally, the depressive/anxiety symptoms was predicted by the attitude to the work situation (R^2=14%) and psychosocial work factors (+3%, p<0.001).

In general, the attitude questions could predict the health measures and explained more variance than the more specific questions about work demands, influence over work tasks and psychosocial work climate or support.

3.2   Study 2: three-shift workers

The means and the correlations with attitude to work hours and attitude to work situation are presented in table 4. Significant correlations with the attitude to work hours were found for KSS, SQI, both social indices and SRH. A negative attitude to work hours was associated with a high level of sleepiness, poor sleep, insufficient time for social interaction and social activites, and poor health. These variables and age were included in a stepwise MRA with the attitude to work hours as the dependent variable. KSS became the only significant predictor ($R2=43\%$, beta=-0.66, $p<0.001$). Thus, a high level of sleepiness predicted a negative attitude to work hours. As indicated by the MRA, KSS was highly correlated with the other predictors (SQI, r=-0.67, $p<0.001$; social interaction, r=-0.55, $p<0.01$; social activities, r=-0.64, $p<0.01$; SRH, r=-0.46, $p<0.05$). A high level of sleepiness is associated with poor sleep, insufficient time for social activities and social interaction and poor health.

The attitude to the work situation showed only two significant correlations, except the expected correlation with attitude to work hours. Thus, a negative attitude to the work situation was associated with low influence over work tasks and insufficient time for social interactions. When these two variables were included in the MRA (together with age, marital status, children <7 years and the attitude to work hours), the attitude to work hours was the first predictor to enter the regression ($R2=28\%$, beta in the last step=0.48). In the second (and final) step

Table 4. Means, standard error (±se) and correlations (r) with the attitude to work hours and attitude to work situation, respectively (n=22).

variables	mean±se	attitude – work hours (r)	attitude - work situation (r)
Age (years)	38±2	0.03	-0.03
Marital status, % cohabit	64	0.01	-0.09
Children <7 years (%)	32%	-0.08	0.10
Experience of night work (years)	13±1.6	0.27	0.32
Travel time to work (minutes)	34±3	-0.15	-0.34
Karolinska Sleepiness Scale (KSS, 1 alert – 9 sleepy)	4.2±0.16	-0.66***	-0.38
Sleep quality index (SQI, 1 poor-5 good)	4.4±0.09	0.56**	0.16
Well-rested (1 definitely not – 5 yes)	3.4±0.12	0.34	0.13
Sufficient sleep (1 definitely not – 5 yes)	3.7±0.11	0.25	0.01
Ease awakening (1 definitely not – 5 yes)	3.3±0.13	0.12	0.04
DTS (1 evening type – 4 morning type)	2.4±0.10	0.15	0.03
Habitual sleep need (hours)	7.6±0.16	-0.36	-0.03
Self-rated health (SRH, 1 poor – 5 good)	4.3±0.2	0.50*	0.13
Attitude work hours (1 neg. – 5 pos.)	4.4±0.14	-	0.51*
Attitude work situation (1 neg. – 5 pos.)	3.7±0.19	0.51*	-
Work demands (1 low – 4 high)	2.5±0.07	0.29	-0.07
Influence over work tasks (1 low – 4 high)	2.9±0.06	0.11	0.43*
Psychosocial work factors (1 poor-4 good)	3.1±0.09	0.22	0.23
Social interaction index (1 definitely insufficient time – 4 sufficient time)	3.1±0.18	0.60**	0.44*
Social activities index (see above)	3.3±0.13	0.58**	0.39

*=$p<0.05$, **=$p<0.01$, ***=$p<0.001$

influence over work tasks entered and increased the amount of explained variance with 14% (R2 total=42%, p<0.01, beta=0.37). Thus, a negative attitude to the work situation was predicted by a negative attitude to work hours and low possibilities to influence work.

SRH and the SQI was also subjected to a MRA with the following predictors; age, marital status, the attitude questions, work demands, influence over work tasks, and psychosocial work factors. None of the predictors entered the regression for SRH. The SQI was predicted by the attitude to work hours (R2=33%, beta coefficient in the last step=0.59) and by age (R2=+11%, beta=-0.33). These predictors explained 44% of the variance (p<0.01). A poor sleep quality was associated with a negative attitude to work hours and increased age.

4. DISCUSSION

The results demonstrated that the attitude to work hours was strongly associated with insufficient time for social activities and interaction with family and friends. However, poor sleep and high levels of sleepiness were also associated with a negative attitude to work hours. In the group of day-time workers, the social determinants became the strongest, whereas sleepiness was the strongest in the three-shift group. This finding seems logical since the shift workers, due to their irregular work hours, experience higher levels of sleepiness and sleep problems. Thus, as predicted, sleep, sleepiness and insufficient time for social life determined much of the variation in the attitude to work hours.

In the day-time group, age and having children under 7 years also explained some of the variance, although the amount was rather small. Low age and having few children under 7 year were associated with a negative attitude to work hours. The fact that young subjects were more negative could be related to a difference in morning/eveningness. Thus, age correlated strongly with diurnal type (r=0.39, p<0.001) – young subjects were more evening prone and may experience more sleep/wake problems related to the relatively early start time of the work day. Indeed, age also showed several rather strong correlations with sleep/wake problems, for example sleepiness (r=0.43, p<0.001), difficulties waking-up (r=0.45,

p<0.001) and sufficient sleep (r=0.38, p<0.001). Thus, the young workers complained more about sleepiness, difficulties waking-up and insufficient sleep.

The direction of the relation between having children under 7 years and the attitude to work hours was unexpected. One would suspect that having small children must interact with one of the other predictors. Indeed such an interaction was found with age, but not for the other two significant

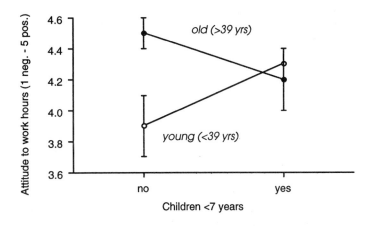

Figure 1. Means and se for the question attitude to work hours. The figure shows the significant interaction etween age and having children under 7 years. Young group=open circles and old group=filled circles.

predictors. The interaction between having children under 7 years and age (p=0.05) is presented in figure 1. The difference within the "older" group (39 years or more) between those having small children and those without small children was small, whereas a clear effect was found within the "younger" group – those who had no children had a more negative attitude to work hours. Within the "younger" group, those who had no small children rated more problems with insufficient time for social interaction (mean: 1.8±0.2) compared with the young subjects who had small children (mean: 2.6±0.2, p<0.01). Thus, it may be that the work hours for the young subjects who had no small children interfered with their (probably more active) social life.

In the introduction, we hypothesised that gender and family situation could be important social determinants for the attitudes to work hours. This was not confirmed in the present analyses. On the other hand, the number of women in the study was small. Since the sample was middle-aged, most of the subjects had no young children. It is clear that we could not test whether women, and in particular those who has a high work load at home, may be more negative to work hours and to the work situation. This question, as well as other social factors, should be explored in future studies. Thus, one needs to be cautious with generalising the present results to other occupations where women and younger subjects are dominating.

In the introduction, we suggested that psychosocial work variables and the attitude to work hours should be the major determinants of the attitude to the work situation. The present analyses confirmed this hypothesis. In the day time group, the psychosocial support and climate at the work place became the strongest predictor, whereas in the shift work group attitude to work hours and the possibility to influence work were the significant predictors. It may be that work hours have a stronger impact on the perception of work in general for shift workers. Certainly, shift work is much more difficult to tolerate compared to day work.

In the day-time group, insufficient time for social activities, poor health, and not having any children under 7 years explained a minor amount of the variance in the attitude to the work situation. Again, the contribution of the variable "children under 7 years" was small and in an unexpected direction. However, there was an interaction between having small children and "insufficient time for social activities" (having small children showed no interaction with the other significant predictors). Thus, subjects having no small children and who perceived that work interfered with social activities had a more negative attitude to the work situation. However, the interaction was weak and it can not be ruled out that the finding was spurious.

The relation between health and attitude to work seems more reliable, although it is difficult to judge the most likely direction of the association. According to our point of view, a poor work situation may be a cause of ill health. On the other hand, ill health can also decrease work ability and make it more difficult to tolerate a demanding work situation. The relation between insufficient time for social activity and the attitude to the work situation disappeared when the attitude to work hours was controlled for by forcing it into the regression. This analysis suggests that the relation between attitude to work and insufficient time for social activity was spurious.

In the day-time group, some of the sleep variables also correlated with the attitude to the work situation. However, they did not enter the regression. As one may expect, many of the sleep variables correlated rather strongly with the index of psychosocial support at the work place (e.g. sleepiness, $r=0.33$, $p<0.001$; sleep quality, $r=0.30$, $p<0.01$). Thus, sleep problems had no independent influence on the attitude to the work situation.

The attitude to work hours correlated strongly with the attitude to the work situation. This covariation may be overestimated due to similar methodology (the construction of the questions are very similar and the questions are placed close to each other in the questionnaire). On the other hand, it seems logical to expect that the attitude to work hours also affect the more general attitude to the work situation. Thus, good work hours, a stimulating work task (including high influence over work), and a good social atmosphere (and perhaps also the salary) probably are important prerequisites for work satisfaction.

Another aim was to examine the relation between subjective health and the attitude questions. With respect to sleep, both samples show a consistent pattern. A negative attitude to work hours had a rather strong relation with the perception of poor sleep quality. In the daytime group, the attitude to the work situation also added some explained variance, whereas in the shift work group age explained about 10% of the variance. However, when it comes to the other health measures (pain, mental health – anxiety/depressive symptoms, gastrointestinal problems, and a general rating of health), the attitude to the work situation was the strongest predictor. In the shift work sample, none of the predictors could explain the variation in self-rated health. On the other hand, the shift work sample was small and the item "self-rated health" showed a clear restriction of range since none of the subjects perceived poor health.

Thus the attitude to the work situation was a relatively good predictor of subjective health. Interestingly, the amount of explained variance was larger for the attitude to the work situation, compared to the job strain indices (work demands and influence over work tasks). Job strain and decision latitude (influence over work) have in several epidemiological studies predicted myocardial infarction, pain complaints, high blood pressure etc. (Theorell et al. 1998) and is considered to be a very powerful psychosocial measure. One may speculate whether a simple question of the attitude to work may predict future disease. We are not aware of any epidemiological studies which have tested this. However, if the perception of the work situation integrates various components of work strain (e.g. the psychosocial and physiological work demands), the simple attitude question might possibly explain work-related diseases and perhaps the risk of having work accidents.

A recent study on the attitude to work hours suggests that a negative attitude to the work schedule may influence biological stress markers. Male three-shift workers who disliked their work hours had a lower testosterone level, except for having more sleep problems and being more sleepy at work (Axelsson et al. 1998). Testosterone is regarded as a physiological stress marker that, possibly, mirrors long lasting strain and represents the general level of anabolic activity (Theorell et al, 1990; Karasek et al, 1982). The decreased testosterone may be interpreted as an early indicator of impaired recuperation, which could be part of a stress related mechanism towards disease. In another study on shift workers, the attitude to work hours entered as a relatively strong predictor (when controlling for age) of the cholesterol level – a poor attitude was associated with a high cholesterol level (Kecklund et al. 1992b). This finding supports the suggestion that the attitude to work hours may be associated with biological stress markers.

In summary, the attitude to work hours was related to insufficient time for social activities and social interaction, as well as to sleep/sleepiness problems. The attitude to the work situation, on the other hand, was mostly determined by psychosocial factors (mainly social support and possibility to influence work) at the work place, and the attitude to work hours. The attitude to the work situation also predicted subjective health, whereas the attitude to work hours predicted sleep problems.

REFERENCES

Åkerstedt, T., 1996, Arbetstider, hälsa och säkerhet. Karolinska Institutet, *Stressforskningsrapporter (in Swedish)*, **270**, 1-121.

Åkerstedt, T., and Gillberg, M., 1990, Subjective and objective sleepiness in the active individual. *International Journal of Neuroscience*, **52**, 29-37.

Åkerstedt, T., Hume, K., Minors, D., and Waterhouse, J., 1994a, The meaning of good sleep: a longitudinal study of polysomnography and subjective sleep quality. *Journal of Sleep Research*, **3**, 152-158.

Åkerstedt, T., Hume, K., Minors, D., and Waterhouse, J., 1994b, The subjective meaning of good sleep - a intraindividual approach using the Karolinska Sleep Diary. *Percepeptual and Motor Skills*, 79, 287-296.

Åkerstedt, T. and Kecklund, G., 1995. Prediction of the attitudes to work and work hours. *Shiftwork International Newsletter*, 12, 64.

Åkerstedt, T., Westerlund, M., and Andersson, G., 1996, Mot bättre tider: en utvärdering av några av vårdens arbetstidsmodeller med avseende på välbefinnande och hälsa. Karolinska Institutet, *Stressforskningsrapporter* (in Swedish), 271, 1-26.

Alfredsson, L., and Theorell, T., 1983, Job characteristics of occupations and myocardial infarction risk effects of possible confounding factors. *Social Science and Medicine*, **17**, 1497-1503.

Axelsson, J., Kecklund, G., Åkerstedt, T., Lowden, A., Atterfors, R., and Lindquist, A., 1998, Sleep, alertness, performance and the attitude to work hours. *Journal of Sleep Research*, **7**, **supplement 2**, 11.

Costa, G., 1996, Effects on health and well-being. In W. P. Colquhoun et al. (ed.) *Shiftwork.. Problems and solutions.* (Peter Lang GmbH, Frankfurt am Main), 113-139.

Karasek, R.A., Russel, R.S., and Theorell, T., 1982. Physiology of stress and regeneration in job related cardiovascular illness. *Journal of Human Stress*, **8**, 29-42.

Kecklund, G., and Åkerstedt, T., 1992a, The psychometric properties of the Karolinska Sleep Questionnaire. *Journal of Sleep Research* **1, suppl 1**, 113.

Kecklund, G., Åkerstedt, T., Göransson, B., and Söderberg, K., 1992b, Omläggning av skiftschema: konsekvenser för välbefinnande, hälsa och arbetstrivsel. Karolinska Institutet, *Stressforskningsrapporter (in Swedish)*, **234**, 1-29.

Knutsson, A., Åkerstedt, T., Jonsson, B. G., and Orth-Gomér, K., 1986, Increased risk of ischemic heart disease in shift workers. *Lancet*, **ii**, 86-92.

Kundi, M., Koller, M., Stefan, H., Lehner, L., Kaindlsdorfer, S., and Rottenbücher, S., 1995, Attitudes of nurses towards 8-h and 12-h shift systems. *Work and Stress*, **9**, 134-139.

Lowden, A., Kecklund, G., Axelsson, J., and Åkerstedt, T., 1996, Övergång från 8 till 12 timmars skift. Karolinska Institutet, *Stressforskningsrapporter* (in Swedish), **268**.

Tenkanen, L., Sjöblom, T., Kalimo, R., Alikoski, T., and Härmä, M., 1997, Shift work occupation and coronary heart disease over 6 years of follow-up in the Helsinki Heart Study. *Scandinavian Journal of Work Environment and Health*, **23**, 257-265.

Theorell, T., 1991. Psychosocial cardiovascular risks - on the double loads in women. *Psychotherapy and Psychosomatics*, **55**, 81-89.

Theorell, T., Karasek, R.A., and Eneroth, P., 1990. Job strain variations in relation to plasma testosterone fluctuations in working men - a longitudinal study. *Journal of Internal Medicine*, **227**, 31-36.

Theorell, T., Perski, A., Åkerstedt, T., Sigala, F., Ahlberg-Hultén, G., Svensson, J., and Eneroth, P., 1988, Changes in job strain in relation to changes in physiological state. *Scandinavian Journal of Work, Environment and Health*, **14**, 189-196.

Theorell, T., Tsutsumi, A., Hallquist, J., Reuterwall, C., Hogstedt, C., Fredlund, P., Emlund, N., and Johnson, J. V., 1998, Decision latitude, job strain, and myocardial infarction: A study of working men in Stockholm. *American Journal of Public Health*, **88** , 382-388.

Torsvall, L., and Åkerstedt, T., 1980, A diurnal type scale. *Scandinavian Journal of Work, Environment and Health*, **6** , 283-290.

EMOTIONAL EXHAUSTION, DEPERSONALIZATION AND HEALTH IN TWO SWEDISH HUMAN SERVICE ORGANIZATIONS

Marie Söderfeldt
National Institute of Working Life, Stockholm, Sweden

Abstract: Emotional exhaustion and depersonalization are usually considered to be parts of the burnout phenomenon, which has been the object of much research. There is however a lack of serious attempts to relate burnout to health. The objective of this paper was therefore analyze emotional exhaustion and depersonalization, investigating their relation to different aspects of health, on a large research material from two Swedish human service organizations. The relations between emotional exhaustion, depersonalization and three health indicators, psychological, musculoskeletal, and gastrointestinal health, were analyzed in regression analyses. The results showed different patterns for the two burnout components in relation to health. Emotional exhaustion was related to all three health indicators, primarily to psychological health, while depersonalization was insignificant for this health aspect. Depersonalization was positively related to musculoskeletal and gastrointestinal health. One interpretation of this result could be that depersonalization independently act as a form of coping mechanism for and therefore could be beneficiary for some health aspects. The results indicate that it is meaningless to discuss in terms of burnout and health. If burnout is a common entity of the two components, there should be a similar pattern for them in relation to health. This should be considered in future studies

1. INTRODUCTION

Emotional exhaustion and depersonalization are usually considered to be parts of the burnout phenomenon, which has been the object of much research during the last 25 years. Burnout is described as an adverse effect of work in human service organizations (Maslach and Schaufeli 1993), i.e work where the core is the relation to other human beings (Hasenfeld 1992). In later years, there have been attempts to widen the burnout concept to denote a general psychological condition (Maslach, Jackson et al. 1996).

Going into the burnout literature, there is an amazing number of reported correlates. In a recent book, Schaufeli and Enzmann present a list of 132 affective, behavioral, physical, motivational, and cognitive symptoms of burnout (Schaufeli and Enzmann 1998) ranging from warts to sexual

Health Effects of the New Labour Market, edited by Isaksson *et al.*
Kluwer Academic / Plenum Publishers, New York, 2000.

problems. Most of the associations to burnout are obtained by simple bivariate correlational methods. There is a surprising lack of serious attempts to relate burnout to health; surprising in the light of the enormous attention devoted to burnout - in 1998, Schaufeli found 5500 references in various databases. Studies that in a more systematic way relate the different burnout components to health are rare.

There are thus indications of positive correlations between especially emotional exhaustion and self-reported psychosomatic complaints (Schaufeli and Van Dierendonk 1993). Self-reported heart problems and circulatory disturbances have been shown to be weakly associated with emotional exhaustion, while there was a stronger relation to self-reported neurasthenic symptoms (Keliber, Enzmann et al. 1998). Emotional exhaustion has also been associated with self-reported cold and flu, but with no relation to cholesterol levels (Hendrix, Steel et al. 1991). A self-report frequency illness measure has been connected to emotional exhaustion and depersonalization (Corrigan, Holmes et al. 1995), but weakened when controlling for social support. The relation to depersonalization disappeared in another similar report (Bhagat, Allie et al. 1995). Landsbergis has found positive relationships between self-reported coronary heart disease symptoms, emotional exhaustion and depersonalization (Landsbergis 1988). To my knowledge, these observations more or less exhaust scientific reports about burnout and health.

The objective of this paper is therefore to extend the analysis of two of the burnout components, emotional exhaustion and depersonalization, investigating their relation to different aspects of health. This will be done on a large research material from two Swedish human service organizations. The analyses will be done on three self-report health related measures, using multivariate analysis, where an array of possible confounders will be controlled.

2. MATERIAL AND METHODS

The study was done on the Social Insurance Organization (SIO) and the Individual and Family Care sections (IFC), which are subsections of the Social Welfare Agencies. The SIO is the main agency in Sweden for the general welfare policies with a coordinating responsibility for rehabilitation. The IFC comprises local income maintenance and social services. The two organizations differ in many respects, but they have the human service orientation in common for most work tasks. Their personnel are responsible for care and rehabilitation of individual clients.

In 1993, a questionnaire was mailed to all personnel in the two organizations in a random sample of 100 communes with 8296 persons employed. The response rate of the questionnaire was 69.1 %, yielding a study sample of altogether 5730 persons, predominantly women (83 %). An aggregate analysis of non-response concluded that the response rates of local units were random. Details of the study can be found elsewhere (Söderfeldt, Söderfeldt et al. 1996).

The response variables were based on a measure of self-reported health (Andersson 1986; Härenstam 1989), especially developed for a healthy working population. There were altogether 12 items. Six items (nervousness, restlessness, anxiety, tiredness, sleeping problems and sadness) indicated psychological health. Three items (stomach pain, upset stomach and heart burns) were interpreted as indicators of gastrointestinal health, and three items (back, neck and shoulder pains, pain in other joints and numbness and creeps) were regarded as indicators of musculoskeletal health.

The measure has been extensively used in occupational health practice in Sweden. It was chosen because it offered comparison possibilities to many other occupational groups. It has not been systematically validated, but has functioned well in practice. However, the items on psychological health are very similar to the mental part of the GHQ (Goldberg and Hillier 1979). Principal components analysis yielded a clear-cut three factor solution, and the items were summed into three simple indices called "psychological health", "gastrointestinal health", and "musculoskeletal health" respectively. Clear relations have been shown between these index variables and known occupational health risk factors (Söderfeldt and Söderfeldt 1997; Söderfeldt, Söderfeldt et al. 1997).

Emotional exhaustion and depersonalization were - as usual in the literature - measured by two subscales of the Maslach Burnout Inventory (MBI). The emotional exhaustion subscale contains nine items, assessing feelings of being emotionally overextended by the work. The depersonalization subscale contains five items measuring unfeeling and impersonal attitudes towards the recipients of the services (Maslach, Jackson et al. 1996). The MBI has shown very good psychometric properties in a variety of studies in different countries (Yadama and Drake 1995; Söderfeldt, Söderfeldt et al. 1996). Also here, the items were summed into two indices.

A set of other independent variables that might influence self-perceived health were also included in the analyses as possible confounders: gender, marital status, age and education. Further, the variable emotional strain was included, developed from the demand-control model (Karasek and Theorell 1990). It was a composite index of high emotional demands and low job control. Emotional demands was measured by three questions concerning perception of emotionally demanding work tasks, feelings of too much responsibility and unability to switch off thoughts of work during free time. Job control was measured by five items capturing its two dimensions skill discretion and decision authority (Härenstam, 1989; Karasek and Theorell, 1990). Emotional strain has been shown to be very important for self-reported health among human service workers (Söderfeldt and Söderfeldt 1997).

The relations between emotional exhaustion, depersonalization and the health indicators were analyzed in bi- tri and multivariate regression analyses, where the multivariate analysis included the possible confounders. For the analyses, all continuous variables were transformed to range between 0-100 in order to allow interpretation in terms of per cent. Age and education were treated as dummy variables. Statistical significance is indicated in the tables with stars: (*) p_0.10, * p_0.05, **p_0.01, *** p_0.001.

3.   RESULTS

The first analyses were done with psychological health as dependent variable. The analyses were done in three steps, starting with investigation of the bivariate relations. The result is shown in table 1.

Table 1. Bivariate regression models with psychological health as dependent variable.

	b	
Emotional exhaustion	-0.54	***
R^2=0.42		
Depersonalization	-0.29	***
R^2=0.10		

There were strong relations between both burnout components and psychological health, especially for emotional exhaustion. Since the variables were transformed to range between 0-100, the result should be interpreted so that one per cent increase in emotional exhaustion decreases psychological health by 0.54 per cent units. The model explained 42 % of the variance for psychological health, which is substantial in a bivariate model including this kind of variables. The relation to depersonalization was weaker, although the regression coefficient was relatively high. This model however explained only 10 per cent of the variance, and the residual plot was heteroscedastic, indicating that the model was not fully specified (Studenmund, 1992).

In the second step, both emotional exhaustion and depersonalization were included as independent variables in a trivariate model of psychological health. The result is shown in table 2.

Table 2. Trivariate regression model with psychological health as dependent variable.

	b	
Emotional exhaustion	0.53	***
Depersonalization	0.00	n.s.

$R^2 = 0.42$

Here, the independent relation between emotional exhaustion and depersonalization and psychological health disappeared, while it remained stable for emotional exhaustion. The bivariate relation to depersonalization was thus spurious in relation to emotional exhaustion. The explained variance in this model was the same as in the bivariate model for emotional exhaustion which also indicates that depersonalization does not add anything for the explanation of psychological health.

The third step was to include a set of other possible confounders in a multivariate model. The result is shown in table 3.

Table 3. Multivariate regression model with psychological health as.dependent variable.

	b	
Emotional exhaustion	-0.47	***
Depersonalization	-0.02	n.s.
Emotional strain	-0.18	***
Gender - woman	-1.43	***
Marital status - single	-1.04	***
Age _35 years	1.12	***
Age 36-49 years (ref.cat)	-	-
Age _ 50 years	-2.11	***
Education, junior high school	-0.17	n.s.
Education, high school (ref.cat)	-	-
Education, college degree	-0.34	n.s.

$R^2 = 0.44$

The relations between the two burnout components and psychological health remained almost the same as in the trivariate model. The regression coefficient for emotional exhaustion decreased from -0.53 to -0.47 and there was no relation to depersonalization . All the other variables except education showed independent relations to psychological health. The relation between emotional strain and psychological health was stable in relation to previous analyses (Söderfeldt and Söderfeldt 1997), but less than half as strong as the coefficient for emotional exhaustion.

The second health indicator to be analyzed was musculoskeletal health. Also here, the relations to emotional exhaustion and depersonalization were first analyzed in bivariate regression models. The result is shown in table 4.

Table 4. Bivariate regression models with musculoskeletal health as dependent variable.

	b	
Emotional exhaustion	-0.26	***

R^2=0.06

Depersonalization	-0.03	*

R^2=0.00

Compared to previous analyses, the relations were much weaker here. Emotional exhaustion showed an independent relation with musculoskeletal health, but the model only explained 6 per cent of the variance. Residual analysis indicated heteroscedasticity. The model for depersonalization did not explain any variance, which means that this model fails to say more about musculosceltal health than the simple sample mean. Also the regression coefficient was almost 0, although statistically significant. In a large material, as the present one, even trivial relations become significant.

The relations were further analyzed in a trivariate regression model where both emotional exhaustion and depersonalization were included as independent variables. The result is stated in table 5.

Table 5. Trivariate regression model with musculoskeletal health as dependent variable.

	b	
Emotional exhaustion	-0.33	***
Depersonalization	0.14	***

R^2=0.07

When including both burnout variables in the model, the regression coefficient for emotional exhaustion increased somewhat so that one per cent increased exhaustion worsened health by 0.33 per cent units. For depersonalization the opposite pattern was revealed. The bivariate analysis showed almost no relation between depersonalization and musculoskeletal health, but in the trivariate analys something happened. The regression coefficient became reversed and should be interpreted so that for each per cent increase in depersonalization, musculoskeletal health was *improved* by

0.14 per cent units. This unexpected result was also stable in the multivariate analysis as shown in table 6.

Table 6. Multivariate regression model with musculoskeletal health as dependent variable.

	b	
Emotional exhaustion	-0.29	***
Depersonalization	0.08	***
Emotional strain	-0.10	***
Gender - woman	-5.50	***
Marital status - single	-0.16	n.s.
Age _35 years	4.08	***
Age 36-49 years (ref. cat)	-	-
Age _ 50 years	-3.78	***
Education, junior high school	-2.32	***
Education, high school (ref.cat)	-	-
Education, college degree	3.42	***

R^2=0.13

In this model, the relations between emotional exhaustion and health was about the same as in the bi-and trivariate models. The reversed pattern for depersonalization remained although the regression coefficient became weaker as compared with the trivariate analysis. All the other included variables had independent significant effects, especially gender and age. Emotional strain had a relatively weak independent relation. The model explained 13 % of the variance in musculoskeletal health, which is considerably less compared to the model of psychological health.

The third health indicator to be investigated was gastrointestinal health. Also here, the relations to emotional exhaustion and depersonalization were first assessed in bivariate models. The results are stated in table 7.

Table 7. Bivariate regression models with gastrointestinal health as dependent variable.

	b	
Emotional exhaustion	-0.32	***
R^2=0.10		
Depersonalization	-0.14	***
R^2=0.02		

As in all previous models, the relation between emotional exhaustion and health was stronger than the one for depersonalization. The regression coefficients were significant but similarly to the models for musculoskeletal health, explained variance was rather low. Also here, a trivariate model was analyzed and the result is stated in table 8.

Table 8. Trivariate regression model with gastrointestinal health as dependent variable.

	b	
Emotional exhaustion	-0.33	***
Depersonalization	0.04	**

$R^2=0.10$

When introducing both burnout components in a trivariate model, the relation to depersonalization also here became reversed, indicating that increased depersonalization improves health. Still, the regression coefficient was very low, but the same pattern as for the musculoskeletal health indicator was shown. The regression coefficient for emotional exhaustion remained stable compared to the bivariate analysis.

Finally, a multivariate model was analyzed also for gastrointestinal health. The result is shown in table 9.

Table 9. Multivariate regression model with gastrointestinal health as dependent variable.

	b	
Emotional exhaustion	-0.31	***
Depersonalization	0.03	(*)
Emotional strain	-0.10	***
Gender - woman	1.00	n.s.
Marital status - single	0.08	n.s.
Age _35 years	-0.96	n.s.
Age 36-49 years (ref.cat.)	-	-
Age _ 50 years	-1.53	**
Education, junior high school	-1.48	**
Education, high school (ref.cat.)	-	-
Education, college degree	1.53	**

$R^2=0.10$

Again, the pattern from the trivariate analysis was confirmed. The regression coefficient for emotional exhaustion was almost the same as in previous analyses. For depersonalization the reversed pattern was still there, but the regression coefficient was weakened and barely significant. Concerning the other included variables, education, and emotional strain had independent relations to gastrointestinal health. Also the oldest age group showed somewhat worse health as compared to the reference category. The model explained only 10 per cent of the variance in gastrointestinal health, similar to the models of musculoskeletal health.

In sum, there were different patterns for the two burnout components in relation to health. Emotional exhaustion was related to all three health indicators, primarily to psychological health, while depersonalization was insignificant for this health aspect. The reversed pattern for depersonalization in the tri- and multivariate models of musculoskeletal and gastrointestinal health was an unexpected finding. One interpretation of this result could be that a depersonalization independently act as a form of coping mechanism for these two health aspects, and therefore could be beneficiary for health.

4.   DISCUSSION

The result of this study is in line with other studies of burnout and health (Schaufeli and Enzmann, 1998). The strong relations between emotional exhaustion and psychological health should however be discussed and cannot readily be interpreted so that such emotional exhaustion worsens psychological health. There are at least two possible alternative explanations of this result, either that there is a common underlying factor rendering the relation spurious, or that the results are due to common method variance, building on self-reports as they are.

In the literature, negative affectivity as a personality construct is an often suggested candidate for spuriousity of associations between many social psychological constructs, *nota bene* between stressors and their effects (Jex and Spector, 1996). It may be possible that people with a personality making them prone to emotional exhaustion also tend to report more psychological complaints.

There is another methodological problem related to the spuriousity problem, namely the common method variance problem (Spector, 1987). Contemplating the items constituting the emotional exhaustion scale, the possibility of an interpretation for the respondent in terms of psychological complaints cannot be excluded. Consequently, the strong associations with emotional demands found in the models of psychological health might be due to this similarity. A third possibility in could be that emotional exhaustion is a part of psychological health. Eventually, the strong relations between emotional exhaustion and psychosomatic health end up as methodological artefacts.

The different patterns for emotional exhaustion and depersonalization was an interesting finding here. In my opinion, this indicates that it is meaningless to discuss in terms of burnout and health. If burnout is a common entity of the two components, there should also be a similar pattern for them in relation to health. In a previous study, I have shown that the empirical connections between the burnout components are problematic. Further, I have shown that there are different mechanisms behind emotional exhaustion and depersonalization, making it questionable to consider burnout as a syndrome. There is no "burnout syndrome", but there are emotionally exhausted and depersonalized human service workers (Söderfeldt 1997). This should be considered in future studies. The interpretation of depersonalization as a form of coping mechanism for two of the health aspects, can not be an argument in the discussion of a burnout syndrome. The relations are weak and they also represent independent relations irrespective of emotional exhaustion.

A weakness of this study is the cross-sectional design, but I am presently working on longitudinal data in order to deepen the results of the relations between emotional exhaustion, depersonalization and health.

ACKNOWLEDGEMENT

This work was funded by the Swedish Work Environment Fund, grant no AMFO 91-0864.

REFERENCES

Andersson, K. (1986). Utveckling och prövning av ett frågeformulär rörande arbetsmiljö och hälsotillstånd. Stiftelsen för yrkesmedicinsk och miljömedicinsk forskning och utveckling i Örebro.

Bhagat, R., Allie, S., & Ford, DL. (1995). Coping with stressful life events: An empirical analysis. In *Occupational stress: A handbook* (R. Crandall and P. Perrewe, eds.), Taylor & Francis, Philadelphia, pp. 93-112.

Corrigan, P., Holmes, E., & Luchins, D. (1995). Burnout and collegial support in state psychoatric hospital staff. *J Clin Psych* 51: 703-710.

Goldberg, D. & Hillier, VF. (1979). A scaled version of the General Health Questionnaire. *Psych Med* 9: 139-145.

Hasenfeld, Y. (1992). The nature of human service organizations. In *Human services as complex organizations* (Y. Hasenfeld, ed.); Sage, Newbury Park, pp. 3-23.

Hendrix, WH., Steel, RP., Leap, TL., & Summers, TP. (1991). Development of a stress-related health promotion model: Antecedents and organizational effectiveness outcomes. *J Soc Beh and Pers* 6:141-162.

Härenstam, A. (1989). PhD Thesis *Prison personnel - working conditions, stress, and health.* Karolinska Institute, Stockholm.

Jex, S., & Spector, P. (1996). "The impact of negative affectivity on stressor-strain relations: a replication and extension. *Work and Stress,*10: 36-45.

Karasek, R. & Theorell, T. (1990). *Healthy work - stress, productivity and the reconstruction of working life.* Basic Books, New York.

Keliber, D., Enzmann, D., & Gusy, B. (1998). *Skalenhandbuch zur Streß- und Burnoutforschung im medizinisch-psychosozialen Bereich.* Verlag für Psychologie, Göttingen.

Landsbergis, P. A. (1988). Occupational stress among health care workers: A test of the job demands-control model. *J Org Beh* 9: 217-239.

Maslach, C., Jackson, SE., & Leiter, M. (1996). *Maslach Burnout Inventory* (research manual, third edition). Consulting Psychologists Press, Palo Alto.

Maslach, C., & Schaufeli, W. (1993). Historical and conceptual development of burnout. In *Professional burnout: Recent developments in theory and research* (W. Schaufeli, C. Maslach & T. Marek,eds.), Taylor & Francis, London, pp. 1-18.

Schaufeli, W. & Enzmann, D. (1998). *The burnout companion to study and practice.* Taylor &Francis, London.

Schaufeli, W. & Van Dierendonk, D. (1993). The construct validity of two burnout measures. *J Org Beh* 14: 631-647.

Söderfeldt, B., & Söderfeldt, M. (1997). *Psykosocial arbetsmiljö i människovårdande organisationer. En undersökning av personal i Försäkringskassan och socialtjänstens Individ- och Familjeomsorg.* Socialhögskolan, Lunds Universitet 1997:3, Lund.

Söderfeldt, B., Söderfeldt, M., Jones, K., O'Campo, P., Muntaner, C., Ohlson, CG., & Warg, LE. (1997). Does organization matter ? A multilevel analysis of demand, control, and health in human services. *Soc Sci Med* 44: 527-534.

Söderfeldt, B., Söderfeldt M., Ohlson, CG., & Warg, LE. (1996). Psychosomatic symptoms in human service work - a study on Swedish social workers and social insurance personnel. *Scand J Soc Med* 24: 43-49.

Söderfeldt, M. (1997). PhD Thesis, *Burnout ?* Lund University, School of Social Work.

Söderfeldt, M., Söderfeldt, B., Warg, LE., & Ohlson, CG. (1996). The factor structure of the Maslach Burnout Inventory in two Swedish human service organizations. *Scand J Psych* 37: 437-443.

Spector, P. (1987). Method variance as an artefact in self-reported affect and perceptions at work: myth or significant problem? *J Appl Psych* 72: 438-443.

Studenmund, A. (1992). *Using Econometrics.* NY, Harper Collins, New York.

Yadama, G. & Drake, B. (1995). Confirmatory factor analysis of the Maslach Burnout Inventory. *SocWork Res* 19: 184-194.

OPPORTUNITIES AND CONSTRAINTS IN THE LABOUR MARKET

THE POLARIZATION OF THE LABOUR MARKET AND THE EXCLUSION OF VULNERABLE GROUPS

Duncan Gallie
Nuffield College, Oxford, UK

Abstract: Since the 1980s there has been an increased differentiation of labour market experiences in most European labour markets. For those in middle and higher level occupations, there has been a marked rise in skill levels, whereas for those in lower manual occupations skill development has been limited and there has been a sharp increase in the risk of unemployment. Recent research has provided a clearer picture of the implications of these trends for the quality of people's lives. Both developments raise significant issues with respect to the health and well-being of those in the labour force. The rise in skill levels has ambivalent consequences for the quality of work life. It is linked to more intrinsically interesting work, but at the same time to an intensification of work effort. Unemployment has strong negative psychological consequences in all European societies. However, the severity of its implications differ from one society to another. The risk that it will lead to poverty is affected by the nature of the welfare institutions of a society, while the likelihood that it will be associated with social isolation is conditioned by the prevailing patterns of household organisation and of sociability.

1.   INTRODUCTION

An influential perspective on the labour market has emphasised the role of skill change in generating increased polarization between sectors of the workforce. It is widely believed that changes both in technology and in managerial philosophies of work organisation have had the effect of raising skill requirements at work. However, there is considerable disagreement about how general such processes have been. To the extent that upskilling was restricted to certain occupational categories rather than others, it may have accentuated social differentiation and increased polarization in the labour market. In particular, if it was focused primarily on those in more highly qualified occupations, it may have increased the employment vulnerability of those with low skill levels. But until recently the empirical evidence on such trends has remained very thin.

Health Effects of the New Labour Market, edited by Isaksson *et al.*
Kluwer Academic / Plenum Publishers, New York, 2000.

This paper draws on the results from several recent research projects to address the issue of how extensive the rise in skill levels has been and how far it involved a polarization of experiences. Further, it considers the implications of such changes both for well-being of those at work and for the lives of those for whom it has implied labour market marginalisation. Does the raising of skill levels imply an unambiguously better quality of working life for those who benefit from skill development? Are those who lose out from skill change and suffer unemployment necessarily destined to longer-term social exclusion or is their vulnerability to marginalisation mediated by the institutional and cultural frameworks of particular societies?

2.   TRENDS IN SKILL

We still lack any reliable comparative evidence about trends in skill, but there has now been significant work carried out within particular countries. Given these constraints and the complexity of issues involved, I confine the assessment here to the evidence that has become available for Britain. A first approach is to consider the changing distribution of occupational classes. The matching of occupations to classes by consistent criteria is exceedingly complex. The most rigorous attempt to date for Britain was that of Guy Routh (1980, 1987), whose schema has been updated to the 1990s (Gallie, 1999b). This provides a rather clear picture of the broad pattern of occupational change. In the first half of the century, the most striking development was the growth of the class of clerical employees. Whereas in 1911 they represented 4.5% of the working population, by 1951 the figure was 10.4%. There was a continued but less rapid increase in the second half of the century. Over the century as a whole, but particularly in the second half of the century, there was a marked increase in the proportion of the population in professional work (higher and lower) and in managerial jobs. The expansion of these occupational classes was counterbalanced by a massive decline in the proportions employed in manual work. Between 1911 and 1991 manual work fell from three-quarters to just over a third of all jobs (74.6% to 37.7%).

An analysis based on trends in occupational structure, however, can be criticised on the grounds of the potentially misleading character of job titles. The number of people with a given job title might stay stable or increase over time, but, over the same period, the actual content of the work might change significantly. For instance, it has been argued that, with feminisation, the skill content of clerical work was drastically reduced, so that clerical work has become increasingly similar to manual work (Braverman, 1974; Crompton and Jones, 1984; Lane, 1988).

It is necessary, then, to look more closely at the experience of skill change within occupations. We are now in a position to make direct comparisons of the development of skill trends from the mid 1980s. In 1992 a nationally representative survey - the Employment in Britain survey - was carried out, providing a sample of 3, 477 employees aged 20-60 (Gallie *et al.* 1998). The survey was designed to include a number of indicators that would allow for comparison with a survey that had been carried out in the mid-1980s: the Social Change and Economic Life Initiative, involving a sample of 6,111 people. In order to assess trends, we adopted several different measures of skill. These included the qualifications required for jobs, and the frequency and duration of training and on-the-job experience. Finally, we examined people's own perceptions of whether or not skills have increased over recent years, leaving them free to define skill in the way most relevant to them.

In practice, the broad trends that emerge are very similar across the different measures. There had been a clear increase over the period in the overall level of qualifications required for jobs. Between 1986 and 1992, jobs requiring no or low level qualifications have declined (Figure 1), whereas those requiring higher level qualifications increased. The proportion of jobs where no qualifications were required was 6 percentage points lower in 1992, whereas jobs requiring A Level or more had increased by the same amount. A very similar pattern emerged with respect to training and on-the-job experience. Whereas, in 1986, 52% of employees had received no training for the type of work that they were doing, by 1992 this was the case for only 42%. The requirement for on-the-job experience was measured with a question asking how long it had taken after the employee first started the type of work to do the job well. In 1986, 27% had said that it had required less than a month, whereas by 1992 this was the case for only 22%. This pattern of change in skill levels over time can be seen within each occupational class, although it was more marked for some classes than for others. The change in qualification requirements and in training was particularly strong among lower non-manual employees.

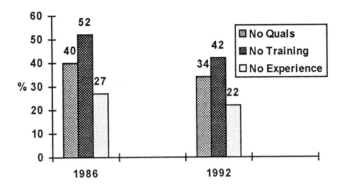

Figure 1. Changes in Qualifications, Training and On-the-Job Experience
Requirements 1986-1992

Source: Gallie et al. (1998: 33)

This increase in the skill demands of work is confirmed by people's own accounts of *changes* over the last five years in the skills required for their jobs. A majority of employees (63%) reported that the level of skill they used in their job had increased over the previous five years (Table 1). In contrast, only 9% said that the skills they used at work had decreased[i]. A majority of employees at all job levels experienced an increase in their skills, with the exception of semi and non-skilled manual workers. The increase was particularly marked among professional and managerial workers (74%), technicians and supervisors (73%) and lower non-manual workers (70%). But it was also the case that 64% of skilled manual workers thought that the skills involved in their work had increased. The proportion experiencing an increase in their skills was however considerably lower among semi and non-skilled manual workers (45%), suggesting that some degree of skill polarisation was indeed occurring in the workforce.

The view that the experience of upskilling reflects important changes in the content of jobs is reinforced when changes over time are examined (Table 1). Compared to the mid 1980s, the process of upskilling appears to have extended to a substantially wider sector of the workforce. Survey data for 1986 also showed a general tendency for skills to have increased at all job levels. But the proportion that experienced an increase in their skills has gone up from 52% in 1986 to 63% in 1992. This increase had been particularly sharp among technicians and supervisors, lower non-manual workers and skilled manual workers. In contrast, the proportion that had experienced a decrease in their skills was unchanged at 9%.

Table 1 Skill Change in the job in last 5 years, percentage experiencing an increase in skill

	1986	1992
	cell percentages	
Professional/Managerial	67	74
Lower Non-Manual	55	70
Technician/Supervisory	56	73
Skilled Manual	50	64
Semi & Nonskilled manual	33	45
All Employees	52	63

Source: Gallie et al. (1998:34)

Did these trends in skill effect men and women in a similar way? There were still very clear differences between men and women in the skill level of jobs in the early 1990s. Women were more likely to be in jobs where no qualifications were required and they were less likely to have prior training. They were also less likely than men to report that the skill requirements of their work had increased over the previous five years (60% compared with 66%). Nonetheless, if the relative position of men and women is compared to the situation in the mid-1980s, the notable point is that the gender differential had declined sharply. Over the decade the skill requirements of women's jobs had become very much more like those of men.

The overall picture is a clear one. The dominant trend has been an increase in the level of skills. This was the case not only for those who had been upwardly mobile, but also for those who had remained in the same job over the five years. This strongly suggests that a major factor behind the rise in skill levels has been the restructuring of work tasks. The rise in skills was remarkably general across occupational classes. However, there was one important exception. In contrast to those in other class positions, only a minority of people in semi and non-skilled occupations had experienced development of their skills over the previous five years, indicating that they were being left behind in the general process of in-career upskilling. This was likely to increase their vulnerability to unemployment in a period of rapid economic restructuring and to make much more difficult subsequent re-entry to the labour market.

3.   SKILL CHANGE AND THE EXPERIENCE OF WORK

3.1   Skill Change and Intrinsic Job Interest

What was the impact of upskilling on people's experience of the quality of their work? The relationship of skill change to the intrinsic quality of the work task was explored with respect to four dimensions: the variety of the work, the extent to which people feel that they can utilise their skills, the opportunities the job provides for self-development and finally their degree of involvement in the work.

There were two measures in the survey relating to the repetitiveness or variety of work. The first asked people whether the variety of their work has increased, stayed the same or decreased over the last five years; the second the extent the work involved short repetitive tasks. There were separate items for whether people felt they could use most of their previous skills in their work and whether they felt that they could keep on learning new things in the work. Finally, there were three measures of job involvement that sought to tap the amount of discretionary effort that people were prepared to put in, the extent to which the work was experienced as boring and the level of job interest.[ii]

An overall measure of intrinsic job interest was created from the seven items discussed above.[iii] As can be seen in Figure 2, there was a strong linear relationship between skill change experience and the overall score of intrinsic job interest. A range of other factors were also associated with these aspects of the quality of employment - such as people's age and the occupational class of their job (although not their sex). Yet, the striking fact is that, even allowing for the influence of these, the association between skill change experience and the intrinsic interest of the work still emerges very clearly. Further, a more detailed examination showed that skill change had a consistent and powerful effect in improving job quality *within* each occupational class.

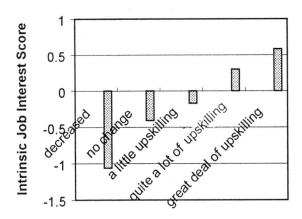

Figure 2. Intrinsic Job Interest and Skill Change

Source: Gallie (1996)

3.2   Skill Change and the Intensification of Work

For pessimistic theorists of skill change, the evolution of work involved not only the increased prevalence of repetitive and uninteresting work, but at the same time the intensification of work effort. In contrast, the theorists that emphasised tendencies for skills to increase had remarkably little to say about the likely implications of such developments for work effort. It has, however, been suggested that upskilling is linked with a tendency to break down the rigidity of traditional skill demarcations, in particular through a growth of multi-skilling or polyvalence. Such a requirement to provide greater flexibility in work could represent a potentially important source of increased work demand.

There were a number of items in the survey that provide information about the level of work pressure.[iv] It was clear from the results for each of these items that, while the rise in skill levels was associated with an improvement in the quality of work task, it led at the same time to a marked

increase in the effort involved in work. A summary picture of the
relationship between skill change and work pressure can be obtained by
creating an overall index of work pressure.[v] As can be seen in Figure 3, work
pressure is least among those that have been deskilled, followed by those
that have experienced no change in their skill level. People whose jobs have
been upskilled a little report greater pressure than those with no change, but
the difference is a modest one. It is above all those that have experienced
either quite a lot or a great deal of upskilling who report much higher levels
of work pressure. This strong relationship between experiences of skill
change and work pressure persists even when account has been taken of
occupational class.

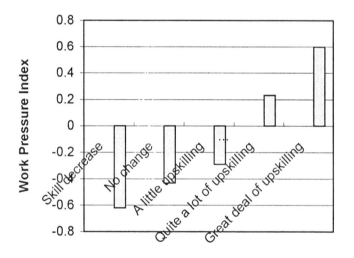

Figure 3 Skill Change and Work Pressure

Source: Gallie (1996)

The process of skill increase was associated not only with greater work
effort but also with greater strain job strain. Our measure of work strain was
derived from a four item question asking people how they felt at the end of
the work day, using for each item a six point scale ranging from 'never' to

'all of the time'. The emphasis on the duration of symptoms of strain is of central importance. Persistent work strain is far more likely to be damaging than a transient spell, and it was such persisting forms of strain that we wished to capture through the measure. The items scaled well and for most of the analysis we have used the overall scale of work strain based on the four items.[vi] The wording of the items was as follows:

'Thinking of the past few weeks, how much of the time has your job made you feel each of the following?

– After I leave my work I keep worrying about job problems.
– I find it difficult to unwind at the end of a workday.
– I feel used up at the end of a workday.
– My job makes me feel quite exhausted by the end of a workday.

A first point to note is that in terms of these measures a substantial proportion of the British workforce would appear to have experienced substantial work strain. Taking the items separately, each symptom of work strain was experienced by at least of third of all employees at least some of the time and, depending on the particular item, between 11 % and 22% experienced it regularly. Each of the items expresses a fairly strong manifestation of work strain. If one takes as an indicator of the prevalence of strain the proportion of those reporting that they experienced at least one of these symptoms much of the time, 31% of all employees experienced a high level of work strain.

There was also a widely prevalent view among employees in British industry that the level of strain involved in the job had increased over recent years. Overall, 53% said that stress had increased, 34% that it had stayed the same and 12% that it had decreased. Increased stress was particularly common among those in professional/ managerial work (67%) and among those in technical/ supervisory jobs (66%). Even among those in lower non-manual work a majority (55%) reported that the stress involved in their work had increased. In contrast, this was the case for only a minority of skilled manual workers (44%) and semi and non-skilled manual workers.

There appeared to be a clear relationship between the skill demands of work and the likelihood that people would experience work strain. A first point to note is that there was a highly significant relationship between class position and work strain. As can be seen in Table 2, those in professional and managerial work had much higher levels of work strain than any other category. Lower non-manual, technical/supervisory and skilled manual work seemed to involve rather similar levels of strain, while semi and non-skilled manual work was the least stressful. The pattern remains remarkably stable even when a wide range of other factors affecting work strain are taken into account.

It was also notable that those who had increased their skill over the last five years had significantly higher levels of work strain. As can also be seen in Table 2, people whose skill level had remained the same had the lowest levels of work strain, followed by those who had been deskilled and those whose skills had increased in a relatively modest way. High levels of work strain were mainly typical of those who had experienced a marked increase in their skill level. This association was principally due to the fact that upskilling was associated with an intensification of work effort. When controls were introduced for the intensity of work and for change in work effort over the previous five years, upskilling itself no longer has a significant effect.

Table 2 Class, Upskilling and Work Strain

	WorkStrain Score *means*	N
Class		
Professional/ Managerial	.33	1155
Lower Non-Manual	-.08	554
Technician/ Supervisory	-.05	149
Skilled Manual	-.11	358
Non-skilled	-.28	1059
Skill Change		
Increased a great deal	.33	702
Increased quite a lot	.09	1033
Increased a little	-.17	320
No change	-.23	919
Decreased	-.20	293

Note: Higher scores indicate greater work strain.
Source: Gallie et al. (1998:221)

In summary, for those whose skills did increase, the trend had ambivalent consequences for the quality of working life. In some respects it was very positive. It was associated with an increased likelihood of intrinsically interesting work, with greater variety, better opportunity to make full use of skills and the possibility of developing skills through their work. But it was also associated with a sharp intensification of the pressures of work, which had implications for levels of work strain.

4.   UNEMPLOYMENT AND SOCIAL EXCLUSION

If upskilling was two-edged even for those who benefited from it, it is clear that its most negative implications have been the increased vulnerability to unemployment of those with low or manual qualifications. Awareness of this has led to growing public concern with the issue of social exclusion. However the use of the term has been rather loose and there has been a tendency to assume that there is a deterministic relationship between unemployment and the risk of social exclusion.

Social exclusion refers to a situation where people suffer from the cumulative disadvantages of labour market marginalisation, poverty and social isolation. The different aspects of deprivation become mutually reinforcing over time, leading to a downward spiral in which the individual comes to lack either the economic or the social resources needed to participate in their society or to retain a sense of social worth. We would argue that there is no simple relationship between unemployment and social exclusion, but rather that it will depend crucially on the specific institutional and social structural characteristics of the society.

In the first place it is likely to depend in an important way on the nature of public welfare provision for the unemployed. Without entering into the continuing debate about whether it is useful to conceptualise such welfare arrangements in terms of different types of 'regime', it is clear that there are major differences between countries in the generosity of provision. The two key factors that affect such generosity are on the one hand the extensiveness of the cover of the unemployed and on the other the extent to which the benefits that are paid protect people against a sharp fall in their living standards. Estimates of the proportion of the unemployed covered by benefits range from less than one in ten in Italy (6.8%) and Greece (8.6%) to over two thirds in countries such Denmark (66.8%), Germany (70.5%) and Belgium (80%). While there are wide variations in estimates of the replacement rates provided by benefits, it is clear that there is a vast difference between a country such as the UK where the estimates tend to be between 25% and 35% and Denmark and Sweden where they over 70%.

These differences in welfare provision are reflected in very different risks of poverty among the unemployed. A recent research programme has compared the experience of unemployment in Denmark, France, Germany, the Netherlands, Ireland, Italy, Sweden and the UK[vii]. National data sets were aligned to provide as rigorous a comparison as possible of the proportions of the unemployed in poverty (Hauser and Nolan, 1999). If poverty is defined in terms of equivalised household income that is less than half of the mean, it is notable that less than 10% of the unemployed are in poverty in Denmark compared to 46% in Italy and around half of the unemployed in Britain (Table 3). If one takes half of the median income as the measure, the gap is reduced but still ranges from around 7% in Denmark to 36% in the UK and 37% in Italy.

Table 3: Poverty ratios of unemployed persons according to different poverty lines in the EPUSE countries in the mid-90s (OECD new equivalisation scale).

Mid-90s	Mean
Mean*	**32.0**
Denmark	7.6
Germany	41.7
France	23.3
Ireland	33.4
Italy	45.7
Netherlands	25.2
Sweden	30.4
UK	49.4

Source: Hauser and Nolan, (1998), a) Figures refer only to West-Germany.

In all of the countries, unemployed men were more vulnerable to poverty than unemployed women. In Denmark, these sex differences were very modest indeed (7.2% for men, compared with 6.7% for women). But in Germany, France, Ireland and the Netherlands the sex differential was ten percentage points or higher. This did not reflect the fact that women were better protected by the welfare system. In many of these countries, benefits are related to the duration and continuity of employment experience and thus tend to be less favourable to women. Rather it was due to the fact that unemployed women, particularly if they were married, were more likely to be in households where living standards were protected by the income of other adults. However, despite the variations in the risk of poverty by sex within countries, the rank order *between* countries remained very similar for men and for women.

An analysis by Nolan et al. (1999) shows that the system of social welfare is of crucial importance in accounting for the country differences in poverty rates among the unemployed. For each country, a comparison was made of poverty rates before and after social transfers. Taking the extreme cases, the pre-transfer poverty rates in Denmark and Britain were not very different: indeed it was slightly higher in Denmark (66.6% as against 61.0% in Britain, taking the 50% of mean income poverty measure). But whereas in Denmark the system of social transfers lifted 89% of the pre-transfer unemployed above the poverty line, in the UK this was the case for only 19% (Table 4).

Table 4: Impact of Transfers on Poverty Rates for the Unemployed in the 1990s, 50% Line

	% of pre-transfer poor unemployed lifted above line	% of all unemployed lifted above line
Denmark	88.6	59.0
France	52.4	25.7
Germany	32.0	17.8
Ireland	58.0	46.2
Sweden	51.2	31.9
UK	19.0	11.6

Source: Nolan et al. (1999)

5. THE SOCIAL INTEGRATION OF THE UNEMPLOYED

It is also clear that there are wide country variations in the likelihood that people will experience social isolation, a factor that lies very much at the heart of the current concern with social exclusion. A picture of the differences between countries can be gained from a cross-sectional survey carried out in all of the EU countries by the European Commission in 1996 (Gallie, 1999a).[viii]

The central concern in discussions of social exclusion is with the extent to which the individual becomes isolated from contact with others. There are two sets of relationships, which are crucial in this respect - those within the household and those that link the household to the wider community. It is important to consider each, since they may be to some degree interchangeable. Those who can rely on support within the household may be less in need of strong links to the wider community, and vice versa.

With respect to social isolation in the household, the central question is whether unemployed people tended to be living on their own or with others. The proportion of people in a position of household isolation depends primarily on the relative balance of people that are single and with partners and on the residential position of those that are single. Table 5 shows the breakdown of the unemployed into four 'household situations': people living on their own, people living with their parents, people living with other adults and people living with partners.

Overall, 20% of the unemployed were in the most isolated situation of living on their own. A further 29% were living with their parents, 45% lived with partners (married or cohabiting) and 7% were living with other adults. The frequency of household isolation varied very little with duration of unemployment, with 21% of the long-term unemployed living on their own compared with 20% of those unemployed for less than twelve months. However, at country level the proportion of the unemployed in the most socially isolated position (adults living on their own) varied very considerably. They constituted more than a half of all unemployed people in Denmark (53%) and the Netherlands (54%) and around a third in 'West' Germany (34%), Finland (32%), Sweden (35%) and Belgium (32%). In contrast, people in this position represented less than 10% of the unemployed in Italy, Spain, Greece and Portugal. The proportions are also relatively low in Britain, Ireland and East Germany.

These differences may not reflect the impact of unemployment *per se*, but rather the interplay between unemployment and cultural differences in household patterns. Are the unemployed in some countries particularly likely to be living on their own?

Table 5: Household Isolation of the Unemployed

	Living on own	Living with parents	Living with partner	Living with other adults
Austria	26.7	15.6	53.3	4.4
Belgium	32.3	26.2	36.9	4.6
Denmark	52.9	2.0	39.2	5.9
Finland	32.1	12.8	48.6	6.4
France	28.6	20.7	49.3	1.4
Germany E	25.9	7.2	61.5	5.4
Germany W	33.6	10.4	50.5	5.5
Great Britain	29.7	21.3	45.3	3.8
Greece	9.1	46.4	32.7	11.8
Ireland	18.9	37.8	29.7	13.5
Italy	1.9	56.3	27.7	14.0
Netherlands	53.5	5.1	37.6	3.8
Portugal	8.8	36.3	42.9	12.1
Spain	5.7	44.4	41.8	8.2
Sweden	34.7	6.9	56.9	1.4
EU15 (N=4565)	20.0	28.5	44.9	6.6

Source: Gallie (1999a)

There are only five countries where the effect of unemployment is distinctive. In Denmark and the Netherlands, the unemployed were more likely to be living on their own than was the case in most other countries, even when account was taken of broader country differences in household living patterns. In contrast, in Austria, Ireland and above all Italy, the unemployed were significantly *less* likely to be living on their own than in other countries[ix]. This general picture remains very similar if age, sex and class differences are taken into account. Overall, there is clearly a general tendency for the unemployed to be more socially isolated in terms of their household position. While the extent to which this is the case varies substantially between the European countries, much of this variation reflects more general societal differences in household patterns rather than country differences in the impact of unemployment per se.

An important conclusion from inter-war research was that unemployment led not only to acute financial difficulty, but also to the breakdown of people's social networks, thereby severing connections with the community and the information channels that could lead to new job opportunities (Jahoda, 1972/1933). Is this still the case in the post-war world, with more generous welfare systems and with lifestyles in which leisure plays a more central role?

To provide basic measures of sociability, people were asked first how often they spent time with relatives other than any they were living with and, second, how often they spent time with friends. Taking the overall pattern, there was little evidence that unemployment led necessarily to higher social isolation. The unemployed were considerably *more likely* to be in the most highly sociable category - meeting people several times a week. Whereas 27% of those in work met relatives several times a week, the proportion among the unemployed was 38%. Similarly, while 40% of those in work met friends several times a week, the proportion among the unemployed was 55%. The increased sociability of the unemployed was evident for both men and women. Men and women who were in work were very similar in the likelihood that they would see friends several times a week (40%). Among unemployed men the figure rose to 57%, while the comparable figure for unemployed women was 54%. It also notable that the pattern was similar for both the shorter and longer-term unemployed. There is no evidence then of any general collapse of social networks accompanying unemployment. Rather unemployment seems to increase the frequency of contact with relatives and friends.

There were, however, important country variations in patterns of sociability that were independent of whether people were in work or were unemployed. For instance, people were particularly unlikely to see their relatives on a weekly (or more frequent basis) in 'East' Germany and

Austria, irrespective of whether they had a job or were unemployed. Similarly, sociability was particularly high for both those in and out of work in Spain, Greece and Italy. These societal variations mean that the unemployed had rather different possibilities of interacting with others outside the work situation depending on the particular country in which they were living (Table 6). These differences were quite substantial: only 23% of unemployed people in Belgium spent time with relatives on less than a weekly basis, while in Austria this was the case for 53% and in 'East' Germany for 55%. With respect to sociability with friends, only 13% of the unemployed in Spain and 7% in Greece did not meet up with friends on at least a weekly basis, while in 'West' Germany this was the case for 29%, in Austria for 31% and in 'East' Germany for 52%.

The notion of network isolation ultimately hinges on whether or not people are deprived of all types of close contact, whether they be relatives or friends. It might be that family and friendship contacts are to some degree compensatory, so that those who have less of one tend to have more of the other. It is possible to create an overall index of integration in social networks by distinguishing those who did not meet *either* relatives *or* friends on at least a weekly basis. These can be regarded as people suffering from a significant level of social isolation. This measure is presented in the last column of Table 6. Overall, 12% of the unemployed had no weekly contacts outside the household with people with whom they felt close. The longer-term unemployed (12 months or more) were a little more isolated, but the difference was very slight (13% compared with 11%).

However, there were striking country differences. The proportion of socially isolated among the unemployed ranges from only 4% in Spain and 5% in Belgium to 20% in 'West' Germany and 33% in 'East' Germany. The other countries where the networks of the unemployed seem to be particularly weak are the Netherlands (18%), Austria (19%), France (18%) and Finland (17%). All of the Southern countries - Spain, Greece, Portugal and Italy - are below average in their proportions of unemployed with infrequent social contacts. In contrast, the Northern countries are closer to the patterns for Germany. They are either close to the average or in the case of the Netherlands and Finland well above it.

Again, a more detailed analysis indicated that these differences in sociability among the unemployed are almost wholly a result of wider societal differences in patterns of sociability[x].

Table 6: Social Isolation outside the Household among the Unemployed by Country
% Sees less than weekly:

	Relatives	Friends	Either
Austria	52.9	30.9	18.5
Belgium	22.7	22.2	5.4
Denmark	25.5	30.9	8.5
Finland	50.6	23.3	17.1
France	44.8	31.2	18.3
Germany E	54.9	51.7	32.9
Germany W	51.8	29.2	20.1
Great Britain	32.2	15.6	7.7
Greece	35.3	7.0	4.9
Ireland	38.7	9.7	7.8
Italy	34.4	9.0	2.7
Netherlands	50.4	31.1	18.0
Portugal	40.2	14.3	7.6
Spain	27.8	13.2	3.7
Sweden	51.8	15.8	10.9
EU15	38.8	22.1	12.1
N=	4581	4580	4586

Source: Gallie (1999a)

With the exception of the Netherlands (and more tentatively Germany), the effect of unemployment on social isolation did not differ significantly between countries. The substantial differences in sociability between the unemployed in different countries relate to the broader patterns of social interaction in these societies rather than to differences in the effect of unemployment itself.

6. LIFE SATISFACTION

Finally, is the relationship between unemployment and psychological well-being a relatively constant one or are there substantial variations in the impact of unemployment between one society and another? It must be recognised from the start that we still lack the ideal type of data for comparative analysis. However some work has been carried out using a measure of life satisfaction available in the series of Eurobarometer surveys (Gallie and Russell, 1998)[xi]. These are carried out in member states of the European Community (EU). A number of items have been asked repeatedly in different surveys and it was possible to examine the pattern over the period 1977 to 1990 for eleven countries.[xii]

The differences by country can be seen from the life satisfaction indices provided in Table 7. These show the relative satisfaction scores, that is to say the ratio of the scores of the unemployed to those of the employed in each country. Since life dissatisfaction may reflect a wide variety of influences, low absolute levels of satisfaction among the unemployed may reflect the influence of factors that lead to demoralisation among most sectors of the society. Taking the measure of the life satisfaction of the unemployed relative to the employed controls for such general influences and highlights the distinctive factors that affect the unemployed.

Table 7 Life Satisfaction: Comparison of Employed and Unemployed in Eleven European Countries

	Belg	Den	Fr	Ger	GB	Gr	Neths	Irel	Italy	Port	Sp
1983-86	0.89	0.92	0.87	0.86	0.79	0.87	0.84	0.76	0.81	0.87	0.93
1987-90	0.89	0.93	0.88	0.86	0.81	0.90	0.87	0.77	0.87	0.90	0.88
1991-94	0.89	0.91	0.88	0.82	0.83	0.96	0.87	0.83	0.90	0.87	0.89
1983-94	0.89	0.92	0.88	0.85	0.81	0.90	0.86	0.79	0.86	0.88	0.89

Source: Gallie and Russell (1998)

A first point to note is that, in all of the countries, the unemployed were markedly less satisfied with their lives than those in employment. In nine of the eleven countries, the ratios are below 0.90. Unemployment reduced life satisfaction for both men and women, although in all countries but Italy the effect was sharper for men[xiii]. Taking the overall picture, the countries can be grouped into three broad categories. There is a group of countries where the relative deprivation of the unemployed is least marked: Denmark, Greece, Spain, Portugal, France and Belgium. These are followed at some remove by Germany, the Netherlands and Italy. Finally, Ireland and Britain stand out as countries in which the impact of unemployment is particularly severe. A regression analysis confirmed the distinctiveness of these two countries even when factors such as the age and sex composition of the unemployed had been taken into account[xiv].

The pattern has been relatively stable over time. The first three rows of the table show the life satisfaction scores of the unemployed relative to those of the employed for three four-year time periods: 1983-86, 1987-90; 1991-94. Very roughly, the first of these was a period of relatively high unemployment, the second a period of recovery and the third a period which witnessed a return of high unemployment. The particularly severe effects of unemployment in Ireland and Britain emerge in each of the time periods across the three periods. Britain and Ireland were the lowest ranked in both the mid and the late 1980s, and shared the second lowest ratios for the early 1990s. In contrast, Denmark was in either first or second place in each of the three time periods. There is, however, some sign that the relative position of the unemployed changed over time in some countries. The life satisfaction ratios became lower in Germany in the 1990s and in Spain after the mid 1980s. In contrast, they improved considerably in the 1990s in Ireland, Italy and Greece.

Why should the cases of Britain and Ireland have stood out in this way? These were countries which approximated what has been called the liberal/minimalist model of the welfare state. They provided relatively wide benefit coverage of the unemployed, but at a very low level indeed. Further, the single largest proportion of the unemployed in these countries were heads of household. In general, the unemployed in the other low welfare societies (particularly those in Southern Europe) were protected to a significant degree by the fact that they were much more likely to be living with their parents and to have access to important sources of alternative support.

Country variations in levels of dissatisfaction are not then a simple reflection of the level of generosity of the public welfare regime. The impact of the welfare regime will depend significantly on the availability of other family sources of support and on the household composition of unemployment. In some countries, a system of 'household welfare' mediates the impact of low welfare provision, while in others household responsibilities may sharply accentuate the pressures deriving from welfare provision.

* * *

Overall, the evidence at least for Britain confirms the view that there has been a very sharp rise in the skill requirements of jobs in recent years, involving a significant polarisation between those in higher and intermediate class positions on the one hand and those in less skilled class positions on the other. This rise in skill requirements has had ambivalent implications for those directly affected. Our evidence suggests that it was generally associated with an increase in the intrinsic interest of work tasks. However, at the same time it led to an intensification of work effort, which was an important factor contributing to higher levels of work strain. This process of skill polarization also in part accounted for the marked increase in the vulnerability to unemployment of those in manual occupations. But the extent to which unemployment led to a risk of social exclusion in the sense of a cumulative impact of poverty and social isolation, varied significantly between societies. It depended not only on the system of welfare benefits but also on the prevailing patterns of household organisation and of community sociability. The 'Northern' European societies were particularly effective in offsetting the risk of social exclusion by providing relatively generous levels of financial support, while the 'Southern' European societies gave a measure of protection through their stronger systems of family and kin support which meant that the unemployed remained more closely integrated into supportive social networks.

REFERENCES

Braverman, H. (1974) Labor and Monopoly Capital. The Degradation of Work in the 20th Century. New York: Monthly Review Press.

Crompton, R and Jones, G. (1984) White-Collar Proletariat. London: Macmillan.

Gallie, D. (1999a) Unemployment and Social Exclusion in the European Union. European Societies, Vol 1, No. 2.

Gallie, D. (1999b) The Labour Force. In: Halsey, A.H., (Ed.) British Social Trends 1900-2000, London: Macmillan.

Gallie, D. (1996) 'Skill, Gender and the Quality of Employment' in R. Crompton, D. Gallie and K. Purcell eds. Changing Forms of Employment. Organisations, Skills, and Gender. London: Routledge.

Gallie, D., White, M., Cheng, Y. and Tomlinson, M. (1998) Restructuring the Employment Relationship, Oxford: Clarendon Press.

Gallie, D. and Russell, H. (1998) Unemployment and Life Satisfaction. Archives Europeennes de sociologie XXXIX, 3-35.

Gallie, D. and Paugam, S. (1998) Employment Precarity, Unemployment and Social Exclusion: An Overview of the Research Programme, Oxford: EPUSE Working Paper No 1.

Hauser, R. and Nolan, B. (1998) Changes in Income Poverty and Deprivation over Time, Oxford: EPUSE Working Paper, No. 3.

Jahoda, M., Lazarsfeld, P., and Zeitel, H. (1972/1933) Marienthal. The Sociology of an Unemployed Community. London: Tavistock.

Lane, C. (1988) 'New Technology and Clerical Work' in D. Gallie ed. Employment in Britain. Oxford: Blackwell.

Nolan, B., Hauser, R., and Zoyem, J.P. (1999) The Changing Effects of Social Protection on Poverty. Oxford: EPUSE Working Paper No 4.

Routh, G. (1981) Occupation and Pay in Great Britain, Cambridge: Cambridge University Press.

Routh, G. (1987) Occupations of the People of Great Britain, London: Macmillan.

Notes

[i] With respect to the validity of the measure, it should be noted that there was a strong relationship between whether or not people said that the skill requirements of their jobs had increased and whether they had received training. Only about a

third of those who had seen no change in their skills or who had been deskilled had received training (32% and 35% respectively). In contrast, among those who had experienced a small increase in skill, 44% had received training in the previous three years, while the figure rose to 61% among those whose skills had increased quite a lot and to 72% among those whose skills had increased a great deal.

[ii] The items asked how much effort people put into their job beyond what was required, how often time seemed to drag on the job and how often they thought about their job when they were doing something else.

[iii] The measure represented a statistically satisfactory scale, with a Cronbach's alpha of 0.64. A principal components analysis showed that the seven items formed a single factor, with an eigenvalue of 2.24, accounting for 32% of the variance. The factor scores have been taken as the measure of intrinsic job interest.

[iv] Two were designed to tap the general level of work pressure, taking account of both physical and mental pressures. People were asked how strongly they agreed or disagreed that 'My work requires that I work very hard' and that 'I work under a great deal of tension'. There were a further two items on the time pressures in work: whether or not people felt they had enough time to get everything done on the job and whether they often had 'to work extra time, over and above the formal hours of the job, to get through the work or to help out'. There was a question asking people whether they were expected to be more flexible in the way they carried out their work than two years earlier. Finally, to get an overall indication of whether or not people felt that there had been a change in the level of effort, they were asked whether, over the last five years, 'the effort you have to put into your job' had increased, stayed the same or decreased.

[v] The six items discussed above form an acceptable scale with a Cronbach's alpha of 0.70. A principal components analysis revealed a single factor, with an eigenvalue of 2.41, accounting for 40% of the various. The factor scores have been taken as the values for the index of work pressure. An anova test of the bivariate relationship between the overall work pressure index and the measure of skill change shows these are associated at a high level of statistical significance ($p < 0.000$).

[vi] The items scaled with a Cronbach's alpha of .82. A principal components analysis produced a single factor, with an eigenvalue of 2.63, accounting for 66% of the variance. The factor score has been taken as the measure of work stress.

[vii] The research project 'Employment Precarity, Unemployment and Social Exclusion' (EPUSE) was funded by the European Commission as part of the

Fourth Framework Programme. It was co-ordinated by Duncan Gallie and Serge Paugam. For details of the themes covered see (Gallie and Paugam, 1998).

[viii] The survey involved a random sample of approximately 1000 people aged 16 or more in each country, together with a random booster sample of approximately 300 people who were without work and seeking work.

[ix] The test involved pooling the sample of the employed and unemployed and carrying out a regression analysis adding, after the main country effects, interaction terms for the effects of unemployment in each country (for full details see Gallie, 1999a).

[x] This again was examined with a pooled regression, including both those in work and the unemployed, which included interaction terms representing the unemployment effect for each country (Gallie, 1999a).

[xi] The principal studies of the impact of unemployment on psychological well-being use a more sophisticated measure (the GHQ or General Health Questionnaire), which has been validated as a predictor of clinically assessed minor psychological morbidity. One of the surveys, however, contains both the standard life satisfaction measure and a six-item version of the GHQ. The overall correlation between the two measures was .49. This was very similar for both men and women. Moreover, the correlation coefficients are reasonable for all of the countries taken individually. The consistent nature of this pattern suggests that the life satisfaction measure is likely to provide an indication of the relative level of psychological distress.

[xii] The main virtue of the surveys is that the cumulative file provides the types of sample numbers needed to examine differences by country, employment status and sex. The analysis has focused on the period since 1983 when data became available for Greece, Spain and Portugal. The most recent member states - Austria, Finland and Sweden - have had to be excluded, given the low sample numbers. For a similar reason, the analysis has been restricted to 'West' Germany throughout the time period. Luxembourg and Northern Ireland were also excluded because of a relatively low number of cases. This left eleven countries for which adequate data were available. the sample numbers for the employed range from 14,722 for Denmark to 9284 for Spain, while those for the unemployed range from 2266 for Ireland to 689 for Portugal.

[xiii] Interestingly, this would not appear to be the case with a more severe measure of psychological distress. A comparative survey carried out in 1996 shows no significant differences between men and women on a six-item version of Goldberg's General Health Questionnaire (GHQ).

[xiv] For details of the analysis, see Gallie and Russell, 1998.

THE QUALITY OF WORK: THE WORK-FAMILY INTERFACE

Roel L.J. Schouteten and Marco C. de Witte
Faculty of Management and Organisation, University of Groningen, The Netherlands

Abstract: Since the early years of this century the characteristics of work and work circumstances in the Netherlands, like in other European countries, changed dramatically. The development of a 24 hour economy, the flexibilisation of work, and a greater participation of women in the labour force are relevant examples in this context. As a consequence of these changes of work and work circumstances, it is no longer evident that the quality of work can be studied from an isolated work perspective. In our view it is worthwhile to study the determinants of well-being at work not only from the perspective of the quality of work, but from an interrelated approach consisting of both a work and life course perspective. Based on data derived from a survey in a home care organisation (309 respondents in the caring profession), we carefully conclude that the definition of the quality of work has to be redefined. Defining the quality of work only in terms of the content of jobs seems to be outdated. In studies of labour it is time to incorporate the family, too.

1.   LABOUR MARKET DEVELOPMENTS IN THE NETHERLANDS: A BIRD'S EYE VIEW

In this article we want to contribute to the discussion of well-being at work from the perspective of two different points of view. First we want to contribute to the discussion from the perspective of different theoretical frameworks, such as the Sociotechnical Systems Theory and the Job Characteristics Model. Second, we want to introduce a more dynamic approach than is commonly used in this discussion. Before we state our research questions in section 3, we will describe the Dutch labour market developments (this section) and the Dutch discussion on the quality of work (section 2). This discussion is rather different from the discussion in other European countries, because the concept of well-being at work plays a more explicit role in the Dutch Work Circumstances Act than it does in most other countries. We come back to this later, first we present a bird's eye view on labour market developments in the Netherlands.

Health Effects of the New Labour Market, edited by Isaksson *et al.*
Kluwer Academic / Plenum Publishers, New York, 2000.

267

1.1   Employment and unemployment

Since the early years of this century the characteristics of work and work circumstances have changed dramatically. First, the employment structure changed from highly agrarian to a service economy. In the agricultural sector the employment rate declined from 31% in 1899 to 4% in 1992[1]. In the services sector, on the other hand, the employment rate increased from 36% in 1899 to 70% in 1992. The employment rate within the industrial sector did not change dramatically. It decreased from 25% in 1899 to 19% in 1992. Over the whole period employment rose quantitatively in terms of man-years, although between 1970 and 1993 the number of man-years did not or hardly increased in the Netherlands (Schmid 1997).

From the beginning of the seventies the unemployment rate rose steadily in the Netherlands. In 1970 the number of unemployed people was 440,000, in 1984 this number rose to 591,000, to diminish in 1996 again to 440,000. The official unemployment rate in 1996 is less than 6 percent[2]. Most striking is the structural character of this unemployment. Since 1984 more than half of the unemployed have been without a job for more than one year. In the second half of the eighties half of all long-term unemployed were in this position for more than three years. Within the total number of unemployed, the share of women, workers between 25 and 54 years of age, people from ethnic minorities and employees with intermediate and higher education have increased strongly (SCP 1998).

1.2   Flexibilisation

The above mentioned (limited) quantitative growth of the employment in the Netherlands was largely produced by the increase in part-time work and the reduction of working hours. To start with the latter, the length of the working week decreased from 60 hours per week in 1910, to 38 hours a week in 1996 (Smulders 1995). In 1998 even a further reduction was an issue on the political agenda. In some sectors a 36 hours working week is already realised and plans for a reduction to 34 hours a week are being discussed.

Like in most industrial countries the number of workers with a flexible labour contract is increasing in the Netherlands (Delsen 1995). Although still more than 80% of Dutch workers hold a job on a permanent contract, the number of flexible workers is growing. When we compare the figures

---

[1] In percentages of the total employment in all sectors.

[2] Using the broad unemployment definition of the OECD the unemployment rate even rises to 24%. More than 2 million people (out of a labour force of 6.7 million) receive social welfare benefits or are active in subsidised jobs.

between 1985 and 1996 this is true for all categories (part-time workers, specific flexible workers, temping agency workers and temporary workers), but especially true for specific flexible and temping agency workers (Steijn 1998). The turnover of employment agencies has set record after record. This often involves externalisation of permanent staff. A mobility policy mainly addressing external outflow and flanked by provisions regarding out-placement and a focus on employability is becoming common property (Oeij et al. 1998). It is important to note that in general women, younger people and the lower educated are overrepresented within the various categories of flexible workers (Dekker and Doorenbos 1997). From these indicators the conclusion can be drawn that in general the Dutch labour market has become more flexible.

1.3   Participation of women

Next to flexibilisation, another major change is the growing participation of women in the labour force, which increased from 23% in 1899 up to 36% in 1987 and 45% in 1996. Between 1985 and 1996 the participation rates for men have grown from 67% to 72%, only 5%. For the year 2000 a participation rate of women of more than 50% has been forecast. Even the number of working mothers increased significantly. In 1988 27% of mothers with minor children had a job. In 1996 already 42% of them worked outdoors (Min. SZW/CBS 1998). Not only the participation rate of women is lower than for men, they work less hours as well. In 1996 the average number of working hours for Dutch men is 36.6 a week and the average for Dutch women is 26.5 hours a week. Women are concentrated in a couple of branches of industry. In the not-for-profit service sector (especially health care and public services) more than half of the employees are female. After 1987 the differences between the branches of industry in this respect did not change (Min. SZW/CBS 1998). As an effect of the participation of women in the labour force the number of double-income households is increasing.

1.4   Increasing workloads

Most analysts interpret the above-mentioned changes as improvements of the quality of work and the conditions of the working life. However, this does not mean that there are no problems left concerning health and work circumstances (Smulders 1995). There are some serious drawbacks as well. One of the most obvious is the increasing workload. The crisis of the Tayloristic labour organisation implies a search for new organisational concepts focussing on guidelines such as flexibility, quality and efficiency (Oeij et al. 1998). Apart from altering the psychological contract between employer and employee, workers run the risk of workloads exceeding the limits (Van Klaveren & Tom 1995, Nijhuis 1995, Kompier 1996).

There are serious indications that this is already the case. A survey of the working conditions of the Statistics Netherlands (CBS), held since 1974, shows minimal reductions of the exposure to physical hazards (noise, polluted air, heat, cold, vibrations, carrying heavy loads and tiring positions). Remarkable, however, is the growing number of employees reporting of working at high speeds and to tight deadlines. In 1977 this was reported by 39%, in 1992 this percentage rose to 56% and in 1997 this was reported by 59% of the workforce. Furthermore, 10% of the workforce shows symptoms of serious psychological fatigue. Especially policemen, teaching staff and people working in the printing industry and health care suffer from high workloads.

Increasing workloads are of course related to the development of the 24 hours economy. The flexibilisation of working hours (even by law) resulted in a more dispersed working day. In 1995 already 55% of the Dutch labour force is confronted with working hours outside the normal '9 to 5' regime, and 48% is confronted with evening, night and weekend shifts (Breedveld 1998).

Another reason for demanding workloads is the increasing employment in the service and knowledge sectors. One of the biggest problems in these sectors is the difficulty in defining the output parameters. When are clients sufficiently satisfied? When is the quality of a policy document, a marketing plan, or a research proposal satisfactory enough? Empowered employees, negotiating with independent and emancipated internal or external clients, have to set their own goals and increasingly determine the quality level of the required output themselves. Because most professionals are intrinsically motivated this determination of output becomes even more problematic. Work that is rewarding produces energy and is at the same time demanding, at least in terms of working hours. With the help of the latest information and communication technology (e.g. faxes, lap top computers, cellular phones) many workers are even no longer constrained by their working place and working time. They can work whenever and wherever they like, which of course blurs the demarcation between working and leisure time, between work and family. A fine example of these trends is of course the growing number of teleworking employees. In this type of work home is the workplace and of course the source of many social pressures. Problems in controlling the natural borders between work and family result in an increasing work pressure.

Although many recent labour developments can be interpreted as improvements of the quality of work and the conditions of the working life, increased workloads is one of the obvious drawbacks. In our view this quality of work and especially the changing interface between work and family needs attention. In the next section we first turn to the debate on the quality of work.

2. THE 'WORK CIRCUMSTANCES ACT', THE QUALITY OF WORK AND THE WORK-FAMILY INTERFACE

2.1 The Work Circumstances Act

As stated, paying attention to work, work circumstances and the workers' health is still called for. This is one of the reasons why the 'Arbowet' (Work Circumstances Act) was introduced in the Netherlands in 1980. This Act prescribes attention to, and improvement of safety, health and well-being at work. It obliges Dutch companies to audit risks related to the workers' safety, health and well-being at work.

Safety and health at work have been widely studied. Well-being at work, on the other hand, is a more complex and less well-known concept. In this field there is not much experience. There are still many questions about the definition of well-being at work, how it can be measured (risk audits), and how it can be improved. In the Dutch research literature the topic of well-being at work is unique and relatively young[3]. Only since the introduction of the 'Arbowet' (in 1980) has the subject of well-being at work aroused interest, although its theoretical background is the same as that of the better known (and older) subject of the quality of work. Therefore, we will use these concepts as synonyms coinciding with the definition of well-being in the 'Arbowet'.

The introduction of the 'Arbowet' in the Netherlands can be seen as a contribution of the Dutch government to the historical trends to improve the quality of work and as an interpretation of the directives of the European Community (89/391/EEG). The basic assumption of the 'Arbowet' is that well-being at work, besides safety and health at work, is an independent part of work circumstances (Jol et al. 1987). Well-being should be treated in the same way as health and safety are dealt with: prevent the occurrence of risks and eliminate existing risks. Standards about work conditions are formulated, and jobs should meet these standards or should alternatively be subject to measures to eliminate the existing risks. In this way well-being becomes a rather normative and prescriptive concept: independent of the

---

[3] Most other European countries do not use the concept of well-being at work in their attempt to improve the work conditions. They just use the concepts of safety and health at work.

worker, jobs are evaluated on risks concerning the well-being at work (Projectgroep WEBA, 1989).

2.2   The quality of work

In the assumptions of the 'Arbowet' a sociotechnical background is recognisable. After all, one of the basic assumptions with regard to sociotechnical interpretation of the quality of work is that it is determined by the characteristics of the work itself. The Sociotechnical Systems Theory is one of the theoretical frameworks frequently used in the Dutch discussion on the quality of work. It states that jobs and organisations that are designed according to certain principles improve the quality of the organisation and the quality of work. These rules are based on the striving for balance between problems in the work (also called control need) and possibilities to deal with these problems (also called control capacity)[4]. To deal with problems an employee should have enough possibilities to solve them conclusively. So there should be enough control capacity located there where the need for control arises[5]. According to the (Modern) Sociotechnical Systems Theory this balance can be achieved by designing the organisation into task groups (teams) which perform 'whole tasks' (a coherent set of tasks within a production cycle). Within these task groups the members have enough control capacity to deal with the problems which can occur during the work. In other words, there is a balance between control need and control capacity (Van der Zwaan 1994). Then control is both effective and efficient. With regard to well-being the benefit of a sociotechnically designed organisation is that the workers perform not just one small, monotonous task in the whole production process (as in Taylorised organisations), but that they perform, and are responsible for, a coherent set of tasks within a production cycle.

This brief sketch illustrates that within a sociotechnical interpretation of the quality of work the focus is on the characteristics of the work and the organisation of labour itself. In these so-called objective evaluations of the quality of work the opinions of those who actually do the jobs are left out.

Other (more psychological) theories frequently used in the Dutch discussion on the quality of work, state that next to job characteristics the fit between the individual and the job is also important to explain the motivation and satisfaction of employees. The fit model that has received the widest attention is the Job Characteristics Model, proposed by Hackman and Oldham (1980). The model identifies five core job characteristics (skill

---

[4] This is the same balance Karasek (1979) described between job demands and decision latitude.

[5] Based on Ashby's Law of Requisite Variety (Ashby, 1969).

variety, task identity, task significance, autonomy, feedback from the work) that influence critical psychological states, such as the experienced meaningfulness of work, the experienced responsibility for the work, and feedback relating to knowledge of results of work activities. Collectively, these critical psychological states affect five outcomes, namely work satisfaction, internal work motivation, work performance, absenteeism and turnover. The central focus of the model is the individual's attitudinal response to the work. In many studies the mediating (intervening) role of the psychological states between job characteristics and personal outcomes is supported (Fried and Ferris 1987).

Existing Dutch risk audit instruments for well-being, such as WEBA and NOVA-WEBA (Dhondt & Houtman, 1992; 1996; Vaas et al., 1995) are developed under the authority of the Ministry of Social Affairs and Employment in order to measure the well-being at work as mentioned in the 'Arbowet'. Since the assumptions in the 'Arbowet' have a sociotechnical background as well, the same applies for WEBA and NOVA-WEBA. Accordingly these instruments focus only on the characteristics of the work itself, and not on the characteristics of the worker or the fit between work and worker. This one-sided interpretation is subject to a great deal of discussion, because apart from the balance between control need and control capacity in the work itself, some analysts state that the balance between the work and the worker is equally important. The goal of this article is partly to contribute to this discussion by analysing simultaneously determinants derived from the (Modern) Sociotechnical Systems Theory and the Job Characteristics Model. This results in our first research question: In what way is well-being at work determined by the characteristics of work and/or the fit between the work and the worker?

2.3   The work-family interface

Because of the changes of work and work circumstances (described in the first section), it is no longer evident that questions of labour are being studied from an isolated work perspective. Next to labour the total number of activities of workers have to be considered, such as leisure time and the care for family members. The need of workers to adapt their work and leisure time to their private circumstances is growing. The sharp division between work and private, originated in the second half of the 19th century, will disappear and become more diffuse. That is why workers increasingly make great demands upon their work in terms of conditions, content and hours. In this sense there is no longer a clear distinction between the quality of work and the quality of life.

This explains the recent debates on the interface between labour and care activities. In general, studies on the quality of work are directed at one field of activity, although recent developments on the labour market point at the increasing inter-relatedness of work and the other fields of activity. As far as we know such an approach to the study of the quality of work does not (yet) exist. At the same time such a new perspective would mean a less static approach. Connecting the study of the quality of labour to, what can be called, a life course perspective implies a more dynamic point of view. What can be considered as highly qualitative work could depend on the stages of life workers are in. The content of a job, the working conditions and the conditions of employment under which the work is executed are traded off differently in alternative stages of life. Highly qualitative work in the beginning of the career can be very stressful in a later stage of the life course, for instance while having a working partner or having responsibilities for the upbringing of children. So, in our view it is worthwhile to study the determinants of well-being not only from the perspective of the quality of work but from an interrelated dynamical approach between work and other fields of activity, e.g. care. Therefore our second research question is: In what way are these determinants of well-being influenced by the stages of life workers are in?

3.   CONCEPTUAL MODEL AND RESEARCH QUESTIONS

As mentioned in the previous sections, the goal of this article is twofold. First we want to contribute to the discussion on well-being at work by analysing simultaneously determinants derived from the (Modern) Sociotechnical Systems Theory and from the Job Characteristics Model. Next to this, we want to investigate in what way these determinants are influenced by the stages of life workers are in. So, to gain knowledge about the determinants of well-being at work the conceptual model focuses on the characteristics of work, the fit between work and worker and the stage of life of workers (see figure 1). First, we analyse the relations between the content of jobs, the fit between work and worker and the experienced well-being at work. Here the assumptions of the Modern Sociotechnical Systems Theory are confronted with those derived from a more psychological fit model. Subsequently, we add the determinants of the stages of the life course into our analysis.

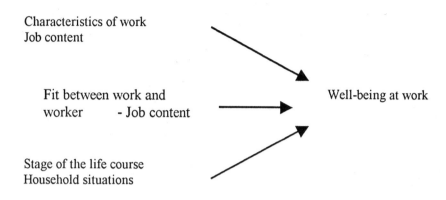

Figure 1: Conceptual model

Since this article is our first attempt to analyse the well-being at work from a life-course perspective, the concept 'stage of life' is predominantly limited to the household situation. We come back to this when we discuss the measurement of the different concepts.

To analyse the assumed relations this article addresses the following research questions:

1. In what way is well-being at work determined by the characteristics of work and/or the fit between the work and the worker?
2. In what way are these determinants influenced by the stages of life workers are in? In other words, does the household situation add extra explaining power compared to a model in which the characteristics of work and the fit between work and worker are taken into account?

4.   METHODS: DESIGN AND MEASUREMENT

4.1   Design

Ideally, our research questions presume a longitudinal design. This kind of design is best suited for connecting studies of the quality of labour to a life course perspective. In essence we want to know whether respondents executing the same jobs judge the well-being at work differently once their life situations have been changed. Since longitudinal data were not available, we had to use a cross-sectional design: varying the different household situations of our respondents. In this way we compared the well-being at work for respondents working in the same jobs with different household situations. The assumption is that these different household situations indicate the effects of the different stages in the life course. So we assume that cross sectional household situations capture a synthetic cohort of changes of the life course. This is a contestable assumption but, considering the available data, the next best solution.

To answer our research questions we analysed data gathered in 1998 in a Dutch organisation for domiciliary care. This case is interesting because the majority of workers are female and it is often found that women value their family more than work. Women especially view work as a means to attain family well-being, or at least both family and work are similarly highly valued (Inglehart 1990, Tausky 1992, Voydanoff 1987, Raabe 1998). Furthermore, most nurses and home helps have flexible working hours, not working from nine to five, but working at early morning hours, evening hours and regularly in the night and in weekends. Reviewing these circumstances the case seems suitable to test our ideas regarding the quality of work from a life course perspective.

From 532 questionnaires distributed among workers in caring jobs[6], 309 were returned (a response rate of 58%). As said, the respondents are mostly female (98,4%). One third of the respondents is between 26 and 35 years of age (see also table 1). 86% lives together with a partner and a little more than half of the respondents (51%) is responsible for the care for children.

Table 1: Age of the respondents (n=308)

Age	Number of respondents
Younger than 26	13
Between 26 and 35	101
Between 36 and 45	95
Between 46 and 55	81
Between 56 and 65	18

---

[6] Management and staff were not included in the risk audit.

Within the organisation eight jobs are divided: home help A (61 respondents), care help B (36), nurse C (80), nurse D (21), qualified nurse E (10), district nurse I (34), district nurse II (30), weekend help (35). The average length of the working week is 20.4 hours (minimum is 1 and maximum is 37 hours per week). The average level of experience of the nurses and home helps (the time that the respondents work in this organisation) is 11 years (minimum is 0.5 year and maximum is 28 years). The average level of experience in the job (the time the respondents work in their current job) is 9 years (minimum is 2 months and maximum is 31 years). Most nurses and home helps are qualified on a lower vocational training level or on a secondary education general level. The distribution of the respondents with regard to their educational level is shown in table 2.

Table 2: Educational level of the respondents (n=307)

Educational level	Numb. of respondents
Primary education	14
Lower vocational training	69
Secondary education general level	42
Secondary vocational training	129
Secondary education advanced level	13
Higher professional education	40

4.2   Measures

In order to measure the concepts within the conceptual model, we studied a great diversity of instruments based on the different theoretical backgrounds of the model (Fruytier & ter Huurne, 1983). From these instruments we derived a new questionnaire consisting of already existing and validated scales. To answer our research questions we only used a part of the questionnaire. In the next sections we present the measures used in this article.

4.2.1   Characteristics of work.

The characteristics of work are measured with the following scales: 1. difficulty of the work, 2. completeness of the work, 3. monotony of work, 4. autonomy, 5. interaction potential, 6. organising tasks, and 7. information. These scales are derived from NOVA WEBA[7].

---

[7] Because we want to test the assumptions of the sociotechnical systems design, the scales of the NOVA WEBA questionnaire are included anyway.

4.2.2   The fit between work and worker.

Although the characteristics of the worker will not be used in this article, it is important to explain how they are measured, because there is a direct relationship with the way the fit is measured. To measure the characteristics of the workers, some questions were asked regarding educational level, age, marital status, care for children, and job experience. In addition to these variables, and most important, we measured the workers' orientations (need strength) on job content, work circumstances, work relations, or terms of employment. The orientations are measured by asking how important certain characteristics of the work are. The answer gives an impression of which categories of scales are important in the workers' jobs (according to those workers) (Ten Horn 1989).

The same categories are used to measure the characteristics of the relation (fit) between the work and the worker. But here the question was not how important a certain characteristic is, but the worker's satisfaction with the present work situation with regard to that characteristic. This is a question about how the worker experiences the characteristics of the work. It reflects the worker's perception of the work. Two examples of questions in the questionnaire can explain the difference between a measurement of a characteristic of the worker and a measurement of a characteristic of the relation between work and worker. The following questions from the questionnaire are questions 173 and 174.

173.   How important is good co-operation with your colleagues?

174.   How satisfying is the co-operation with your colleagues?

The first question is about someone's need strength for good co-operation. This can be seen as a personal characteristic. The second question asks how someone's need strength is satisfied in the present work situation. This is a measurement of the relation between the work (how is the situation) and the worker (what is important). In our conceptual model for this article only the second type of questions with regard to the job content are used in the analysis.

Furthermore the fit is measured by looking at the utilisation of the workers' educational level and the workers' job experience. So the following scales measure the fit between work and worker: 1. perception of the job content, 2. utilisation of the worker's educational level, and 3. utilisation of the worker's job experience.

4.2.3   Household situation.

To measure the characteristics of the household situation we constructed three variables: 1. stage of life, 2. regularity of working hours of the respondents and their partners, and 3. the total amount of working hours of the respondents and their partners.

Following Tijdens et al. (1994), we distinguished 6 stages of life:
1. Living alone (32 respondents)
2. Living together with a partner and no children (114)
3. Living together with partner and youngest child 0-4 (56)
4. Living together with partner and youngest child 5-12 (30)
5. Living together with partner and youngest child 13-18 (44)
6. Living together with partner and youngest child 19 or older (18)

To measure the regularity of working hours of the respondents and their partners, we asked whether the respondents and their partners work at hours between 8 am and 5 pm. This leads to a division of four categories:
1. Both work at regular working hours (99 respondents)
2. The respondent works at irregular hours and the partner at regular hours (46)
3. The respondent works at regular hours and the partner at irregular hours (53)
4. Both work at irregular working hours (33)

The third variable, used as an indicator for the household situation, is the total amount of working hours of the respondents and their partners. This variable is constructed simply by adding the respondents working hours to those of their partners.

4.2.4   Well-being at work.

Finally, the effects of well-being were measured with scales from different already existing and validated questionnaires. The different scales used are (between brackets the name of the instrument the scale is derived from[8]) 1. workload (NOVA WEBA) 2. need for recovery after work (VBBA), 3. work satisfaction (VBBA), 4. commitment (VBBA), 5. intention to turnover (VBBA), 6. health (VOS-D), and 7. mental and physical state during work (VOS-D).

Since the use of many (dependent) variables in a regression analysis is not useful, a reduction of the variables is desirable. There are two ways to do this, a theoretical way and a statistical one. A disadvantage of the statistical way is that the results need to be interpreted, which can become very difficult. However, a factor analysis on the dependent variables, being the

---

[8] VBBA = Vragenlijst Beleving en Beoordeling van de Arbeid (Questionnaire Experience and Judgement of Work; Van Veldhoven and Meijman 1994). VOS-D = Vragenlijst Organisatie Stress-Doetichem (Questionnaire Organisational Stress-Doetichem; see Kompier and Marcelissen 1993).

effects of well-being, distinguished four factors. Table 3 shows the results of the principal axis factoring with varimax rotation and Kaiser normalisation.

Table 3: Results of the factor analysis

	Factor			
	1	2	3	4
Need for recovery	.073	-.131	**.295**	.152
Satisfaction	-.020	.069	-.075	**.716**
Commitment	-.071	**.536**	-.020	-.134
Intention to turnover	-.107	**.330**	.001	.067
Health	**.194**	-.134	.059	.094
Mental/physical effects	**.763**	.097	-.195	-.208
Workload	-.106	.053	**.654**	-.125

These factors can be interpreted as follows. The first factor is 'mental and physical effects of work'. It contains the scales 'health' and 'mental and physical state during work'. The second factor can be called 'commitment'. It contains the scales 'commitment' and 'intention to turnover'. The third factor is 'workload'. It contains the scales 'workload' and 'need for recovery after work'. The fourth factor is 'job satisfaction' and consists of the scale with that name.

However, the skewness of all four factors is rather high. This is probably due to a lack of variance in the scores per scale, e.g. most respondents report that they are (very) satisfied with their work. To reduce this skewness problems we constructed a variable 'overall effects' in which all dependent variables are added together. This results in a more normal (or Gaussian) distribution. We used only this variable ('overall effects') as dependent variable. To construct this variable the scores on the dependent variables were recoded to a score between 0 and 1 and added together. This gives an impression of the overall effects the work has on the person.

4.3   The reliability of the scales

The reliability of the scales is assessed by Cronbach's alpha. Apart from means and standard deviations we present in table 4 the reliability coefficients per scale. Although only validated existing scales were used, Chronbach's α yielded some reliability coefficients that are only just reasonable. The reasons for this need to be investigated further. One of the possible reasons is that the respondents are mostly women in caring jobs. This is not a representative sample of all working people and this may cause the deviation in the reliability of the scales.

Table 4: Means, standard deviations and Chronbach's alpha per scale

Scale	Mean	Std. Deviation	Cronbach's α
Characteristics of work			
Difficulty of the work	.560	.294	.81
Completeness of the work	.408	.196	.78
Interaction potential	.394	.227	.54
Monotony of work	.314	.265	.43
Autonomy	.337	.233	.67
Organising tasks	.317	.328	.75
Information	.278	.205	.70
Fit between work and worker			
Perception of job content	3.148	1.000	.88
Utilisation of educational level	.153	.360	(1 question)
Utilisation of job experience	.169	.375	(1 question)
Well-being at work			
Work load	.321	.211	.75
Recovery need after work	.278	.304	.89
Work satisfaction	.092	.167	.78
Commitment	.358	.247	.76
Intention to turnover	.221	.300	.77
Health	.106	.112	.88
Ment./physical effort	.247	.119	.80
Overall effects	1.911	.065	.69

Explanation: the scores for the characteristics of the work and the effects of well-being are standardised between 0 and 1. A high score (close to 1) indicates a risk on that characteristic. The score for the perception of job content can range between 1 and 7. A high score (close to 7) indicates a low satisfaction (perception) with regard to that characteristic. The score for the overall effects can range between 0 and 4. A high score (close to 4) indicates a great deal of problems concerning the overall effects of well-being at work.

With regard to the effects of well-being at work the scores are excellent. None of the scales gives reason to expect high risks for the well-being of the employees. If we look at the scales representing the characteristics of the work, we can see two scales with rather high scores (>.5): difficulty of the work and physical strain. This may indicate that the work is mentally and physically exhausting. The workers have to work hard and fast, and the work demands a great deal of attention and attentiveness. But until now this has not lead to high scores on the scales that measure the well-being effects.

5.   ANALYSIS

To answer our research questions we executed several regression analyses in SPSS. To find out what variables are the most important determinants of well-being we executed stepwise regression analyses to test three different models. In the first step we entered the characteristics of work. The model then consists of well-being as dependent variable and work characteristics as independent variables. This is the sociotechnical model in which only characteristics of work are important determinants of well-being. In the second step we entered, following the framework of the Job Characteristics Model, the characteristics of the fit (as additional independent variables in model 2). In the final step we entered the variables regarding the household situation as additional independent variables (model 3). This is meant as a test of our ideas about the fundamental change of the work-family interface. It should be noticed that the indicators of the household situation are entered as dummy variables.

As mentioned, within the first analysis we used as the dependent variable 'overall effects'. The results of this regression analysis are shown in table 5. The results of the regression analyses on the other dependent variables are not fully presented in this article, because they show similar outcomes. However, the tables presenting these results can be obtained from the authors.

Furthermore, we checked for interaction effects of the household situation with the other independent variables. But using general linear modelling did not result in significant interaction effects. So these are not taken into consideration in the regression analysis. Therefore, only the direct relations between household situation and well-being are used in the analysis.

Table 5 shows that the characteristics of work are important determinants of the dependent variables in the model. However, the characteristics of the fit and the household situation add extra explanatory power. This is shown by the values of R^2 that increased significantly by adding these variables to the model. With this result we are able to answer our research questions.

The first question was: in what way is well-being at work determined by the work characteristics and/or by the characteristics of the fit between work and worker? From the comparison between model 1 and model 2 we can conclude that adding the characteristics of the fit increases the model fit (R^2). So we should use the second model to tell what determines well-being at work. This is also shown in an earlier analysis on the same data. This analysis showed that the characteristics of the work are the most important determinants of well-being at work (this confirms the sociotechnical assumption), but that the characteristics of the fit are important as well.

Especially the perception of control capacity (in that analysis a characteristic of fit) is important, even more important than control capacity (as a work characteristic) (Schouteten 1998).

Table 5: Regression analysis of different independent variables on 'overall effects'

Variables	Model 1 Beta	Model 2 Beta	Model 3 Beta
Characteristics of work			
Difficulty of the work	.207**	.183*	.155*
Completeness of the work	-.142*	-.166*	-.166*
Interaction potential	-.020	-.047	-.002
Monotony of work	.136#	.124#	.118
Autonomy	.104	.073	.053
Organising tasks	.104	.077	.061
Information	.408***	.343***	.341***
Fit work-worker			
Perception of job content		.280***	.271***
Utilisation of educational level		-.080	-.049
Utilisation of job experience		-.099	-.135#
Household situation			
Household situation = living together			-.075
Household situation = youngest child 1-4			-.085
Household situation = youngest child 5-12			-.004
Household situation = youngest child 13-18			-.061
Household situation = youngest child > 18			-.160
Amount of working hours of both partners			.131#
Working at regular hours = partner irregular			-.059
Working at regular hours = self irregular			.058
Working at regular hours = both irregular			.089
R^2	.310***	.373***	.430***
N=160			

# $p < .1$ / * $p < .05$ / ** $p < .01$ / *** $p < .001$

The second question was whether the household situation would add extra explanatory power to model 2. Comparing models 2 and 3 shows that adding the household situation to the model significantly increases the model fit. So these are also important determinants of well-being at work. This is an important conclusion because it confirms our idea that the sharp division between work and family is disappearing among the women in this study and that it is worthwhile to study the determinants of well-being not only from the perspective of the quality of work but from an interrelated dynamical approach between work and other fields of activity.

This conclusion can be verified by looking at the different dependent variables (see table 6).

Table 6: Model fit (R^2) of the different models.

R^2	Overall effects	Satisfaction	Workload	Commitment	Ment./ phys. effects
Model 1	.310	.148	.254	.168	.184
Model 2	.373	.188	.313	.201	.231
Model 3	.430	.249	.373	.239	.302

Explanation: in Model 1 only characteristics of the work are included, in Model 2 characteristics of the fit are added to Model 1, and in Model 3 characteristics of the household situation are added to Model 2.

This table illustrates that for each dependent variable R^2 increases significantly when variables from model 3 are added into our second model. But we have to be careful in our conclusions because the values of beta in table 5 do not state our conclusion. It is remarkable that most values of beta are not significant while R^2 is so high. Although, there are some values that are close to significance (p<.1, see Wanous 1974). This means that the influence of the individual variables in the model is limited. A possible explanation is that the variance within the variables (especially the dependent variables) are limited (see also table 4). This means that there is a small effect size and, hence, that there is not a great amount of variance that can possibly be explained. Therefore it is difficult to find variables that have a significant influence on the dependent variables.

The fact that there is little variance in the dependent variables can be due to the background of the respondents. The respondents are mostly female and working in the health care sector. This is not a representative sample of all working people. Workers in the health care sector are highly intrinsically motivated to perform their jobs. Therefore they hardly complain about problems in their work; they just try to perform as well as possible to serve their clients. Therefore it is advisable to do the same analysis on data gathered in another population in which the variance in the dependent variables is bigger.

6. CONCLUSIONS AND DISCUSSION

In the last decades far-reaching changes have occurred in the labour market situation in the Netherlands. Like in other European countries, the work itself and the work circumstances have changed radically. These transformations can be interpreted, as an improvement of the quality of work and the conditions of the working life in general. Beside improvements some serious drawbacks are easy to mention. One of the most obvious is the quick increasing pressure of work. The development of a 16 hour economy combined with the growing possibilities especially for empowered professionals to work whenever and wherever they like, the work-family interface becomes a field of tension. However, most studies of well-being at work focus merely on the field of paid labour, or to be more specific the characteristics of the work itself. To the best of our knowledge an approach of well-being at work focussing on the work-family interface does not exist. In our view it is worthwhile to study the determinants of well-being from an interrelated dynamical approach between work and family, especially care activities.

The results of our analysis are summarised in table 5. The findings illustrate clearly that the characteristics of work are the most important determinants of well-being. Especially the difficulty of work, the completeness of work and the amount of information are significant factors. To date, this confirms the sociotechnical assumption especially. However, the characteristics of the fit between work and worker are also relevant. Especially the perception of the job content by the worker contributes significantly. Finally, even the household situation of the respondents adds extra explaining power to our model. Remarkable however is that, although the model fit increases significantly, none of the variables is significant separately. However, the influence of the total amount of working hours of both partners is close to significance.

Summing up, it is not legitimate to conclude that the characteristics of work are the only important determinants of well-being. After all the fit between work and worker and even the household situation of the respondents adds extra explaining power to our models. Because this article is our first attempt to study well-being at work from an integrated approach focussing on the work-family interface, definite conclusions are rather premature. But we carefully conclude that definitions of well-being at work based solely in terms of job characteristics have to be revisited. Because of the developments within the advanced industrial economies and more specific in modern workplaces, an approach of well-being focussing primarily on job characteristics is outdated. In our view the work-family interface is increasingly important. In studies of labour it is time to bring in the family, as well.

6.1   Future research

Because our data set is not based on a representative sample of the Dutch labour force, we have to be careful in generalising our conclusions. It is necessary to find out whether our conclusions will stand up to future evidence. More analyses, within different organisations, are required to explore the sociotechnical assumptions. And in those case studies we will add also several personal traits of the workers, like the employee growth need strength. In that way a full test of sociotechnical assumptions and for instance assumptions derived from the Job Characteristics Model become possible. To do so, it takes more than just linear regression analysis. It is likely that the personal characteristics of the workers have non-linear or indirect effects on the well-being at work. In that case LISREL analyses are asked for.

Of course, the work-family interface is relevant for future research. Studying the quality of work from a life course perspective implies a more dynamic approach. This approach asks for longitudinal research designs and data sets including both women and men, that make it possible to measure the well-being at work of the same respondents in different stages of their life course. The demarcation between the life spheres of work and family becomes increasingly blurred. That is why it is worthwhile to study well-being at work starting theoretically and empirically by focusing on the work-family interface. Our first findings suggest that this is indeed an interesting area of future studies.

REFERENCES

Ashby, W.R., 1969, "Self-regulation and requisite variety", in F.E. Emery (ed.), *Systems thinking; selected readings*, Harmondsworth, Penguin Books, pp. 105-124.

Breedveld, K., 1998, Illusies van een 24-uurs economie. Ontwikkelingen in gespreid werken en verschillen in zeggenschap, *Tijdschrift voor Arbeidsvraagstukken,* vol. 14, nr. 1, pp. 23-36.

Dekker, R. and R. Doorenbos, 1997, Flexibel werk aan de onderkant van de arbeidsmarkt, Tijdschrift voor Arbeidsvraagstukken, vol. 13, nr. 2, pp. 103-112.

Delsen, L., 1995, *Atypical Employment: An International Perspective,* Groningen: Wolters Noordhoff.

Dhondt, S. and I. Houtman, 1992, *NIPG onderzoeksvragenlijst arbeidsinhoud: constructie en eerste toets op betrouwbaarheid en validiteit,* Leiden, TNO, rapportnummer 92.088.

Dhondt, S. and I. Houtman, 1996, *De WEBA-Methode. NOVA-WEBA handleiding. Een vragenlijst om welzijnsknelpunten op te sporen,* Leiden, TNO Preventie en Gezondheid, rapportnummer 96.027.

European Community (89/391/EEG), "Richtlijn van de Raad van 12 juni 1989 betreffende de tenuitvoerlegging van maatregelen ter bevordering van de verbetering van de veiligheid en de gezondheid van de werknemers op het werk", in *Publicatieblad van de Europese Gemeenschappen,* nr. L183/1-8, 19.6.89.

Fried, Y. and G.R. Ferris, 1987, The validity of the job characteristics model: a review and meta-analysis, *Personnel Psychology,* vol. 40, pp. 287-322.

Fruytier, B. and A. ter Huurne, 1983, *Kwaliteit van de arbeid als meetprobleem; een vergelijkende literatuurstudie,* Tilburg, IVA.

Hackman, J.R. and G.R. Oldham, 1980, *Work Redesign*, Addison-Wesley Publishing Company.

Horn, L.A. ten , 1989, *Your work...and what you think of it. Questionnaire for the measurement of variables related to the quality of jobs*, Delft, University of Technology.

Inglehart, R., 1990, *Culture shift in advanced industrial society,* Princeton: Princeton University Press.

Jol, J.A. et al., 1987, *De inhoud van het welzijnsbegrip in artikel 3 van de Arbowet,* Voorburg, Directoraat-Generaal van de Arbeid, Directie Sociaal Arbeidsbeleid.

Karasek, R.A., 1979, "Job demands, job decision latitude, and implications for job redesign", in *Administrative Science Quarterly,* vol. 24, pp. 285-307.

Klaveren, M. van and T. Tom, 1995, All-round groepswerk: doen of doen alsof? *Tijdschrift voor Arbeidsvraagstukken,* vol. 11, nr, 1, pp. 21-33.

Kompier, M.A.J. and F.H.G. Marcelissen, 1993, *Handboek werkstress; Systematische aanpak voor de bedrijfspraktijk,* Amsterdam, NIA.

Kompier, 1996, *The best of both worlds. Arbeids- en organisatiepsychologie tussen theorie en praktijk,* Nijmegen: Katholieke Universiteit Nijmegen (oratie).

Ministerie van SZW/CBS, 1998, Jaarboek Emancipatie 1998. Tijd en ruimte voor arbeid en zorg, Den Haag: Vuga.

Nijhuis, F.J.N., 1995, De paradoxale gezondheidseffecten van arbeid. Van gezondheidsbedreiging naar gezondheidsbevordering, Maastricht: Rijksuniversiteit Limburg (oratie).

Oeij, P., B. Fruytier, and I. van den Broek, 1998, Research Into the Quality of Work, in: G. Evers, B. van Hees, J. Schippers, *Work, Organisation and Labour in Dutch Society. A State of the Art of the Research,* Dordrecht/Boston/London: Kluwer Academic Publishers, pp. 105-138.

Projectgroep WEBA, 1989, "Functieverbetering en Arbowet", in *Gedrag & Organisatie,* vol. 2, nr. 4/5, pp. 361-382.

Raabe, P.H., 1998, Women, work, and family in Czech Republic and comparisons with the West, Community, Work & Family, Vol. 1., nr. 1, pp. 51-64.

SCP, 1998, Sociaal en Cultureel Rapport 1998, Rijswijk: Sociaal en Cultureel Planbureau.

Schmid, G., 1997, *Jobwunder Niederlande. Eine Moderne Arbeitsmarkt- und Beschäftigungspolitik,* WZB-Mittielungen, vol. 36, pp. 3-6.

Schouteten, R., 1998, *Determinants of well-being at work: conceptual model, questionnaire and the first results.* Paper for the Weswa Conference 1998, Rotterdam, 25 November.

Smulders, P.G.W., 1995, "Arbeid en gezondheid: inleiding", in P.G.W. Smulders and J.M.J. op de Weegh, *Arbeid en Gezondheid: Risicofactoren,* Utrecht, Lemma, pp. 19-41.

Steijn, A.J., 1998, Career chances to become unemployed of flexible and permanent workers. Proof of a segmented labour market?, Paper Weswa Conferentie, Rotterdam, 25 november 1998.

Tausky, C., 1992, Work is desirable/loathsome, *Work and Occupations,* vol. 19, nr. 1, pp. 3-17.

Tijdens, K., H. Maassen-van den Brink, M. Noom, and W. Groot, 1994, Arbeid en zorg; Maatschappelijke effecten van strategieën van huishoudens om betaalde arbeid en zorg te combineren, Den Haag, OSA.

Vaas, S. et al., 1995, *De WEBA-methode, deel 1: WEBA-analyse handleiding*, Alphen aan den Rijn/Zaventem, Samsom Bedrijfsinformatie.

Veldhoven, M. van, T. Meijman, 1994, *Het meten van psychosociale arbeidsbelasting met een vragenlijst. De Vragenlijst Beleving en Beoordeling van de Arbeid (VBBA),* Amsterdam, NIA.

Voydanoff, P., 1987, *Work and family life,* Newbury Park, CA: Sage.
Wanous, J.P., 1974, Individual differences and reactions to job characteristics, *Journal of Applied Psychology*, vol. 59, no. 5, pp. 616-622.
Zwaan, A.H. van der, 1994, *Engineering the work organization*, Assen, Van Gorcum.

FROM SCHOOL TO WORK IN THE 1970s, 1980s AND 1990s FOR EARLY SCHOOL LEAVERS

Åsa Murray
Department of Special Education, Stockholm Institute of Education
P.O.Box 47308, 100 74 Stockholm, telephone +46 8 737 56 53,
email: asa.murray@lhs.se

Abstract: The aim of the study is to investigate the route from school to work in the 1970s, 1980s and 1990s for early school leavers in Sweden. How has their situation on the labour market developed during this period in relation to young people with a 2-year vocational education and training from upper secondary school? The research material consists of three large scale follow-up studies of school leavers who were investigated seven years after they had left compulsory school at the age of 23 by Statistics Sweden. The first study was conducted in 1978, the second in 1986 and the third in 1995. Employment rates for 16-year-old school leavers were studied for the 7-year follow-up period and were compared to school leavers with a 2-year vocational education and training. Only small differences in employment rates were found between the young men irrespective of whether they had vocational training or not. In the 1990s only men with building and construction training had a much lower employment rate than the male 16-year old school leavers. Differences in employment rates were also rather small between the compared groups of young women. However, in the 1990s these differences widened and the 16-year-old leavers had the lowest employment rate. Thus, an upper secondary education seems to have become a more important prerequisite for young women to get a job during the investigated period but hardly so for young men.

1.   EDUCATIONAL POLICY IN SWEDEN

Educational policy in Sweden since the end of the war has been to raise the educational attainment of young people and this is still the current policy. In the 1960s a nine-year compulsory comprehensive education was implemented. In 1971 a reformed upper secondary school was introduced which also incorporated vocational education. These were 2-year vocational programmes and included some general education. The academic programmes leading to higher education were mainly 3-year programmes. Another reform of the upper secondary school has been implemented all over the country in 1995/96. In this reform the vocational programmes have also become 3-year programmes and include more general education. The aim is to give general competence for higher education.

Health Effects of the New Labour Market, edited by Isaksson *et al.*
Kluwer Academic / Plenum Publishers, New York, 2000.

The background of this policy was an increasing demand for more education among young people after the war. To provide all young people with equal educational opportunities, a nine-year comprehensive education was a natural political solution. When unemployment among young people increased in the 1970s the political solution was an expansion of upper secondary education. In the 1980s a slogan 'an upper secondary school for everybody' was introduced and the political aim was to enrol all young people in the upper secondary school. This is still the political aim in the 1990s, as well as to extend the 2-year programmes into 3-year programmes and to raise the academic standard of the vocational programmes. In all political documents about education for young people an upper secondary education is considered a necessary minimum level of competence for young people.

Compared to many other European countries the Swedish educational policy has been successful in raising the educational attainment among young people. Sweden had one of the highest enrolment rates for 17- and 18-year olds in secondary education in 1996 (OECD, 1998).

However, the extension of upper secondary education has not been without problems. Many young people are fed up with school and would leave if they had a job. An investigation of students in upper secondary school found that 16 per cent of the students were critical, discontented or unhappy with school (Andersson, 1996). An expansion of further education and training can also create special problems for the early school leavers in the labour market. This has been found in Ireland and in the Netherlands (Hannan & Hovels, 1995). One explanation for their difficulty in getting a job is 'credentialism' or 'qualification inflation' (Bowles & Gintis, 1976). The employers adjust their recruitment criteria upwards as a reaction to the shift in supply of young workers with further education and training.

The vocational education in upper secondary school has also been criticised for being a monopoly in vocational education and training. A competing system of vocational education and a recreation of a labour market for young people has been considered a necessary alternative. Year after year in school which seems hopeless and degrading should not be the only alternative for young people (Pettersson, 1997). It is therefore of interest to investigate employment of early school leavers in Sweden. How has this changed during the last decades in relation to school leavers *with* a vocational education from upper secondary school?

2. UPPER SECONDARY EDUCATION AND THE LABOUR MARKET IN SWEDEN

The demand for low-skilled workers has been falling in all industrialised countries since the 1970s. The expansion of higher and further education in the industrialised countries has also reduced the supply of low-skilled workers. But, since the beginning of the 1980s, the demand seems to be falling faster than the supply (Nickell & Bell, 1995). In the less regulated US economy these effects have been reflected in falling real wages for the low-skilled workers. In the more regulated European economies it is argued that the wages of the low-skilled were kept high but at the cost of increasing unemployment (OECD, 1994). Before 1990 Sweden had high employment and low unemployment in an international perspective. Differences in unemployment rates between people with varying educational attainment were also rather small in the 1970s and 1980s. In 1990 the economic recession changed this picture. Unemployment increased dramatically and differences in unemployment rates between people with varying educational attainment widened (Fig 1).

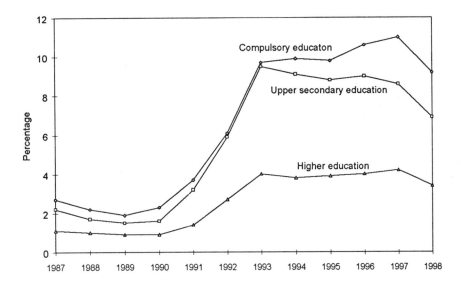

Figure 1. Relative unemployment by educational attainment in Sweden. Source: Labour force survey, Statistics Sweden

The risk of unemployment became higher for men and women with only compulsory education or an upper secondary education than for men and women with higher education. The risk of unemployment also increased more for those with compulsory education than for those with an upper secondary education.

International unemployment statistics from industrialised countries for *young* people have also shown differences in unemployment between young people with and without further education and training. High unemployment was found among those without qualifications beyond compulsory schooling (OECD, 1985, 1998). The labour market position of those young people has also deteriorated. Employers and the labour market have increasingly tended to exclude those young people with only a minimum of qualifications in Ireland, in the Netherlands and in the UK (Hannan & Hovels, 1995). Differences in unemployment have also been found in Sweden between young people with and without an upper secondary education (Statistics Sweden, 1980, 1987, 1996; Forneng, 1987; Arnell-Gustafsson & Skjöld, 1990; Jonsson, 1991). However, some investigations have not been able to show an impact of an upper secondary education on the labour market position for young people. In a study of the job quality of school leavers, Schröder (1995) found no effect of a 2-year vocational upper secondary education on subsequent job quality, 10 years after leaving school during the period of 1970-1991. A study from 1992 did not show any greater chance of getting a job for young men with a vocational upper secondary education than for young men with only compulsory education among long term unemployed men (Blomskog & Schröder, 1997).

There are a number of factors that should be considered when studying the impact of an upper secondary education on young people's labour market situations. Age is for example an important factor. Sixteen and 17-year-olds generally have more difficulty in getting a job on the open labour market than 18-19-year-olds or young adults (age 20-24). On the other hand few teenagers have been unemployed since 1984 as they have got 'youth jobs", i.e. publicly subsidised jobs for young people, instead. It is also important to take into account the time needed to become established on the labour market. Young people who left school at the age of 16 have had another two years on the labour market than young people with a 2-year vocational upper secondary education. Most difficult to take into account is the varying background of young people with different educational attainments (OECD, 1985; Härnquist, 1993; Erikson & Jonsson, 1996). Their background can be a factor explaining their different positions on the labour market.

In order to make comparisons as fair as possible between young people with and without an upper secondary education it is necessary to take these factors into account. As there have been great changes on the labour market during the 1990s in Sweden, it is also of interest to study the early school leavers during a long period, to find out whether the changes in the 1990s are a trend over several years or if they have appeared more recently.

3. AIMS

The aim of this study is to investigate the labour market position of young people without an upper secondary education in the 1970s, 1980s and 1990s. Their position on the labour market will be compared with that of young people *with* a 2-year vocational upper secondary education who have a similar social background to them. How is their position on the labour market compared to young adults with a 2-year vocational training? How has it changed during the investigated period? Have the changes been the same for men and women?

4. METHOD

The research material consists of three large scale and nationally representative investigations of school leavers from compulsory school, conducted by Statistics Sweden in 1978, 1986 and 1995 (Statistics Sweden, 1980, 1987, 1996). The sample sizes were 13 000, 14 000 and 16 000 respectively. The school leavers were investigated seven years after leaving compulsory school at the age of 23 with a questionnaire sent to them by mail. A sample of those who did not respond were contacted by telephone. The non-response rate was estimated as 16 per cent in 1978, 18 per cent in 1986 and 21 per cent in 1995. In the latest investigation all immigrants of the same age cohort as the school leavers were included in the follow-up as part of a special study. By weighting they have, however, the same impact on the results as in a random sample.

The investigation group in the present study consists of young people who did not continue to upper secondary school but left after compulsory school at the age of 16 (16-year-old leavers). The comparison groups are young adults with a 2-year vocational upper secondary education and training (men/women with vocational training). The men are from two large vocational programmes, 'metalwork' and 'building and construction', with low entrance requirements in upper secondary school. The women are from two large vocational programmes with a female profile 'home economics' and 'office work', also with low entrance requirements.

Young people attending these programmes have similar home backgrounds and experiences of compulsory education as those who left school at age 16 (Murray, 1997), and these programmes were a realistic alternative for many young people with low achievements in compulsory education. Other programmes had entrance requirements which many of the early school leavers could not meet. The number of persons who answered the questionnaire at the age of 23 in the investigation group and the comparison groups are presented in Table 1.

Table 1. Investigation group and comparison groups in three follow-up studies of school leavers from compulsory school

Men	1978	1986	1995	
			Sw	Immigr
Investigation group				
16-year-old school leavers	867	811	204	159
Comparison groups				
Metalwork programme	160	233	180	103
Building and constr. programme	183	219	194	127
Women	1978	1986	1995	
			Sw	Immigr
Investigation group				
16-year-old school leavers	745	463	191	144
Comparison groups				
Home economics programme	184	445	143	65
Office work	173	342	175	216

The questionnaires asked similar questions of the young persons in all three investigations about their main occupation (employment, studies, unemployment or other occupations) for every autumn in the first follow-up study and every autumn and spring in the following two. They also had a question about their job situation at the time of the investigation, a special week in March 1978 and in February in 1986 and 1995 when the questionnaire was sent out. The answers to the questionnaires about their employment and job situation in the three different investigations will be compared in the present study.

5.   RESULTS

The student flows through upper secondary school in the three seven-year follow-up studies are presented in Table 2.

Table 2. Educational attainment at age 23 in three age cohorts in 1978, 1986 and 1995. Percentages

Men	1971-1978	1979-1986	1988-1995
Academic programme	35	35	39
Vocational programme	30	37	44
Dropouts	12	8	10
Not enrolled in upper secondary school	24	20	7
Total	100	100	100
Women	**1971-1978**	**1979-1986**	**1988-1995**
Academic programme	37	40	49
Vocational programme	29	35	36
Dropouts	12	7	9
Not enrolled in upper secondary school	21	17	7
Total	100	100	100

Table 2 shows an increasing proportion continuing to upper secondary school. In the first cohort 24 per cent of the men and 21 per cent of the women did not enrol in upper secondary school but left school at the age of 16. In the last cohort this proportion was reduced to only a third of this number. We can also see that the vocational programmes have absorbed most of the growing number of young men enrolled in upper secondary education, while the women more often enrolled in the academic programmes. In the last cohort a minor proportion participated in the reformed upper secondary school with 3-year curriculum. Most of them, however, received the old 2-year curriculum. In a cohort aged five years younger, who left compulsory school in 1993, most young people attended the reformed upper secondary school with the new curriculum. Four years later they had achieved the following educational attainment (Table 3).

From Table 3 we can see that most young people leaving compulsory school in 1993 continued to upper secondary school. Only three per cent did not continue. We can also see that an increasing proportion of young men and women received a vocational education and training compared to the age cohort which completed compulsory school five years earlier, especially among women.

Table 3. Educational attainment at age 20 (1997) among the age cohorts leaving compulsory school in 1993. Percentages

	1993-1997	
Upper secondary education	Men n=2198	Women n=2087
Academic programme	37	42
Vocational programme	46	42
Dropouts of upper secondary school or not yet finished	15	14
16-year-old school leavers	3	3
Total	100	100

Source: Panels of pupils for longitudinal studies, Statistics Sweden

The proportion with a vocational education increased from 36 to 42 per cent among them. As all programmes have a 3-year curriculum in Table 3 and the follow-up period is four years and not seven years as in Table 2, the proportion of dropouts also includes many young people who had not yet finished their programme.

5.1   Employment

The most important criterion of young people's labour market situation is whether they have got a job or not. Wages are not very low for young people as the unions and employers have agreed to equal the minimum wage irrespective of age for the same kind of job in Sweden. There are also minimum wages for most jobs. Thus, on the open labour market there are no special wages for young people. Instead young people have more difficulty in getting a job on the open labour market, compared to adults of working age (Wadensjö, 1987).

The development of the unemployment rate in Sweden for the whole labour force 1970-1998 is presented in Fig 2.

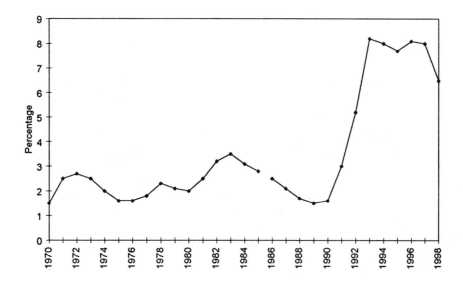

Figure 2. Unemployment Rate in Sweden 1970-1998.

The unemployment rate varied between 1.5 to 2.8 during the 1970s and 1980s. But in the 1990s it increased to 8.2 in 1993 and it has continued to be high since then, although a reduction has taken place in 1998. Thus, unemployment in the labour force did not vary much in the follow-up periods in 1971-1977 and 1979-1985 compared to the dramatic increase in the follow-up period of 1988-1995.

Fig's 3-8 illustrate the proportion of school leavers whose main occupation was employment on the open labour market during the autumn each year of the follow-up period and finally at the end of the investigation period (the measurement week). At the beginning of the investigation period the school leavers were 16 and at the end they were 23 years old. During the first two years of every follow-up study the school leavers with vocational training attended upper secondary school. Not until the third year of the follow-up period did they enter the labour market.

5.1.1 Men

The employment rates on the open labour market for the male 16-year-old leavers and for men who have completed a 2-year training course in metalwork and building and construction in 1971-1978 are presented in Figure 3.

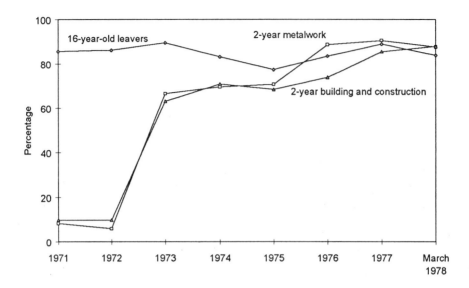

Figure 3. Employment rates for school leavers (men) with and without a 2-year vocational training from age 16-23 in 1971-1978.

A similar employment rate is found among the comparison groups at the end of the investigation period (Fig 3). The employment rate of men with two years of metalwork training overtook that of the 16-year-old leavers in the autumn of 1976, while the men with building and construction training did not reach this level of employment until March 1978, in the final year of the investigated period.

The employment rates in the next follow-up study in the 1980s are found in Fig 4. The employment rate was slightly lower for the 16-year-old leavers in the 1980s, compared to the earlier follow-up study from the 1970s (Fig 4). They were also lower for the comparison groups with vocational training, with the exception of the final years of the investigated period. Thus, the employment rates were rather similar for the men in the investigation group and the comparison groups, but they deviated slightly more in the 1980s investigation than in the former survey, the men in the comparison groups having somewhat higher employment rates.

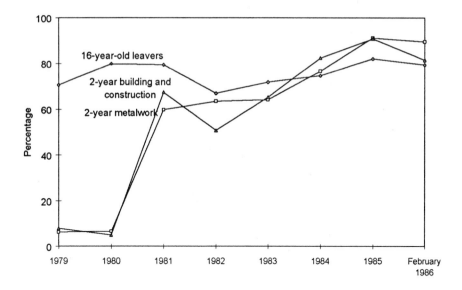

Figure 4. Employment rates for school leavers (men) with and without a 2-year vocational education and training from age 16 to 23 in 1979-1986.

In the third follow-up study the employment rate among the 16-year-old leavers from 1991 onwards was lower than in the earlier two studies (Fig 5). The employment rates for the men with vocational training were similalrly lower. The employment rate for the men with metalwork training did not pass the rate of the 16-year-old leavers until the final year of the investigation period and the men with building and construction training did not reach the same employment rate at all. They had a much lower employment rate than the other two groups at the end of the investigation period.

Thus, the employment rate for the male 16-year-old leavers decreased in every investigation. The decrease was greater from the 1980s to the 1990s than from the 1970s to the 1980s. The employment rate at the time of the investigation was 84 per cent in March 1978, 79 per cent in the February 1986 and 66 per cent in February 1995.

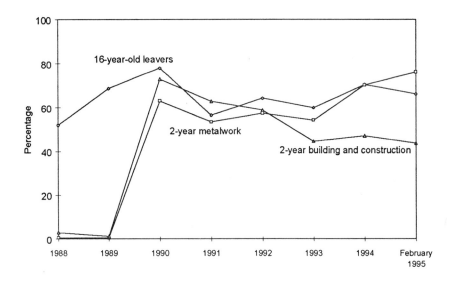

Figure 5. Employment rates for school leavers (men) with and without a 2-year vocational
training from age 16 to 23 in 1988-1995.

The employment rates for the comparison groups were also lower in the second investigation compared to the first, but only during the first years of the investigated period, and not in the final years. This implies a widening gap between the employment rates of men with and without a vocational upper secondary education between the 1970s and 1980s. In the 1990s the employment rates decreased to the same extent for the 2-year metalwork group as for the 16-year-old leavers but even more for the men with building and construction training, which means a narrowing gap between men with and without a vocational upper secondary education.

5.1.2   Women

The employment situation for women who left school at the age of 16 and the comparison groups with two years of vocational training (home economics and office work) are presented in Fig 6.

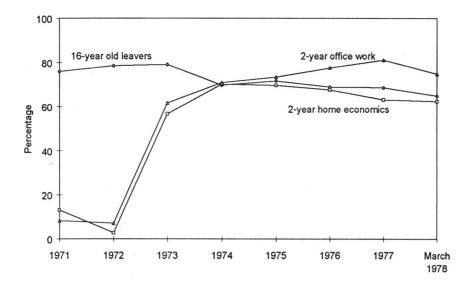

Figure 6. Employment rates for school leavers (women) with and without 2-year vocational training from age 16 to 23 in 1971-1978.

The employment rate for the women who left school at age 16 was lower than for the men with the same educational background during the whole period 1971-1978. It was below 70 per cent for women but over 80 for the men in the last years of the investigated period. Compared to the women with two years of home economics training, the employment rate did not deviate much, but women with two years of education in office work had a higher employment rate than the 16-year-old leavers in the last years of the investigation period. In 1977 it was 81 per cent while it was 69 per cent for the 16-year-old leavers.

The employment rates for the women in the investigation group and the comparison groups in the second follow-up study in 1986 are found in Fig 7 and the third in 1995 in Fig 8.

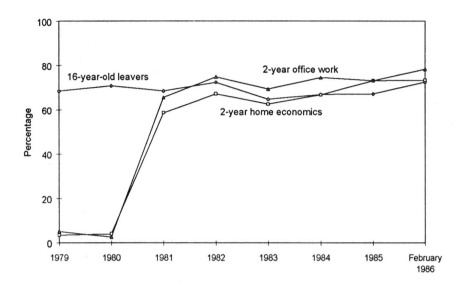

Figure 7. Employment rates for school leavers (women) with and without a 2-year vocational training from age 16 to 23 in 1979-1986.

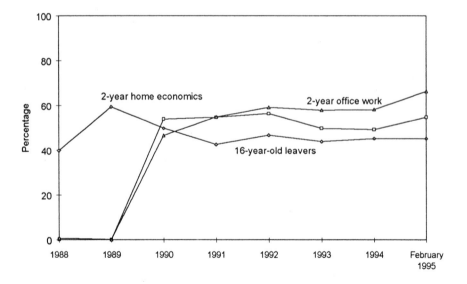

Figure 8. Employment rates for school leavers with and without a 2-year vocational training from age 16 to 23 in 1988-1995.

During the 1980s the 16-year-old leavers (Fig 7) had a slightly lower employment rate than in the former investigation in 1978 at the beginning of the investigated period, but about the same employment rate in the following part of it. The employment rate differed very little from those for the young women in the comparison groups with two years of home economics and office work training from upper secondary school.

In the third follow-up study (Fig 8) in the 1990s the employment rate for the 16-year-old leavers was lower than in the two former follow-up studies. The employment rates for the women in the comparison groups were also lower, but the change was smaller for these women so the gap between them and 16-year-old leavers widened. Thus, the results for the women followed a different pattern than for the men. The employment rates were very much the same in the first two investigations from the 1970s and 1980s but much lower in the 1990s for the 16-year-old leavers, as well as for the women with vocational training, but the change was greatest for the 16-year-old leavers.

Summarising the results for the women we found that the employment rate for the 16-year-old leavers was slightly higher than for women with two years of home economics training in the first investigation in the 1970s. In the 1980s it was slightly lower than for these women. In the 1990s the gap between these groups widened. The women with two years of office work training had a higher employment rate than the 16-year-old leavers in all three follow-up studies, but the difference was greatest in the last one, in the 1990s.

5.1.3   Wages

Wages of those young adults who had a job at the time of the investigation were divided into five classes in the first two investigations and for consistency this was done also in the third. Table 4 shows the proportion of men with 'high' wages (within the two highest intervals) and the proportion of men with 'low' wages (within the two lowest intervals) among the 16-year-old leavers and the men with vocational training.

The proportion of men with 'high' wages was greater among those with vocational training than among the 16-year-old leavers in the first two investigations but not in the third investigation in 1995 (Table 4). In 1995 the proportion with 'high' wages was almost the same (57-58 per cent) in all three groups. The proportion of men with 'low' wages was also smaller among the young men with vocational training than among the 16-year-old leavers in the first two follow-up studies. In 1995 these differences had diminished.

Table 4. The proportion of men with 'high' and 'low' wages. Percentages

Men with 'high' wages	1978	1986	1995
16-year old school leavers	58	28	57
Metalwork programme	64	34	58
Building and construction programme	71	54	57
Men with 'low' wages	**1978**	**1986**	**1995**
16-year old school leavers	8	41	21
Metalwork programme	3	26	17
Building and construction programme	2	20	19

The proportion of women with 'high' and 'low' wages are presented in Table 5.

Table 5. The proportion of women with 'high' and 'low' wages. Percentages

Women with 'high' wages	1978	1986	1995
16-year old school leavers	16	7	11
Home economics programme	34	4	11
Office work programme	26	2	10
Women with 'low' wages	**1978**	**1986**	**1995**
16-year old school leavers	39	64	69
Home economics programme	24	68	67
Office work programme	13	77	53

The proportion of women with 'high' wages was much smaller than among the men irrespective of educational background in all three investigations. The smallest proportion of 'high' wages was found amongst the 16-year-old leavers in the first investigation, but in the last one the proportion with 'high' wages was almost the same as in the comparison groups. The proportion of women with 'low' wages was, as expected, greater among the women than among the men irrespective of their educational background. It was also greater among the 16-year-old leavers than among the women in the comparison groups in the first investigation in 1978. In the following second and third investigation only women with office work training differed from the other two groups of women, but not systematically in the same direction. Thus, the wage differences also seem to be decreasing between the women in the investigation group and the comparison groups.

5.2   Occupations

The jobs the young men and women had at the time of the three investigations were classified into different vocational sectors. The sectors in which most of the male 16-year-old leavers had a job are presented in Table 6. It shows the percentage of men working in each sector.

Table 6. The percentage of men working in different vocational sectors

Manufacturing	1978	1986	1995
16-year-old school leavers	26	27	27
Metalwork programme	10	19	26
Building and construction programme	10	11	9
Metalwork	1978	1986	1995
16-year old school leavers	22	21	18
Metalwork programme	61	55	46
Building and construction programme	18	16	16
Building and construction	1978	1986	1995
16-year old school leavers	10	11	19
Metalwork programme	11	4	6
Building and construction programme	53	56	55
Transport	1978	1986	1995
16-year old school leavers	11	9	6
Metalwork programme	3	6	2
Building and construction programme	7	6	10

The most common type of job among men who left school at age 16 was in the manufacturing sector (Table 6). Twenty-six -twenty-seven per cent of these men had such a job in all three investigations. Jobs in the manufacturing sector were hardly frequent among men with metalwork training in 1978 but they became increasingly more common in 1986 and in 1995 among these men. About ten per cent of the men with building and construction training had a job in manufacturing in all three investigations. Jobs in the metalwork sector were also common among the 16-year-old leavers but, as expected, metalwork jobs were most frequent among men with some training for these type of jobs. These jobs became, however, less frequent among such men. In the first follow-up study 61 per cent of them had a metalwork job, but in the last follow-up study only 46 per cent had this type of job.

Jobs in the building and construction sector were as expected most frequent among the men with some training for these jobs. Slightly over fifty per cent of these men had a job in building and construction in all three investigations. Thus, the proportion with these jobs was stable over the studied period. However, a large per cent of the men with building and construction training were unemployed in the 1990s. Among the 16-year-old leavers these jobs became more common. In 1995 they were as frequent as metalwork jobs. Working as a concreter was the most common type of job they had.

Transport jobs were as common as jobs in building and construction among the 16-year-old leavers in 1978 but less common in the later investigations. Instead these jobs became slightly more common among men with some training in building and construction during the investigated period. Only a small proportion of the metalwork-trained men had a job in the transport sector in any of the three investigations.

The results indicate that 16-year-old leavers to a large extent had a job in manufacturing and metalwork in 1978 and in 1995. However, men with metalwork training had increasing difficulty finding a job in the sector for which they were trained, and men with building and construction training were to a great extent unemployed in 1995. Thus, the men with vocational training had increasing difficulty finding a job in the sector for which they were trained.

The women and their job sectors are presented in Table 7. Office work was the most common type of job for 16-year-old leavers in 1978. Twenty per cent of the 16-year-old school leavers had this type of job. Among the women with office work training, over 60 per cent had office-based work. In the following two investigations, office work became less common among 16-year-old leavers as well as among the women trained for office work. In 1995 only 6 per cent of the 16-year-old leavers and 26 per cent of the women with office work training worked in an office. Manufacturing jobs became instead more common among the 16-year-old leavers but not among the women in the comparison groups.

Service jobs were almost as common among 16-year-old leavers as office work in 1978 and even more common in 1986, but in 1995 the proportion with service jobs was reduced to 12 per cent. Women in the comparison groups were increasingly employed in the service sector. It was the most common type of job among the women with home economics training in 1995.

Table 7. The percentage of women working in different vocational sectors

Office work	1978	1986	1995
16-year-old school leavers	20	12	6
Home economics programme	8	7	4
Office work programme	61	41	26
Manufacturing	*1978*	*1986*	*1995*
16-year-old school leavers	18	15	38
Home economics programme	6	6	2
Office work programme	5	7	2
Services	*1978*	*1986*	*1995*
16-year-old school leavers	18	30	12
Home economics programme	20	28	37
Office work programme	1	16	16
Nursing and child care	*1978*	*1986*	*1995*
16-year-old school leavers	16	15	9
Home economics programme	44	29	22
Office work programme	8	8	13
Commerce	*1978*	*1986*	*1995*
16-year-old school leavers	11	10	16
Home economics programme	1	14	12
Office work programme	13	16	34

Nursing and child care jobs were common among women with home economics training in 1978. By 1995 the proportion in this sector had been halved. The proportion of the 16-year-old leavers in this sector was also almost halved.

Finally, commercial jobs became slightly more frequent among the 16-year-old leavers. For women trained for office work, commercial jobs seem to have replaced office work in the 1990s to a great extent.

In contrast to the men who left school at the age of 16, the women with the same educational background changed occupational sector during the investigated period. Office work, manufacturing and service jobs were the most common type of jobs for them in 1978. In 1995 manufacturing jobs seemed to have replaced many office and service jobs, which were less frequent in 1995 among these women. The women in the comparison groups with vocational training also had to change sector. Women with home economics training changed from nursing and child care to the service sector and women with office work training changed from office work to commercial jobs. However, manufacturing jobs did not become more common in either of the two comparison groups.

6.   SUMMARY AND CONCLUSIONS

Only small differences in employment rates were found between 16-year-old school leavers and men with vocational training in the comparison groups in the 1970s and 1980s. In the 1990s the men with building and construction training had a much lower employment rate than the 16-year-old school leavers. Differences in employment rates were also rather small between the compared groups of young women. However, in the 1990s the differences widened and the 16-year-old school leavers had the lowest employment rate. Thus, an upper secondary education seems to have become a more important prerequisite for young women to get a job during the investigated period but not so for young men.

The men with metalwork training had a higher employment rate than the men with building and construction training in 1995. But on the other hand they had increasing difficulty finding a job in the sector for which they were trained. They were instead found in manufacturing, the most common sector for the 16-year-old leavers. The male 16-year old leavers were to a great extent found in the same sectors during the investigated period but the women changed from office jobs to manufacturing. The women with vocational training also had to change occupational sector during the investigated period. In 1995 the proportion of women with office work training who worked at an office in 1995 was only a fraction of what it was in 1978. The women with home economics training had also changed their job sector from nursing and child care jobs to service jobs.

The wage premium for a 2-year vocational education and training course seemed to have diminished during the investigated period. The wage gap between the 16-year-old leavers and the men and women with vocational training had almost disappeared in 1995.

These results are found in a comparison between men and women with and without an upper secondary education. This comparison is fairer than in many other studies for several reasons. First it is made between young people of the same age. Second young people with a similar background are compared. Sixteen-year-old school leavers are compared to young people with a *vocational* instead of an academic education from upper secondary school. Third, the difference in the time for becoming established on the labour market for young people with and without an upper secondary education is taken into account, as the employment rate is investigated each year during the 7-year follow-up period. The follow-up period is also unusually long compared to most studies.

The results do not give a simple picture of the significance of a vocational upper secondary education on the labour market. In 1995 it hardly meant better employment opportunities or a better paid job for the men, but at least it meant better chances to get a job in the sector for which they were trained. The women with vocational training hardly got a better paid job, though this was the case in the earlier decades. But they had somewhat better employment opportunities and access to other jobs, compared to the female 16-year-old school leavers.

ACKNOWLEDGEMENTS

Funding for this study has been provided by the Swedish Council for Social Research. BA Anders Skarlind has helped me with all data work in the study from 1995.

REFERENCES

Andersson, B.E. (1996) Adolescent Perceptions of School. *EERA Bulletin,* No 2, 17-23, 1996.

Arnell-Gustafsson, U. & Skjöld, C. (1990) *Transition from school to work 1973-1985* (in Swedish). Report No 64, Living conditions, Statistics Sweden, Stockholm.

Blomskog, S. & Schröder, L. (1997) *The in-flow of young people into unemployment* (in Swedish). Report to the National Board of Health and Welfare. Institute of Social Research, Stockholm University, Stockholm

Bowles, S. & Gintis, H. (1976) *Schooling in capitalist America: educational reform and the contradictions of economic life.* Basic Books, New York.

Erikson, R. & Jonsson, J. O. (1996) *Can Education Be Equalized? The Swedish Case in a Comparative Perspective. Westview press, Boulder, Colorado.*

Forneng, S. (1987) *From school to work. Tendencies on the labour market* (in Swedish). Report No 2, Information about the labour market, Statistics Sweden, Stockholm.

Hannan, D. & Hovels, B., (1995) 'Early Leavers' from Education and Training in Ireland, the Netherlands and the United Kingdom. *European Journal of Education*, 30, 325-347.

Härnquist, K. (1993) *The social selection to upper secondary and higher education. Analyses from the longitudinal database UGU* (in Swedish). Report No 10. Department of Education, University of Gothenburg, Gothenburg.

Jonsson, J.O. (1991) The early school leavers a new proletariat? *Sociological Research* (in Swedish) No 2, 44-64.

Murray, Å. (1997) Young people without an upper secondary education in Sweden. Their home background and labour market experiences. *Scandinavian Journal of Educational Research*, No 2, 93-125.

Nickell, S. & Bell, B. (1995) The Collapse in demand for the unskilled and unemployment across the OECD. *Oxford Review of Economic Policy*, 11(1): 40-62

Pettersson, L. (1997) Vocational education for economic growth?
Labour market and work life (in Swedish) No 1, 35-44, 1997.

OECD (1985) *Education and Training after Basic Schooling*. OECD, Paris.

OECD (1994) *The Job Study Part I*. Ch.1, OECD, Paris.

OECD (1998) *Education at a Glance*. OECD, Paris.

Schröder, L. (1995) *From school to work. From the 1950s to the 1990s* (in Swedish). EFA, Ministry of Labour, Stockholm

Statistics Sweden (1980) Compulsory school. Follow up in 1978 in the spring. Studies, work etc. seven years after leaving compulsory school in 1971 (in Swedish). *Statistical Report* U 1980:13, Stockholm.

Statistics Sweden (1987) Occupation of young adults after compulsory school. Work, studies, unemployment etc. in 1995 in the spring for young adults who left compulsory school in 1979 (in Swedish). *Statistical Report* U 44 8701, Stockholm.

Statistics Sweden (1996) Occupation of young adults seven years after leaving compulsory school. Work, studies and unemployment in 1995 in the spring for young adults who left compulsory school in 1988 (in Swedish). *Statistical Report* U 82 9601, Stockholm

Wadensjö, E. (1987) The Youth Labour Market in Sweden. Changes in the 1980's. *Economia et Lavaro*, No 1, 97-104.

WORK VALUES AND EARLY WORK SOCIALIZATION AMONG NURSES AND ENGINEERS

Tom Hagström and Anders Kjellberg
[1]National Institute for Working Life, Sweden

Abstract: The objective of the study was to gain knowledge of the early work socialization of 498 nurses and 307 engineers in the light of value changes and work experiences. The two groups were chosen to represent contrasting values and socialization conditions as well as typical and atypical gender influenced occupational choices. Questionnaires were completed at the end of their trainee period and about one and a half a year later. Results showed that nurses emphasized intrinsic qualities of work, e.g. self-realization and altruism higher than did the engineers, who, in turn, put more emphasis on extrinsic/instrumental aspects, e.g. benefits. Among male engineers and female nurses the results mainly conformed with the gender stereotypes, but male nurses showed comparatively high preferences for self realization and altruism. Post-materialistic values did not change much and the changes were not significantly related to the work conditions studied. Work values were less stable and the changes showed some relations to work experiences. Increased preferences for benefits were, e.g. related to mental strain at work among the nurses but not among the engineers. A need for a more differentiated perspective on work values beyond the intrinsic/extrinsic dimension and gender stereotypes is stressed.

1. BACKGROUND

Work values are of interest to study for at least two reasons. First, there are reasons to suppose that work values are related to work motivation and goal directed behavior. Knowledge of what goals that are considered as valuable and worth striving for in relation to work therefore is of interest in strategic planning both in the school system and in the working life sector, *e.g.* when recruiting personnel and in the planning of human capital resources. Knowledge of what motivates the employees is of vital interest in structuring work tasks and work organizations in a rational way with respect both to the effectiveness of the work organization and the mental health of

Health Effects of the New Labour Market, edited by Isaksson *et al.*
Kluwer Academic / Plenum Publishers, New York, 2000.

311

the working force. Second, from a basic research point of view, it is of interest to analyze the socialization process leading to the internalization of value systems as well as their stability and change in the development from childhood to adult life, *e.g.* to what extent work values are internalized already in the primary socialization, and how the value system is influenced by work experiences.

On a more long term macro level there are indications of a broad structural shift of the value systems in the post-industrial societies, often referred to as a shift from materialistic to post-materialistic value preferences. This shift is described by Ingelhart (1977, 1990, 1997) as a slow change of the value structure implying a higher priority to quality of life, self realisation and altruism and less emphasis on materialistic and security values. This development is said to be especially evident among young and highly educated people. However, these conclusions are not undisputed. Inglehart's results have been debated regarding the direction of value change (Easterlin and Crimmins 1991), the dimensionality of the concept of post-materialism (Flanagan 1982) as well as the causal mechanisms (Graaf and Evans 1996)

From a social psychological perspective there seems to be, some consensus considering values as forming attitudes and guiding actions although not prescribing any particular type of actions. Action is understood in a wide sense including, e.g. evaluations, judgements and decisions (Van Deth and Scarbrough 1995). Value systems are generally viewed as rather stable and consistent. Thus, work values seem to be more stable than work attitudes and more generalisable over work tasks and work organizations (Dose 1997, George and Jones 1997). Work values held before entering the labor force have been found to have long term effects on subsequent labor-market experiences and rewards (Lindsday and Knox 1984) both directly and indirectly, through their effects on education (Marini *et al* 1996).

However, there are still reasons to investigate the stability of work values. Results indicate that although educational choices are affected by initial work values, the educational experiences also affect work values as well as occupational selection (Lindsday and Knox 1984). Work values have been found to be changeable, but it is possible that some work values are less stable than others. Furthermore, the boundaries and relations between basic value system, work values and attitudes remain unclear. The stability of work values in the transition to working life needs to be further clarified, as well as the role of different work experiences for the development of values. Thus, there is a need for research about young people's work values as well as the relationship between these values and their work experiences. This research can also be regarded as studies of young people's socialization into working life since work socialization involves the internalization of work values.

The increasing emphasis on personal development at work that has been reported from many European countries during the eighties, especially in Sweden (Zanders 1994) may be viewed as an indication of strengthened post-materialistic values. Young people's work values are also often discussed in terms of the materialistic–post-materialistic dimension: Are young people, *e.g.* mainly guided by traditional extrinsic, security and materialistic work values and work goals, or by intrinsic, non-materialistic values and goals such as quality of life, self realization and altruism? Issues like these initiated a research program in Sweden in the early 90's. Results from cross-sectional studies among students at secondary schools indicated that non-materialistic kinds of work values and attitudes, for example preferences for interesting jobs and the social aspects of work, were highly rated (Hagström and Gamberale 1995). Furthermore, these work values were only slightly affected by the dramatically changing market conditions in Sweden during this period (Gamberale *et al* 1995).

1.1   Aim of the study and research issues

To illuminate issues described above, men and women in two occupational groups, nurses and engineers, were followed in coordinated longitudinal studies (Hagström *et al* 1995, Hagström and Sconfienza 1996, Hagström and Westerholm 1998). The groups were chosen to represent contrasting gender influenced occupational choices. Both groups, thus, contain subgroups representing gender typical and atypical occupational choices.

The aim was to gain knowledge about early work socialization among men and women in these two groups as reflected in their work values and value changes in the transition from school to working life. Another aim was to relate value changes to work experiences. The main issues thus were the following ones:
- What work values did male and female nurses and engineers declare at the end of their occupational training?
- How did these values change in the transition into working life?
- Did their work experience differ characteristically between male and female nurses and engineers?
- What were the relations between work experiences and value changes?

2.   METHODS

The study of student nurses started in 1993 and the study of engineer students started in 1995. Both groups answered a questionnaire twice, when they were to leave school, and about one and half a year later.

2.1   Participants

At the first measurement occasion (*t1*), 719 nurse- and 428 engineer students, mainly in the Stockholm area, answered a questionnaire. The present study group was formed by the 498 nurses and 307 engineers (Table 1) who also answered the questionnaire at the second measurement occasion (*t2*). The mean age was somewhat higher in the nurse group (M=30.4 y) than among the engineers (24.6 y).

In some cases comparisons are made with a representative sample of 1117 Swedish youth (528 men and 589 women) between 20 and 26 years of age (Gamberale *et al.* 1996).

Table 1. Number of participants in the four subgroups.

	Male	Female	Total
Engineers	252	55	307
Nurses	50	448	498
Total	302	503	805

2.2   Measures

Measurements were made of post-materialistic value preferences, work centrality and seven other aspects of work values as well as of different aspects of work experiences after school.

Post-materialistic values were measured by a scale constructed on the basis of questions earlier used to measure post-materialistic orientation (Inglehart 1990, Inglehart 1997). The respondents were asked to choose 6 out of 12 items. Six of those items refer to post-materialistic and six to materialistic preferences. A post-materialism score was determined as the number of post-materialistic items chosen.

One question with a 7-point scale (0=one of the least important thing in my life, 6=one of the most important things in my life) was used to measure *Work centrality.*

Work values were measured by indices based on theoretical considerations and a factor analysis of a 40-items questionnaire concerning what characterizes an ideal job. Seven indices were constructed entitled *Social relations* (4 items, *e.g.* friendly work mates), *Benefits* (4 items, *e.g.* good pay and materialistic benefits), *Influence* (4 items, *e.g.* make important decisions) *Altruism* (4 items, *e.g.* useful to society) *Self realisation* (4 items, *e.g.* develop one's personality), *Work conditions* (4 items, *e.g.* good physical environment, secure job a regular income) and *Independence* (4 items, *e.g.* decide oneself what to think and do).

Work experiences were measured by ten indices based on factor analyses of answers to questions about their work experiences between the two measurement occasions. Three indices concerned different aspects of mental strain: *Physical threat* (five items, *e.g.* worries about violence at work, accident risks, hurting someone else), *Unemployment threat* (four items, *e.g.* worries about personnel reductions or rationalizations at the work place) and *Strain* (seven items, *e.g.* time pressure, work load and fatigue after work). Three indices concerned the psychosocial climate, namely *Work mate support* (2 items, friend with work mates, socially accepted), *Psychological climate* (six items, *e.g.* personnel policy, possibilities to express different opinions) and *Shared values* (three items, *e.g.* sense of "togetherness", feeling of pride and respect of the organization). Two indices concerned learning at work, namely *Stepwise learning* (four items, *e.g.* possibilities and support to learn more difficult tasks) and *Feedback by boss* (three items, *e.g.* feedback from boss informing how well the work tasks are performed, good advice from chief). Two indices, covered different aspects of control: *Control* (five items, *e.g.* possibilities to decide what to do at work and how to do it), and *Task complexity* (five items, *e.g.* job variation, skills necessary to handle the work task).

2.3 Statistical analyses

Differences between work values and post-materialism in the four groups at the first measurement occasion (*t1*) were tested with 2*2 two-way analyses of variance (occupational group * gender). Three-way analyses were made of changes between measurement occasions (occupational group * gender * measurement occasion). In all these analyses age was entered as a covariate since the nurses were about seven years older than the engineers.

The relations between work experiences and the changes between *t1* and *t2* of work values and post-materialistic preferences were analyzed with hierarchical multiple regression analyses with the value index score at *t2* as dependent variable. The independent variables were entered in three blocks. In the first block the score at *t1* was entered.

The second block contained the ten work experience indices. A variable indicating whether their first child had been born between *t1* and *t2* was also

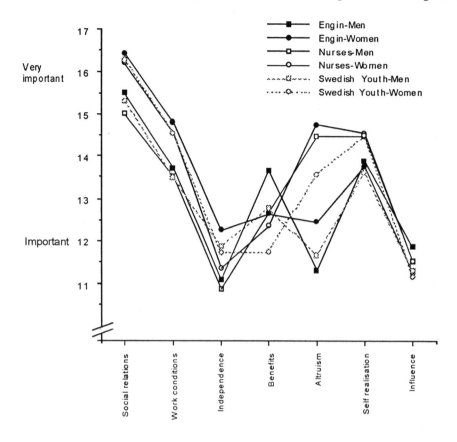

Figure 2. Rating levels of indices among male and female nurses and engineers concerning what characterizes an ideal job. Ratings made at the end of their trainee period (t1).

3.2   Changes between the two measurement occasions.

As shown by Figure 3 ratings of *Post-materialistic values* showed a slight decreasing trend among the nurses and the male engineers, whereas the female engineers showed the opposite development. This yielded a nearly significant interaction between group and time (F(1,681)=3.65, p=.059).

Work centrality did not show any significant systematic changes between the measurement occasions.

Three of the seven work value indices (*Influence, Work conditions* and *Altruism*), did not change significantly.

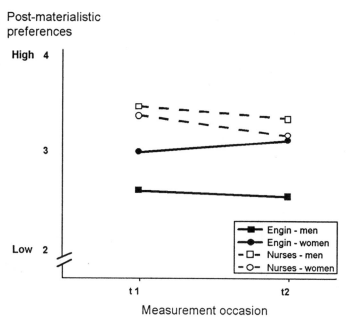

Figure 3. Rating levels concerning *Post-materialistic preferences* among male and female nurses and engineers at the end of their trainee period (t1) and 11/2 year later (t2).

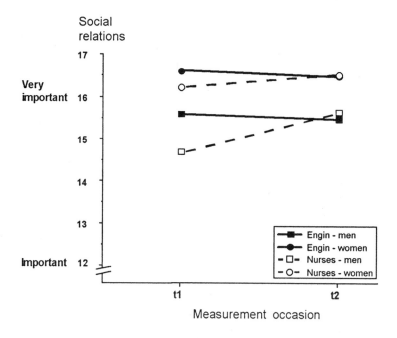

Figure 4. Rating levels of *Social relations* as characterizing an ideal job among male and female nurses and engineers at the end of their trainee period (t1) and 1 1/2 year later (t2).

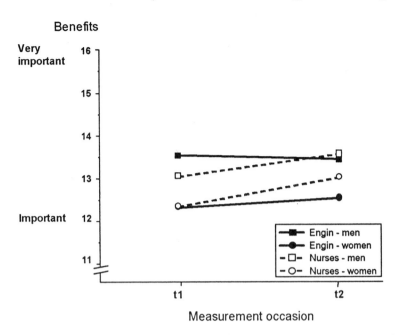

Figure. 5. Rating levels of *Benefits* as characterizing an ideal job among male and female nurses and engineers at the end of their trainee period (t1) and 1 1/2 year later (t2).

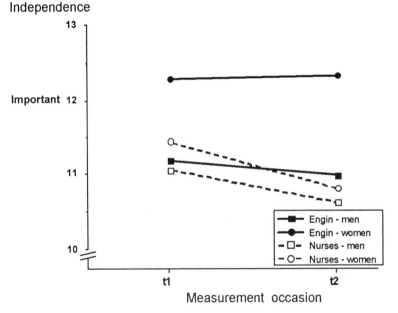

Figure 6. Rating levels of *Independence* as characterizing an ideal job among male and female nurses and engineers at the end of their trainee period (t1) and about 1 1/2 year later (t2).

The nurses' valuation of *Social relations* was strengthened (Figure 4) to the extent that the occupational difference at the first measurement occasion was eliminated (interaction occupation and time: $F(1,785)= 6.53$, p=.011). The ratings of *Benefits* showed a similar pattern (Figure 5), which was confirmed by a significant interaction between occupation and time $(F(1,781)=5.54; p=.019)$.

The *Independence* ratings (Figure 6) showed an overall decrease $(F=(1,758) =4.03, p=.045)$. This development appeared to be stronger among nurses, but the interaction between group and time did not reach a significant level.

3.3   Work conditions

The group was reduced to 659 persons in analyses of questions dealing with work experiences after school. All nurses but only 171 engineers had been working during the 18 month period after school. Figure 7 shows the mean ratings of different aspects of work conditions in the four subgroups.

Nurses had reported higher levels of physical $(F(1,652)=29.11; p<.001)$ and unemployment threats $(F(1,651)=16.83; p<.001)$ as well as higher strain $(F(1,615)=314.04; p<.001)$ than did the engineers. Irrespective of group, women's ratings were higher than those of men in these three respects $(F=3.21, 3.84$ and 6.36, respectively, $p= .074, .050$ and $.012$, respectively). Furthermore, nurses reported more support from work mates

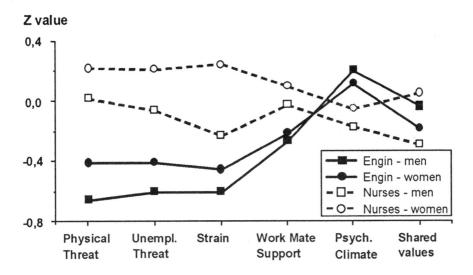

Figure 7. Rating levels (z-values) of six indices concerning different aspects of mental strain and psycho social climate at work among male and female nurses and engineers 11/2 year after their trainee period (t2).

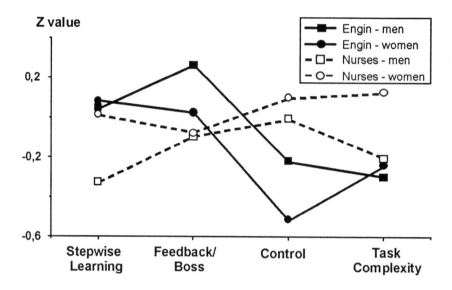

Figure 8. Rating levels (z-values) of four indices concerning perceived learning and control possibilities at work among male and female nurses and engineers 1 1/2 year after their trainee period (t2).

(F(1,640)=9.85, p=.002) and a less favorable psychological climate (F(1,599)=4.21, p=.041) than did the engineers. Shared values tended to be experienced to a larger extent by the "majority gender" in the two occupational groups, as confirmed by the nearly significant interaction between gender and occupation (F(1,641)=3.46, p=.063).

Figure 8 shows that there was a tendency for nurses, especially the female ones, to have experienced more of complex work tasks (F(1,647) =3.47, p=.063) and control at work than had the engineers (F(1,640) = 9.85, p=.002). No systematic group differences were found for *Stepwise learning* and *Feedback by boss*.

3.4   Value changes and work conditions

The results of the hierarchical regression analyses of the relation between work experiences and value changes are shown in Table 2. As can be seen from the r^2 values of the first block, all index scores were fairly stable between *t1* and *t2*. This was especially true of the *Altruism* and the *Benefits* scores. The R^2 change values for the second block indicate that the *Post-materialism* and *Independence* indices were very little affected by the work experiences covered by the variables in this block,

Table 2. Standardized regression coefficients (sign, p<.05 in bold types) and R^2 values from hierarchical regression analyses of the relation between work experiences between the two measurement occasions (*t1* and *t2*) and work values at *t2*. Since the score at *t1* is entered in the first block the coefficients shows the strength of the association between the work experiences and the change of work values between *t1* and *t2*.

Independent variables	Dependent variables (work values)								
	Soc. relat. (n= 525)	Self act. (n= 521)	Wor k cond. (n= 525)	Altru -ism (n= 522)	Ben- efits (n= 523)	In- dep. (n= 500)	Influ ence (n= 527)	Post mat. (n= 455)	Work centr. (n= 518)
Block 1									
Same variable at t1	**.538**	**.529**	**.585**	**.658**	**.635**	**.525**	**.567**	**.589**	**.399**
r^2	.290	.280	.342	.433	.403	.276	.321	.348	.159
Block 2									
Stepwise learning	.046	.047	.054	.025	.045	.083	.021	-.084	-.035
Feedback by boss	.038	.022	.002	**.142**	**.090**	.055	.069	-.028	.050
Control	.008	.079	.087	.000	**.079**	.051	**.132**	-.032	-.044
Task complexity	.068	.080	**-.100**	.018	-.023	-.095	-.082	.070	.073
Psychosocial climate	-.006	.028	.011	.058	.009	.036	.057	.086	.005
Shared values	-.020	.020	.010	-.027	**-.100**	-.049	-.079	-.039	**.130**
Unemployment. threat	.014	-.016	.033	.058	.028	-.030	.040	-.012	.015
Physical threats	**.108**	.032	**.139**	**.178**	**.129**	.030	.060	.030	.046
Strain	.047	.035	.059	-.016	**.102**	.057	**.093**	.023	.019
Work mate support	**.085**	-.040	.033	.001	.033	.023	-.037	.012	-.058
First child after t1	**.072**	-.025	.059	.028	-.027	-.035	**-.103**	-018	-.020
R^2 change	.047	.036	.042	.062	.054	.022	.048	.011	.041
Block 3 Interactions									
Single*1st child after t1	**.079**	-	-	-	-	-	-	-	-
Grp*Physical threat	**.053**	-	-	-	-	-	-	-	-
Grp*1st child after t1	-	-	-	**.113**	-	**-.122**	-	-	-
Grp*Task complexity	-	-	-	**-.085**	-	-	-	-	-
R^2 change	.010	.000	.000	.018	.000	.009	.000	.000	.000
R^2	.347	.316	.384	.495	.457	.303	.369	.359	.200

and that the *Altruism* and *Benefits* scores were the ones most strongly related to these work experiences. *Altruism* scores were strengthened among those who said that they had received support from their manager and among those that had experienced physical threats. These factors also seem to have influenced the evaluation of *Benefits* and career, which, in addition, was positively associated with experiences of *Control*, *Strain* and negatively associated with *Shared values*.

In most respects the work variables had the same relation to value changes in the nurses and engineers groups as shown by the sparse significant interactions (no further interactions were significant in the first step of the stepwise selection of variables).

Among the work variables the experience of *Physical threat* seems to have had the widest and deepest impact on the work values. This is a problem primarily in the nurses' group, and the significant interaction between group and *Physical threat* for *Social relations*, reflects that physical threats did not affect the rated importance of social relations among engineers, but strengthened it among the nurses. The judged importance of *Social relations* was also strengthened by the birth of the first child (especially among singles) and by the feeling of having been accepted by the work group.

It is also to be noted that the work experiences generally are associated with a strengthening of work values as shown by the few negative regression coefficients. One exception was that *Task complexity* was associated with a reduction of the judged importance of work conditions. Furthermore, the experience of *Shared values* and the birth of the first child had such a negative relation with the change of the evaluation of benefits and influence, respectively.

4.   DISCUSSION

The results presented showed some characteristic occupational differences. Nurse students, as compared to engineers, had a more post-materialistic value orientation, regarded work as a somewhat less central part of their lives and put more emphasis on self-realization and altruism in their description of the ideal job. Furthermore, nurses more often reported work experiences of strain, physical threats and threats of unemployment, and they had not experienced a beneficial psychological climate to the same extent as engineers although they also reported more support from their work mates. Values were rather stable among engineers, whereas nurses tended to become less post-materialistically oriented. Among the nurses, social relations and benefits had become more important at the second measurement occasion.

The gender differences in values were generally more striking than the differences between the two occupational groups. In most cases the differences conformed to the gender stereotypes. Notable exceptions were that women regarded work as playing a more important part in their lives, and that they put more stress on independence in their ideal job.

The gender typical characteristics were rather apparent among the "majority subgroups" in both occupations. The male engineers seem to have internalized a traditionally "male-oriented" and materialistic value structure, rather closely related to a conventional conception of their occupational role. The female nurses also seem to represent gender typical values and a high degree of work role integration. The gender typical values and work experiences among the "minority-subgroups" have been illustrated. Male nurses rated *Benefits* as an ideal higher than female nurses and *Social relations* lower. The female engineers, in turn, differed from the male engineers in a gender typical way concerning for example higher ratings of *Social relations* and *Altruism*. Work experiences did not differ considerably compared with the male engineers except slight tendencies towards higher mental strain and lower control at work.

However, the differentiation of values was not delimited to the gender differences. The value profiles of the four subgroups also differed in ways that was not gender typical. The male nurses had, *e.g.* a somewhat higher mean in the post-materialism scale compared with the female nurses and seem to represent more atypical gender value preferences in some important respects, indicated of, *e.g.* their comparable high ratings of *Altruism*. In spite of this, the results indicate a "gender gap" concerning lower perceived learning possibilities and shared values at work compared with the female nurses. The preferences among the female engineers for independence as characterizing an ideal job were higher than in any other subgroup.

These tendencies refer to the differentiation of value profiles, work experiences and different patterns of relations between those parameters. Results of this kind are of interest in applied research in at least two ways. First changing values, considered as motivational forces and guidelines for actions, also indicate changing perceived work rewards. The increased preference for benefits among nurses, which was related to mental strain at work illustrates this aspect. The highest rating of mental strain was found among female nurses. This may be due to or at least accentuated by the personnel reductions and rationalizations in the Swedish health care sector. Another conclusion is that the change in this direction in the transition from school to work, also may reflect a "natural" phase in the socialization from "idealistic" norms in education to the realities in working life as other results indicate (Day *et al* 1995). This occupational socialization process may be of a different character among the engineers whose status as "professionals" has been discussed (Kerr and Von Glinow 1977). Second, the differences found between subgroups show the risk of considering big cohorts like young people and occupational groups as having a homogeneous value orientation. Mean values may not be representative for the value preferences neither in subgroups, nor in the studied group as a whole.

Other issues are more related to the mechanism behind the socialization of value systems, *e.g.* when values are internalized in the individual's development and the stability of the value systems. That post-materialistic ratings did not change much during the period studied support the idea that these preferences reflect a rather stable and basic value system. This stability is also supported by the fact that changes of post-materialistic values were not significantly related to the work conditions. This is in accordance with Inglehart's theory of the "silent revolution" (Inglehart 1997) and a prediction, which could be made from the "socialization hypothesis": The post-materialistic value structure is considered to be a basic one, which is not likely to change much after the teenage period. However, it should be noted that the attrition rate was much higher for this variable than the others, and, thus, that the power of the statistical testing also was lower.

Work values were more changeable than post-materialistic preferences, which supports the idea of work values as less basically internalized. However, work values changed to different degrees and the changes were related to different work conditions. Thus, *Influence* and *Self-realization* seemed to be less changeable by work conditions, than, for example, *Benefits* and *Altruism*. Furthermore some of the work values, as mentioned, were more strongly associated with gender than with occupation, *e.g. Social relations* and *Work conditions*. The preferences for social relations may be internalized in primary socialization in a gender typical way as indicated in other studies (Beutel and Marini 1995, Marini et al. 1996). Other work values, such as *Altruism* and *Self-realization*, were rated as about equally important by both sexes within each occupation group. This indicates a greater influence of secondary socialization in internalizing these work values, for example in education and through occupational selection (Lindsday and Knox 1984).

The results support the importance of applying a "differentiation perspective" in work psychology and work motivation research area. The main approach taken in the distinction between intrinsic orientation (meaning of work itself) and extrinsic orientation (instrumental rewards *e.g.* security, salary, prestige) seem to be insufficient. As found in some previous research, intrinsic work motivation can be divided in different kinds of motives and motivation: Interests in using one's abilities and being creative can be distinguished from altruistic and social rewards. Extrinsic rewards, in turn, such as income and prestige, can be distinguished from rewards related to security, stable work conditions, power orientation and independence/ autonomy (Marini *et al* 1996). As Feather (1984) has pointed out, there seems to be a need for developing the analysis of the socialization of values to reach beyond traditional gender related distinctions such as that between *agentic/instrumental* and *communal/expressive* values. The former male value pattern stands for accomplishment and for being ambitious, independent and more agentic, while the latter female pattern refers to values such as mature love and being helpful.

REFERENCES

Beutel, A. M., and Marini, M. M., 1995, Gender and values. *Am. Sociol. Rev,* **60**: 436-448.

Day, R. A., Field, P. A., Campbell, I. E., and Reutter, L., 1995, Students' evolving beliefs about nursing: from entry to graduation in a four-year baccalaureate programme. *Nurse Educ. Today,* **15**: 357-364.

Dose, J. J., 1997, Work values: An integrative framework and illustrative application to organizational socialization. *J. Occup. Organiz. Psychol.,* **70**: 219-240.

Easterlin, R. A., and Crimmins, E. M., 1991, Private materialism, personal self-fulfillment, family life, and public interest. The nature, effects, and causes of recent changes in the values of American youth. *Public Opinion Quart.,* **55**: 499-533.

Feather, N. T., 1984, Masculinity, femininity, psychological androgyny, and the structure of values. *J. Person. Soc. Psychol.,* **47**: 604-620.

Flanagan, S. C., 1982, Changing values in advanced industrial societies. Inglehart's silent revolution from the perspective of Japanese findings. *Comp. Pol. Stud.,* **14**: 403-444.

Gamberale, F., Sconfienza, C., and Hagström, T. (1996). *[Attitudes towards work and work values among young people in Sweden. A description of a representative sample]* (Arbete och Hälsa 1996:19). Solna, Sweden : National Institute for Working Life. In Swedish.

Gamberale, R., Bracken, R., and Mardones, S. (1995). Work motivation among high school students before and during the economic recession in the Swedish labour market. *Scand. J. Psychol.,* pp. 287-294.

George, M. J., and Jones, R. G., 1997, Experiencing work: Values, attitudes and moods. *Hum. Rel.,* **50**: 393-416.

Graaf, N. D., and Evans, G., 1996, Why are the young more postmaterialist? A cross-national analyses of individual and contextual influences on postmaterial values. *Comp. Pol. Stud.,* **28**: 608-635.

Hagström, T., Gamberale, F., Sconfienza, C., and Westerholm, P. (1995). *[Early experiences of work and the working environment among nurses. A survey at the end of the trainee period]* (Arbete och Hälsa 1995:8). Solna, Sweden : National Institute for Working Life.In Swedish.

Hagström, T., and Sconfienza, C. (1996). *[Values and attitudes towards work among young engineers. A survey at the end of the trainee period]* (1996:21). Solna, Sweden: National Institute for Working Life. In Swedish.

Hagström, T., and Westerholm, P. (1998). *[Nurses work experiences and values. A follow up study 11/2 years after nursing college examination]* (Report No 6). Solna: Arbetslivsinstitutet. In Swedish.

Hagström, T. , and Gamberale, F., 1995, Young people's work motivation and value orientation. *J. Adolesc.,* **18**: 475-490.

Inglehart, R., 1977, *The silent revolution. Changing Values and Political Styles Among Western Publics.* Princeton University Press, Princeton, New Jersey.

Inglehart, R., 1990, *Culture Shift in Advanced Industrial Society.* Princeton University Press, New Jersey.

Inglehart, R., 1997, *Modernization and Postmodernization. Cultural, economic and political change in 43 societies.* Princeton University Press, Princeton, NewJersey.

Kerr, S., and Von Glinow, M. A., 1977, Issues in the study of "professionals" in organizations: the case of scientists and engineers. *Organiz. Beh. Hum. Perform.,* **18**: 329-345.

Lindsday, P., and Knox, W. E., 1984, Continuity and change in work values among young adults: A longitudinal study. *Am. J. Sociol.,* **4**: 918-931.

Mannheim, B., 1988, Social background, schooling, and parental job attitudes as related to adolescents' work values. *Youth & Soc.,* **19**: 269-293.

Marini, M. M., Fan, P. L., Finley, E., and Beutel, A. M., 1996, Gender and job values. *Sociol. of Educ.,* **69**: 49-65.

Tolbert, P., and Moen, P., 1998, Men's and women's definitions of "good" jobs. *Work & Occupat.,* **25**: 168-194.

Van Deth, J. W., and Scarbrough, E., 1995, The concept of values. In *The impact of values* (J. W. Van Deth and E. Scarbrough, Eds.), Oxford University Press, Oxford, pp. 21-46.

Zanders, H., 1994, Changing work values. In *The Individualizing Society. Value Change in Europe and North America* (P. Ester, L. Halman, and R. de Moore, Eds.), Tilburg University Press, pp. 129-153.

OCCUPATIONAL HAZARDS IN THE INFORMAL SECTOR – A GLOBAL PERSPECTIVE

Dr René Loewenson,
Training and Research Support Centre, Zimbabwe

Abstract: This paper draws on reported global experience and a 1997 survey of 1 585
              informal sector workers in Zimbabwe (Loewenson 1997b). The growth of the
              informal sector is largely attributed to the inability of the formal sector to
              provide adequate incomes or employment, leading to the poor consumer
              markets and capital starvation of the informal sector. Various informal sector
              workplaces are described, including home based enterprises, displaying a wide
              range of poorly controlled work hazards, particularly welfare and hygiene,
              ergonomic and chemical hazards, worsened by poor work organisation, and
              poor community environments and social infrastructures. The generally hidden
              but substantial burden of ill health in informal sector work is described.
              Improving occupational health in the sector can be done through implementing
              existing knowledge, but demands efforts to confront the underlying risk
              environments that undermine the application of such knowledge. Such efforts
              include building social capital and organisation within the sector, enhancing
              collective support systems and public infrastructures, supporting multisectoral
              community based approaches, and ultimately confronting the underlying
              economic marginalisation of informal sector work.

1.   INTRODUCTION

The weak understanding of the occupational hazards of informal sector work, and even more importantly of the control measures for these hazards is without doubt the Achilles heel in the body of occupational health. It is a heel that threatens to dominate the body in size, as three in every four jobs globally are found in small, unregistered or unregulated enterprises.

The informal sector is usually taken to include small enterprises, generally with less than 10 employees, unregistered in company law, often without formal contracts of employment.

The International Labour Organisation defines the `informal sector' as:

" ... very small-scale units producing and distributing goods and services, and consisting largely of independent, self-employed producers some of whom also employ family labour and/or a few hired workers or apprentices; which operate with very little capital, or none at all; which utilise a low level of

Health Effects of the New Labour Market, edited by Isaksson *et al.*
Kluwer Academic / Plenum Publishers, New York, 2000.

technology and skills; which therefore operate at a low level of productivity; and which generally provide very low irregular incomes and highly unstable employment to those who work in it. They are informal in the sense that they are for the most part unregulated and unrecorded in official statistics; they tend to have little or no access to organised markets, to formal credit institutions, to formal education and training institutions or to many public services and amenities; Informal sector producers and workers are generally unorganised ... and in most cases beyond the scope of action of trade unions and employers' organisations (ILO quoted in Mhone 1996)

There is some negative connotation of the term `informal sector' that has led to a preference for the sector to be characterised in a more neutral terms, such as `micro-enterprises', or `small-scale enterprises'. This would widen the scope significantly to include the many small enterprises, both registered and unregistered, in industrialised and developing countries. In this paper however, the focus is on both the small scale <u>and</u> unregistered/unregulated nature of the sector. While the paper presents reported experience from different parts of the world, the insights reflect the author's experience and insight from Southern Africa, as well as 1997 survey work on 1 585 informal sector workers in rural and urban Zimbabwe (Loewenson 1997b).

2.   GLOBALISATION AND THE GROWTH OF INFORMAL EMPLOYMENT

Extremely rapid changes are taking place in the global economy. During the last two decades world merchandise trade has tripled and global trade in services has increased more than fourteen-fold (UNDP 1996). While some countries have been able to use these opportunities to compete, globalisation under liberalised markets has generally benefitted the industrialised or strong economies and has marginalised the weak. The share of world trade to the poorest countries has fallen from 4% in 1960 to 1% in 1990, while investment flows have concentrated in about ten countries, mainly in East and South East Asia and Latin America (UNDP 1996), with significant flows of investment funds out of emergent markets more recently. A cycle of diminishing returns is set up where poor countries marginalised from investments and markets do not develop the capacity or exposure to engage investment or trade. Poor countries often compete against each other to capture a small share of the market, driving downwards the returns to trade through economic and labour market concessions. Within many countries, particularly the poorest, this has also set up a cycle of increasing polarisation between enterprises in access to capital and markets and in economic returns.

Privatisation and deregulation of production have been associated with shifts towards flexible employment and increased casual employment. Jobs have shifted from production to service sectors, as the latter has grown under globalisation to 60% of sectoral employment in industrialised countries and 36% in the least developed countries (ILO 1998). In what has been characterised as the second industrial revolution, the application of new information technologies, automation and biotechnology have created new patterns of employment and new types of work organisation, including an increase in self employment and subcontracting, including high skill home based work.

While some of these new forms of employment may reflect economic and technological progress, the growth of the informal sector in the south largely reflects the inability of the formal sector to provide adequate incomes or employment to a rapidly growing labour force. In African countries, formal wage labour occupies only between 0.6% and 51,4% of employment (ILO/JASPA 1992), and under relatively dire economic conditions, informal sector work is often less a means of productive employment and value-added production than a survival mechanism of last resort (Mhone 1996). In Zimbabwe, for example, an estimated two-thirds of small enterprise operators make less profit than the minimum wage for domestic workers and 88% of them make profits below the average earnings of formal sector employees. These enterprises face constraints in both demand and supply, generally service very low income markets, face shortages of finance, material inputs and skills and are generally weakly organised. The informal sector in low income countries is thus a product of the poverty of consumer markets and capital starvation.

Informal sector enterprises are often capitalised from home savings and formal sector wages. While their resilience lies in their small size, lower overheads and greater adaptability to changing environments, it also implies that they provide semi- and unskilled low quality jobs with low and insecure incomes. Most informal sector workers have not undergone any training, gaining their knowledge and skills in service. The terms and conditions of work are generally flexible, often below legal standards in terms of labour relations law and generally without formal written contracts.

These conditions make informal sector employees vulnerable to exploitation. Poor labour conditions arise not only due to poor definition of labour standards, but also due to poor monitoring and to the range of employment patterns found. Self employment is most common, with small family-type businesses common, especially in the initial developmental phase of enterprises. In a 1997 survey of 1 585 informal sector workers in urban and rural Zimbabwe, the greater share of workers were relatively young (more than half under 29 years of age), particularly in rural areas.

3.   WORK ENVIRONMENTS AND OCCUPATIONAL HEALTH

Not surprisingly, the hazards of informal sector work are poorly documented. Information from ad hoc surveys indicate a wide range of hazards in informal sector production, the most common being poor housekeeping, poor lighting, long work hours, inadequate welfare facilities, poor ventilation, poor work postures and work methods, chemical exposure, inadequate provision of personnel protective equipment, poor work place design and low awareness of chemical and other risks. These hazards have been found in urban informal sector workplaces in the Philippines, in Thailand, in Bangladesh, in Tanzania, in India and in Peru (ILO 1990; Institute for Labour Studies 1992b; Lukindo 1993; Manandar 1990, Strassman 1988). The use of complex machinery is not common among informal sector workers, but mechanical hazards have been found due to use of unguarded machinery and sharp hand tools. Chemicals with acute effects are more commonly recognised than those with chronic effects. For example, loss of eye sight is reported in jewellery homeworkers from splashes of acid solutions (e.g. boric, muriatic, nitric acids and caustic soda), while acute reactions have been experienced to powder chemicals (e.g. borax or potassium nitrate) and organic dusts in the handicraft sectors (Das et al 1992; Institute for Labour Studies 1992a, 1992b).

In the 1997 survey of informal sector worksites in Zimbabwe, work organisation, hygiene and ergonomic problems accounted for a significant share of inspected and reported workplace risks across all areas of informal sector work (Loewenson 1997b). Chemical use was present in 40% of workplaces, particularly solvents in urban areas and agrochemicals in rural areas. When asked about their own perceptions of the risks of their work, the most commonly perceived risks in both urban (manufacturing) and rural (agriculture) areas were loads, chemicals and dusts and work postures, comparing closely with the observed risks.

These immediate work environment hazards arise in a wider risk environment arising out of the organisation of work and poor community environments. Piece-rate systems make working hours irregular and work habits unsafe. Long hours without regular breaks, repetitive movement, fixed working positions and prolonged visual concentration were commonplace for simple one-step out-sourced informal sector work tasks, such as gem cutting, net repair, garment gluing and ribbon making (Institute for Labour Studies 1992a, 1992b).

Work is performed in poor residential areas or informal sector worksites where there are inadequate washing facilities, lockers or separate eating areas for workers, no first aid kits and an inadequate supply of clean water.

Few informal enterprises have fire extinguishers. Work spaces are often limited, with emergency exits blocked by cluttered passageways and obstructed by wires and cables. Job-related risk factors are compounded by overcrowding, poor nutrition and other public health problems, inadequate sanitation and the more general effects of poverty. In HBEs, the problems go beyond the worker and involve risks for the worker's family and home environment. The exposure of family members to poor working conditions can lead to their suffering from occupational diseases" even when they are not directly involved in the work.

These conditions are themselves influenced by the underlying risk environment that is characterised by insecurity, poverty and low capital investment in the sector. Economic pressures and low levels of capital are related both to the use of primitive tools and techniques and the tendency to innovate or take short-cuts in production that are necessary for economic survival, even though they pose serious risks to the worker. Informal sector producers are poorly supported by social infrastructures, weakly organised and depend largely on their own internal networks of support. Supportive or regulatory inputs from unions, employer's organisations and the state are absent and workers have poor access to information about hazards, their effects and possible control measures, as well as other aspects of production. Low levels of social capital thus contribute to the risk environment.

The same conditions that generate risk also contribute to the absence of control measures. There is little information in the literature on how these workplace risks are controlled. Even in relation to the 'last line of protection', personal protective equipment, coverage is very low. In the 1997 Zimbabwe survey, there were few in-built safety measures. Personnel protective equipment (PPE) was used by less than 5% of workers, compared to the 55% doing work where it was judged that PPE would be needed (Loewenson 1997b).

Use of PPE is regarded as an additional cost burden in an already under-resourced environment so that hazard control measures are more likely to be implemented where they are linked with inputs for improved production, or yield gains in production. Control strategies would thus more appropriately focus on the worksite design and technologies used and identify in-built design features that would enhance safety so that these are not left to individual implementation. The need for technology support to the informal sector has been raised not only for work safety reasons, but to enhance productivity, implying possibilities of synergy between these goals (Mhone 1996). Low levels of investment in and access to appropriately designed technology thus not only undermines workplace safety but also impacts negatively on the quality and general competitiveness of products from the sector (Mhone 1996).

At a superficial level the workplace hazards are, however, not difficult to control. There is sufficient information, knowledge and technological development to eliminate a vast share of the problems that make informal sector workplaces unsafe. Further, given that occupational risks in the informal sector cluster in common areas of risk in many parts of the world, a significant share of the health burden of occupational risks could be addressed by improving hygiene, ergonomics, work organisation and hand-tool safety, and by reducing exposure to particular chemicals such as solvents and pesticides (Loewenson 1997b). As noted above, control measures would call for a mix of appropriately designed technology, improved organisation of work, improved welfare facilities and general worksite design, including ergonomic features for work benches/ platforms and seats and enhanced information dissemination on risks and their control. The implementation of what are in fact rather clear measures for controlling risks is however confounded by the wider risk environment described earlier, of poor recognition of the sector and the work and employment within it, weak levels of investment and demand on the sector and low levels of social capital and infrastructural support within the sector.

There is almost no formal monitoring or reporting of risks or injury in the sector. In many countries in the South, factory inspectorate systems have inadequate staff and resources to enforce laws, even in the formal sector. Informal sector workplaces are even less likely to be monitored, as they do not fulfil the legal definition of a `factory', are excluded due to their small number of employees or may be excluded due to shortages of inspectors, time and transport (Sitas et al, 1988). In the absence of information on and monitoring of the informal sector, the sector, its risks and the health burden they generate remain largely hidden. Investments in technology and worksite designs that reduce occupational risks is unlikely when the costs of the current systems of production are poorly recognised at national level.

4.   OCCUPATIONAL INJURY AND ILLNESS

Ad-hoc surveys indicate, however, that the health burdens are not small. Informal sector workers in many parts of the world report a common pattern of occupational health problems, including musculoskeletal disorders (shoulder pains, backaches, numbness of hands and feet and rheumatism/arthritis); eye strain and injury, skin irritation and respiratory disorders (Batino 1995, Chatterjee 1987, Chintharia et al 1986; Das et al 1992, Dionisio and Hartati 1993, Loewenson 1997, Tornberg et al 1996). Small enterprises and homework has also been associated with overuse syndrome and stress related disorders (ILO 1998).

This burden of ill health is however generally poorly attributed to work, due to the high background level of ill health low income informal sector workers suffer from due to poor diet, substandard housing, overcrowding and adverse environmental conditions. Their overall vulnerability to ill health increases the possibility of developing work related illnesses. Equally, hazardous and adverse working conditions compound the ill health arising from poor living conditions. Abusive living and working environments lead to stress and social problems, including violence. Informal sector workers are reported to have higher levels of self-treatment of illness using over the counter drugs, including caffeine and analgesics, often for work-related problems such as musculoskeletal pain, eye strain and headache (Loewenson 1997).

While much of the ill health burden of informal sector work is thus hidden, there is evidence that it is substantial. The 1997 Zimbabwe survey found a much higher burden of ill health in the informal sector than is reported recognised in national databases. The survey found reported annual rates of injury and illness in the informal sector of 131 injuries / 1 000 workers and 116 illnesses / 1 000 workers. These rates exceeded those in the formal sector by a factor of 10 in the case of injury and of about 100 in the case of illness, but this is attributable to acknowledged underreporting even in formal sector systems. The distribution of injury between sectors correlated significantly with formal sector rates, with an excess in manufacturing, while illness rates were higher in the agricultural and service sectors. The similar pattern of illness as in the formal sector, the similarity between the ratio of illness and injury to that prevailing in countries with better reporting systems and the fact that under-reporting of injury and illness in the formal sector is widely suspected, signals that the rates found in the informal sector survey in Zimbabwe may be closer to the real health burden than what is formally reported. In particular, the survey found high levels of musculoskeletal and respiratory illness, already reported to be under-detected in routine data systems, but commonly reported in surveys of formal sector workers (Loewenson 1997b, ZCTU 1992). The health problems reported related closely to the occupational risks observed, with musculoskeletal problems from poor work posture and loads; exposure to dusts and chemicals leading to respiratory problems; injury from hand tools and poor housekeeping; and stomach problems linked with the lack of accessible clean water and safe sanitation.

The significant under-detection of occupational morbidity is exacerbated by the almost complete lack of coverage of occupational health services in the informal sector. As informal sector workers are often amongst the poorest in the population, they also have amongst the poorest rates of use of health care, and rely more heavily on self-help, traditional health sectors and primary health care services, where knowledge of occupational health may be poor. It is also difficult to trace illness to its work related origin when people work in a range of insecure and poorly defined jobs. The small size and scattered nature of workforces with high turnover rates and mobility undermine the measurement of both exposure and health outcomes and make work health relationships difficult to detect. Some countries such as Finland, have proposed systems of personal cumulative occupational history monitoring of workers as they move between jobs. Given the general absence of such systems, however, and given that much injury and disease will be hidden in the sector, it appears that greater emphasis should be placed on reducing ill health through reducing risks, rather than relying on (early) detection of disease.

Even traumatic injury, while easier to detect, is poorly reported, recognised or responded to. In the 1997 Zimbabwe survey, 19% of injuries, or 24,8 injuries per 1 000 workers, resulted in some form of permanent disability. In fact while the disability led to job transfer in about one fifth of cases, it did not lead to job loss, indicating that while functional impairment was present, it was not high. While a fifth of these workers were legally eligible for workers compensation in Zimbabwe, only one case was reported and none were compensated. This shortfall in workers compensation coverage in informal sector workers is common across many countries. Hence workers are poorly protected against both the occurrence and consequences of occupational injury. The Zimbabwe survey indicates that many workers continue working after injury albeit at lower levels of productivity, as *even meagre earnings may be a protection against destitution.* However, the survey was not able to trace workers who may have stopped work due to injury, nor the impact of the loss of income associated with it. Informal discussions with workers indicate, however, that injury leaves workers dependent on extended family support, or even on child labour inputs. There is also evidence from surveys of AIDS related losses in the informal sector in Uganda, that illness or injury of workers leads to collapse of the whole business, with wider ripple effects on household wellbeing (ILO-EAMAT 1995).

5.   IMPROVING OCCUPATIONAL HEALTH IN THE INFORMAL SECTOR

As we enter the next millennium, it becomes increasingly inappropriate for occupational health practitioners to ignore a sector in which the majority of people work. It is hardly possible to laud the progress made in the scientific disciplines related to working life, when this progress is inaccessible to the larger and growing share of working people. It is paradoxical that the hazards in the sector cluster in well identified and studied areas of occupational risk, where the immediate hazard control measures are well known, but are poorly implemented in practice.

The major challenge in improving occupational health and the quality of working life within the informal sector thus lies in implementing existing knowledge, and confronting the wider and underlying risk environments that undermine the application of such knowledge. One element of this is, as noted earlier, to more systematically and widely describe, inform and generate social recognition of the work within the sector, and the health burdens it generates.

Efforts to build a safety culture and introduce risk reduction measures into the informal sector quickly confront the fact that it is not a simple matter of extending existing formal sector strategies. The lack of penetration of formal market systems and supports in the informal sector, the low level of formal capital and skills inputs, the weak level of worker organisation and marginalisation from many of the institutional support systems of the formal sector weaken the possibilities of using tripartite systems, production or market incentives or legal provisions to promote occupational health in the informal sector. The success and sustainability of programmes within the informal sector depend on building or supporting organisational networks and linking informal sector producers with non government, private and public sector institutions and infrastuctures that can support their actions. In other words, it means that building social capial within the sector is a vital part of occupational health action.

Hence for example, the lack of security and capacity of individual work-places in the sector calls for strong collective frameworks for risk reduction, and support by more stable, formal institutions. Production inputs, market and capital access and social protection systems would seem to be feasible if organised through collective systems of management, and linked with either public sector institutions or those in the stronger labour, trade and business groups.

The provision by local authorities of appropriate shelters and work stations at agreed sites with adequate toilet, water, electrical, communication and other facilities could provide a framework for wider information and support services, including those supporting risk reduction and management of environmental waste. Coverage with occupational health promotion and workers compensation could be improved if it were linked with other forms of credit and insurance in the sector. Risk assessment and contribution rates for compensation could also be differently formulated for the sector. For example, as in the Netherlands, small enterprises in an area across a range of activities could be pooled for insurance, to create a mutual responsibility system to keep risks and costs down.

It is thus commonly agreed that "alternative approaches" are needed, perhaps more community based than workplace based, more strongly linked with other community based approaches, like primary health care systems, than with an occupational health heirarchy, and certainly linked to support of organisational networks and survival needs in the sector[1]. If these linkages are to be made, then occupational health inputs and actions would need to link with and support

* other programmes aimed at the more general problems of access to infrastructures, capital resources, skills and decision making;

* inputs aimed at improving economic viability and enhanced access to technology, skills, credit and markets

* other production and civic skills;

* community, institutional and media networks for support of social and economic needs;

Occupational health interventions also need to address the underlying economic insecurity and marginalisation that exists within the sector, and to counteract the widening dualism between formal and informal sectors of production. Poor working conditions and poor quality jobs in the sector reflect not only the polarisation of the social benefits from work, but also the polarisation in access to the inputs to work. Hence collective and community based systems for the informal sector need to be interfaced with and supported by formal institutions and inputs, whether through scientific and industrial research centres and larger companies for technology development, through wider industry exchanges and vocational centres for skills and management training, through public and private media for information sharing or through intermediary institutions linking with market finance for capital support.

The profile of the informal sector described in this paper is not one of a small scale sector that integrates with and is a launch pad for the opportunities of national and global economies. It is rather a profile of "survival employment" largely marginal to and isolated from national and global opportunities, markets, capital and skills resources. This socio-economic marginalisation and isolation is perhaps the greatest occupational risk in the sector, and the source of many work environment and work organisation hazards. At the same time, the sector provides evidence of a forceful and often parallel world, where the work done generates the means

---

[1]   This was, for example, articulated in the Bali statement at the ICOH International Conference on Occupational Health in Indonesia in October 1997.

of survival for billions of people. We clearly face a challenge in translating the gains in knowledge of the last century into the practical reality of this survival economy, particularly when formal institutions have so little knowledge of how the sector works and how to work with it. We face an even greater challenge to make unacceptable and confront the patterns of capital investment, production and employment that marginalise an increasing share of the worlds population into this parallel world of insecure, low paid, poor quality and stressful jobs.

REFERENCES

Batino J., 1995, Snapshot of working conditions in the urban informal sector, ILO Interdepartmental Project on the Urban Informal Sector, 1995, Mimeo

Chatterjee M., 1987, Occupational health issues of home-based piece rate workers: three studies of ready made garment, bidi and chikan workers, Ahmedabad: Self Employed Women's Association.

Chintharia A, Desai H, Chatterjee B., 1986, Occupational stresses on women engaged in making beedi. J Soc Occup Med; 36:130-133.

Civic Group Housing Project / Training and Research Support Centre (CGHP/TARSC), 1995, Survey of Home Based Enterprises in Harare, TARSC Monograph. Penguin Printers, Harare

Cooper A, Guthridge S, Riare A., 1992, Occupational health of homeworkers: A study of two villages of Khon Kaen Province in Northeast Thailand. In Lazo L ed. Homeworkers of Southeast Asia: the struggle for social protection in Thailand. Bangkok: International Labour Organisation

Das P, Shukla K, Öry F., 1992, An occupational health programme for adults and children in the carpet weaving industry, Mizapur, India: a case study in the informal sector.Social Science and Medicine 1992;10:1293-1302.

Dionisio A, Hartati D., 1993, Occupational health and safety of homeworkers: the Jelambar Baru Experiment. Jakarta: Save the Children - Jakarta Program, Mimeo

Dulce P, Estrella-Gust D., 1993, Health and safety of child labour. Proceedings of Occupational Safety and Health Congress for the Asian and Pacific region, August 1993. Singapore: International Labour Office

Gilbert A., 1988, Home Enterprises in Poor Urban Settlements: Constraints, Potentials and Policy Options in Regional Development, Dialogue Vol 9 No 4

ILO EAMAT, 1995, The impact of HIV/AIDS on the productive labour force in Africa, EAMAT Working Paper No. 1, Addis Ababa

ILO World Employment Programme / JASPA, 1992, ILO Addis Ababa

International Labour Organisation ILO, 1990, The working poor in Bangladesh. A case study on employment problems, conditions of work and legal protection of selected categories of disadvantaged workers in Bangladesh. Dhaka: International Labour Organisation

ILO, 1997, Yearbook of Labour Statistics 1996, ILO Geneva

IL, 1998, Personal communications with personnel in SEC-HYG Division, Geneva, ILO, Institute for Labour Studies, 1992a, Case studies on the occupational health and safety of homeworkers in the jewellery industry in Manila, Institute for Labour Studies, Department of Labour and Employment, Mimeo

Institute for Labour Studies, 1992b, Case studies on the occupational health and safety of homeworkers in the handicraft industry in Phillipines, Manila, Institute for Labour Studies, Department of Labour and Employment, Mimeo

Jinadu M., 1987, Occupational health and safety in a newly industrialising country Jo Royal Society of Health 107:1: 8-10

Kogi K., 1985, Improving working conditions in small enterprises in developing Asia, ILO, Geneva

Kogi K, Phhon W, Thurman J., 1989, Low cost ways of improving working conditions: 100 examples from Asia, ILO, Geneva

Loewenson R., 1997, Assessment of the health impact of Occupational risk in Africa: Current situation and methodological issues, paper presented at the WHO/ILO Consultation on Health Impact assessment of Occupational and Environmental Risk, Geneva, July 1997

Loewenson R., 1997b, Health impact of occupational risks in the informal sector in Zimbabwe, TARSC Report prepared for the International Labour Organisation, Penguin Printers, Harare

Lukindo J., 1993, Comprehensive survey of the informal sector in Tanzania. African Newsletter on Occupational Health and Safety 1993;3:36-37.

Manandar M., 1990, Study on unorganised / unprotected workers in Nepal in Siddiqui (ed) Labour laws and the working poor, ILO, Bangkok

Mhone G., 1996, (ed) The Informal Sector in Southern Africa, SAPES Books, Harare

Mhone G, Aryee G., 1985, Employment promotion in the informal sector and the current economic crisis- the case of Southern Africa, ILO SATEP

Prompunthum V, Kerdpol C., 1985, Working condition of women piece-rate workers in Thailand. Bangkok: Department of Labour, Ministry of Interior, Mimeo

Sitas F, Davies J, Kieikowski D, Becklake M., 1988, Occupational health services in South African manufacturing industries: a pilot survey, Am J Ind Med 14: 545-557

Strassman W., 1986, Types of Neighbourhood and Home Based Enterprises from Lima, Peru, Urban Studies Vol 22

Strassman W., 1988, Home Based Enterprises in Developing Countries" in Economic Development and Cultural Change. Vol 36 No 1

Tornberg V, Forastieri V, Riwa P, Swai D., 1996, Occupational Safety and Health in the Informal Sector, Afr Newslett on Occup Health and Safety 1996: 6:30-33

Torres A., 1993, Underdevelopment and women in the informal sector: The case of urban workers and rural homeworkers from Women in the Informal Sector: Their contribution, vulnerability and future, International Network for Research and Action on Women in the Informal Sector, UNESCO, Jakarta

Triple A.G., 1993, Shelter as Workplace: A Review of Home Based Enterprises in Developing Countries. International Labour Review. Vol 132 No 4

UNDP, 1996, Human Development Report 1996, Oxford, UNDP

Vilegas G.S., 1990, Home-Work: A Case for Social Protection, International Labour Review. Vol 129 No 4

Zimbabwe Congress of Trade Unions (ZCTU), 1992, Survey of Occupational Health Practices at Workplace Level, Mimeo Report, Harare

INDEX